D0990389

Restructuring Personality Disorders

RESTRUCTURING PERSONALITY DISORDERS

A Short-Term Dynamic Approach

JEFFREY J. MAGNAVITA

Forward by STANLEY B. MESSER

THE GUILFORD PRESS
New York   London

© 1997 The Guilford Press
A Division of Guilford Publications, Inc.
72 Spring Street, New York, NY 10012

Printed in the United States of America

This book is printed on acid-free paper.

Last digit is print number: 9 8 7 6 5 4 3 2 1

Library of Congress Cataloging-in-Publication Data
Magnavita, Jeffrey J.
   Restructuring personality disorders: a short-term dynamic
approach / Jeffrey J. Magnavita.
      p. cm.
   Includes bibliographical references and index.
   ISBN 1-57230-185-6
   1. Personality disorders—Treatment. 2. Brief psychotherapy.
3. Psychodynamic psychotherapy. I. Title.
RC554.M23 1997
616.89'14—dc20   96-44159
                                                            CIP

This is dedicated to those
from whom I draw my inspiration,

Annie, Elizabeth, Emily, and Caroline

Foreword

As recently as 5 years ago, the vast majority of new volumes on psychotherapy made little or no mention of planning out the length of treatment and its focus from the start. Now, hardly a month goes by without a new book on systematic, time-limited therapy coming to my attention. This trend is reflected in the results of surveys indicating that over 80% of clinicians now conduct some brief therapy. The dramatic change has resulted primarily from an economic climate that is increasingly sensitive to cost-effectiveness, not only in the corporate world but in the arena of general and mental health care as well. Insurance companies and managed care entities, for example, typically provide no more than 20 sessions of psychotherapy to their subscribers.

This shift, however, is not due solely to factors external to the field of psychotherapy. Advances in research and theory, along with accumulated clinical experience, have tended to support the value of brief therapy. This has led many clinicians, previously unfamiliar with time-limited therapy, to take a careful look at this modality. For example, in our book on brief therapy (Messer & Warren, 1995), Seth Warren and I concluded, after reviewing the research literature, that time-limited therapy is helpful to a substantial proportion of patients and that its effects are long lasting. Dose–effect relationships indicate that by 13 sessions roughly 50% to 60% of patients are considered improved. We also noted that the percentage of patients who had improved continued to rise with increased sessions, but at a slower rate than in the earlier sessions. A recent *Consumer Reports* survey also confirms that brief therapy of about 6 months' duration can be very helpful even while much longer-term therapy of about 2 years or more can be even more helpful.

In his sophisticated approach to understanding and treating personality disorders in short-term therapy, Jeffrey Magnavita incorporates a wide spectrum of psychodynamic theories of personality and psychotherapy and draws on his 15 years of clinical experience. The result is a sturdy blend of theory and technique that offers a more hopeful approach to treating personality disorders than I have seen to date. Magnavita's writing is exceedingly clear, conveying the major concepts of short-term dynamic therapy in language that is readily accessible. The clinical examples are instructive, and the author's ability to distinguish the more and less treatable personality disorders lends important credibility to this project. That is, the model is sensitive to the considerable differences among the personality disorders (Clusters A, B, and C) and to the range of treatment approaches they call for. It takes into account the considerable resistances and character armor that are among the defining features of this kind of psychopathology. We know from research studies, for example, that some personality disordered patients need longer forms of treatment, and even then, positive outcomes are chancy. Thus, the author stresses the importance of careful assessment through probing interviews, as well as the use, where appropriate, of objective and projective tests.

In the spirit of the brief therapy pioneers—Alexander, French, and Davanloo—Magnavita is admirably flexible in his use of time, sometimes allowing several hours for an interview in order to penetrate to the core of the problem, and at other times, meeting clients on a biweekly basis to give them needed breathing space. He recognizes that there are some patients who need anxiety-dampening cognitive restructuring rather than, or preliminary to, the confrontation of defenses whose aim is to reach their carefully guarded affects. As he states in Chapter 5, in short-term restructuring psychotherapy, "use as much defense analysis as the patient can tolerate and incorporate empathic phases when the patient responds negatively" (p. 85). He expertly lays out the variety and level of defenses one encounters in practice and demonstrates, in a step-by-step fashion, how to work with them.

Magnavita's therapeutic style is refreshingly modest insofar as he offers interpretations in such a way that patients can refuse them. There is a fundamental respect that he conveys to patients even while he challenges their maladaptive defenses and interpersonal patterns. Although the approach is psychodynamically grounded, it has integrative elements that will appeal to the large body of practitioners who regard themselves as integrative or eclectic.

This volume provides a service to mental health clinicians working on the front lines with personality disordered and dual diagnosed patients who want to do more than alleviate crises in their patients. Its value lies in its pointing the way for well-trained clinicians to make significant headway in bringing about characterological change in patients afflicted with a personality disorder.

STANLEY B. MESSER
Professor and Chairman
Department of Clinical Psychology
Graduate School of Applied
 and Professional Psychology
Rutgers University

Preface

My interest in personality disorders grew out of the frustration and help-lessness I experienced when treating patients suffering from some form of comorbid character disturbance. My training in family therapy and eclectic psychotherapy, while useful in other areas of my practice, offered no solutions. I originally felt that traditional psychoanalysis, though lengthy and expensive, was the only in-depth treatment model available that could provide these patients with the help they so desperately needed. Yet I was dismayed by the prospect of being able to treat so few patients and then only those who had the financial means for protracted therapy. In addition, like most practitioners, I was under increasing pressure from insurance companies to provide abbreviated treatment to all my patients. I decided to consider studying short-term dynamic psychotherapy (STDP). The propo-nents of what was then considered a radical school of thought promised in-depth psychotherapy in substantially less time than traditional psycho-analysis. I began intensive work in exploring the history, research, theory, and techniques of STDP.

Over an extended period of time, working with many patients and using audiovisual recordings, I came to develop a model of clinical work. I call this a model because it does not create an entirely new paradigm but, rather, offers a systematic framework for understanding and applying the diverse techniques that various approaches use. I present this approach in this book. This approach encourages flexibility and allows the practitioner to select and use the style and technique that best fit his/her particular case.

Clinicians are now able to provide a wide variety of patients with effective short-term treatment for their personality disorders. Research showing significant, rapid personality change has provided preliminary validation. Convincing evidence was shown with case reports offered by early pioneers including Ferenczi, Rank, Balint, Reich, Alexander, Malan, Davanloo, Sifneos, Mann, and Beck. More recently, systematic research has supported these clinical observations about the efficacy of STDP for personality disorders.

My treatment approach is an integrated model that emphasizes three restructuring methods: *defensive, affective,* and *cognitive.* Given the entrenched nature of most personality disorders, defensive restructuring is the cornerstone of this approach, especially in the early phase of treatment. In my experience, this emphasis on defense restructuring enhances the potency to treat refractory disorders in relatively brief periods. Most psychotherapists are comfortable with affective and cognitive restructuring and feel most comfortable with an empathic style. Anxiety-provoking techniques and defense challenging may seem harsh but, if used correctly, they actually increase patients' ability to experience intimacy.

In the process of writing this book, I found that there was little published on the subject of short-term psychotherapy of personality disorders. For example, there is only one chapter devoted to the brief treatment of personality disorders in Budman and Gurman's (1988) *Theory and Practice of Brief Psychotherapy* and, more recently, two chapters on this topic in Stadter's (1996) *Object Relations Brief Therapy.* The best of what has been written recently, although not on brief treatment, includes Millon's (1981) *Disorders of Personality* and his most recent book, *Disorders of Personality: DSM-IV and Beyond* (Millon & Davis, 1996). In these books, Millon has done an excellent job of integrating research, theory, and practice. Also, Stone's (1993) book *Abnormalities of Personality* has broken new ground in bringing together the seemingly divergent lines of research and clinical knowledge.

It is my hope that practitioners interested in the treatment of personality disorders will find herein a new way to work with the most challenging patients. I hope you will find fresh ideas to help you better formulate tough cases, get at core issues, and stay attuned to your patients. As with any system of psychotherapy, this does not represent a static, finished product but, rather, is a step in the evolution of systematizing what we as psychotherapists are attempting: meaningful change in the shortest possible period of time.

The volume is divided into two parts. Part I, *The Framework,* reviews the pertinent material required to conceptualize the approach and learn the assessment and treatment techniques. Chapter 1 begins with a presentation of the evidence of quantum change. Background information is then offered. In Chapter 2, the treatment approach is briefly described and essential theoretical background material is discussed. This is followed by a detailed presentation of the elements of the approach, reviewing the contributions of many of the major figures in the field. Essential constructs that will be used in the assessment phase and to guide the treatment process are presented. Chapter 3 follows with an overview of the assessment process emphasizing the need for a comprehensive structural understanding of the patient, using anxiety to activate the defense system. Various flexible treatment formats emphasizing extended sessions are offered that set the stage for the treatment process discussed. Chapter 4 is devoted to the topic of how to formulate the core issues, an essential aspect of treatment that determines outcome. This is one of the most difficult aspects of treating patients with personality disorders because of the multifoci of the core issues and the level of repression or acting out typically present.

The integrated techniques used in short-term restructuring psychotherapy (STRP) are presented in Chapter 5, including anxiety-provoking techniques used to accelerate the process and anxiety-reducing techniques used to strengthen the alliance and the ego. The importance of keeping the anxiety high while balancing with empathy is discussed. An in-depth presentation of the three restructuring approaches incorporated in STRP are presented in Chapter 6. These include defensive restructuring, which is emphasized in the early stage of treatment for many personality disorders, as well as affective and cognitive restructuring approaches. Part I ends with Chapter 7, which provides the reader with an overview of the treatment process showing the various elements in the three stages of treatment.

Part II, *Process and Technique*, begins with Chapter 8, which presents clinical case material on the Cluster C personality disorders. Chapter 9 focuses on the Cluster B personality disorders, and Chapter 10 addresses the Cluster A disorders. Case material is presented showing the process of change and the techniques of the approach. Treatment pitfalls that are commonly encountered with personality disordered patients are discussed in Chapter 11. An important aspect of this approach is measuring therapeutic effectiveness, which is described in Chapter 12. Finally, Chapter 13 summarizes and discusses future challenges in this exciting and promising application of short-term dynamic methods to the refractory personality disorders once considered the realm of long-term analysis.

Acknowledgments

Writing this book was a challenging and a rewarding undertaking. Its evolution from my initial murky and fragmented thoughts to the final product was the result of a team effort. First and foremost, I am indebted to my wife, Anne Gardner Magnavita, M.Ed., for her encouragement and support. She generously spent countless hours reviewing and altering my early drafts. More importantly, she read the manuscript with a critical eye and strove to maintain the book's focus.

I especially want to thank my editor, Kitty Moore, who brought this book from a crude outline to the finished product. Her clear editorial thinking forced me to focus on my goals, and her encouragement of me to find my own voice was effective and empowering. I thank her for her patience and guidance.

A good friend who deserves thanks is Susan Uber, Ph.D., who unselfishly edited early drafts of this manuscript, taking time away from her busy clinical practice to read and respond with detailed editorial notes. She provided the important perspective of a seasoned clinician willing to try new approaches.

I also want to thank Valerie Vick, J.D., for her fine editorial assistance and consistent optimism. She eagerly revised numerous drafts with a flair for expressing concepts eloquently and organizing the material coherently.

My interest and passion for conducting psychotherapy have been stoked by a core group of dedicated depth psychotherapists who have generously shared their ideas, excitements, and failures. Our work together, conducting live interviews and reviewing videotapes, often resulted in heated discussions and lively debates. These colleagues include Vincent Stevens, M.D., whose intuitive knowledge and passion for the power of psychotherapy is always inspiring. His enthusiasm prompted my early interest in the study of short-term dynamic psychotherpay (STDP). Frank W. Knoblauch, M.D., a psychoanalyst, has added a level of intellectual rigor to our group and has provided assistance in the form of suggested readings and discussions on related analytic topics. I want to thank William C. Alder, M.D., who generously made accessible his extensive library, thereby providing me with many of the sources that I needed. We spent hours together hiking and discussing clinical cases.

Early in the process, Stanley B. Messer, Ph.D., provided the first outside review of the first half of the manuscript. His suggestions and ideas were very helpful to me in my conceptualization of the model.

A substantial contribution was made by two anonymous reviewers who challenged my thinking and made me reconsider my presentation. A heartfelt thanks is especially due the reviewer who provided copious detailed comments.

I would also like to thank Marc A. Rubenstein, M.D., who gave me my first exposure to my own unconscious and impressed upon me the value of psychoanalysis. My personal development was also advanced by Manuel Trujillo, M.D., whose work with me was immensely beneficial.

Finally, I owe a great debt to the patients I have had the privilege of treating. I have learned a great deal from knowing them and witnessing their courage to pursue intensive short-term psychotherapy. I am especially grateful to all those patients who have allowed me to videotape their treatment so that I, as well as others, can learn to do our work more effectively.

Contents

xviii Contents

PART I

THE FRAMEWORK

The first part of this book supplies the theoretical groundwork for the clinical material that follows. I strongly believe that clinicians should be theoretically grounded before they proceed with clinical work, especially when working with complex personality disorders. This half of the book also describes the techniques and methods which are used to mobilize powerful affective reactions in the restructuring. As I advise throughout the book, those clinicians without sufficient experience and supervision should attempt such techniques with the greatest caution.

The model I have developed has been useful in orienting me and guiding my clinical work. Psychotherapy is entering a new frontier where clinical utility and efficacy will determine which forms of psychotherapy will be practiced in the next millennium. Based on my own and others' observations of the efficiency of short-term dynamic psychotherapy (STDP), I hope that STDP will be given sufficient research attention so that its effectiveness can be further documented.

Readers who are eager to sample the clinical work may prefer to go directly to Part II and observe the flow of the clinical process in a few cases before returning to Part I to study the theory and technical aspects. In writing this book I have assumed the reader has a basic understanding of psychodynamics; less knowledgeable readers may also want to review the other sources mentioned throughout the book to provide a foundation.

CHAPTER 1

Quantum Change for Personality Disordered Patients?

*If radical and sudden shifts in personality do indeed occur, they pose
a puzzle of great potential. Nearly all of current scientific psychology
is focused on describing, understanding, or influencing gradual
incremental change. . . . Quantum transformations, however, suggest
at least a different magnitude of change.*
                                   —MILLER AND C'DEBACA (1994, p. 257)

Is quantum change for the personality disordered patient possible? If so, are
there methods of treatment that can facilitate these changes? People with
personality disorders have deeply embedded pathological patterns of thinking, feeling, behaving, and relating to others that are largely unconscious
(Millon & Davis, 1996). Given the entrenched nature of personality
disorders, and their pervasive influence in the individual's experience of the
world and him/herself, they are considered highly resistant to most forms
of psychotherapeutic and psychopharmacological intervention. The general
consensus, as noted by William James (1890/1981), has been that personality is "set like plaster" early and remains quite stable over time. Yet if
personality is not malleable, then there is not much hope that patients
entering any type of psychotherapy will be able to make dramatic changes
(Heatherton & Nichols, 1995). If this is truly the case, how can anything
short of years or decades of intensive treatment transform personality?

   In this chapter, I begin with some background material on personality disorders including prevalence and etiology. Then I review the evidence that supports "discontinuous transformational experiences" or quantum change occurrences. Next, I discuss some of the factors that are useful to set the stage for major transformations. Finally, I end with a discussion of the elements that distinguish STDP from other forms of psychotherapy.

PERSONALITY DISORDERS: WHAT ARE THEY?

Personality disorders are defined in the fourth edition of the *Diagnostic and Statistical Manual of Mental Disorders* (DSM-IV) as "an enduring pattern of inner experience and behavior that deviates markedly from the expectations of the individual's culture, is pervasive and inflexible, has an onset in adolescence or early adulthood, is stable over time, and leads to distress or impairment" (American Psychiatric Association, 1994 p. 629). These are extreme variants of normally occurring traits that have reached psychopathological proportions (Millon & Klerman, 1986). DSM-IV classifies personality disorders in three clusters based on descriptive similarities. The paranoid, schizoid, and schizotypal personalities comprise Cluster A. These patients are characterized by an odd or eccentric style. The antisocial, borderline, histrionic, and narcissistic personalities make up Cluster B, and they are characterized by their erratic, emotional and dramatic presentation. Patients in Cluster C, which includes the avoidant, dependent, and obsessive–compulsive personality disorders, usually show signs of anxiety and fearfulness.[1]

Each personality disorder is characterized by a circumscribed pattern of defenses, interpersonal expectancies, and core conflicts that can be useful in guiding the clinician in the treatment process. For example, in the Cluster A disorders, the obsessive–compulsive is on some level struggling with the following core issue: "If only I were perfect, I would be accepted and loved; having strong feelings or destructive impulses is a sign of my unworthiness."

PREVALENCE OF PERSONALITY DISORDERS

Although data on the prevalence of personality disorders are limited (Weissman, 1993), it is estimated that approximately one out of 10 adults in the general population and over half of the patients in treatment suffer from a personality disorder (Merikangas & Weissman, 1986). Widiger and Costa (1994) reviewed a number of studies on the prevalence of personality disorders and report the substantial presence of compulsive, histrionic, and antisocial personality traits in urban areas. Consequently, mental health professionals, whether working on an inpatient unit or in an outpatient facility, are routinely faced with these patients in their clinical practices. If the statistics presented are at all accurate, and there is no reason to believe they are not, then this diagnostic group alone accounts for the largest percentage of mental health visits. In my 15 years of practice, as well as in the practices of colleagues, this 50% figure represents an underestimation.

Not surprisingly, there is a high degree of comorbidity,[2] as high as 40%, between Axis I disorders, such as panic disorder (McGinn & Sanderson, 1995), anxiety, and depression, and personality disorders (Pollack, Otto, Rosenbaum, & Sachs, 1992; Seivewright, Ferguson, & Tyrer, 1992). Optimal treatment often requires that the personality disorder be addressed as well as coexisting Axis I disorders. As Reich (1945) pointed out, work on the character armor[3] must occur immediately except when there is severe anxiety or clinical depression, which indicates that the character defenses have already broken down. In a National Institute of Mental Health (NIMH) collaborative study of depression, 74% of the patients diagnosed with major depression had coexisting personality disorders (Shea et al., 1990). Most personality disordered patients, if not encouraged to enter therapy by significant others, are compelled to seek treatment because of symptomatic distress usually attributable to concurrent Axis I disorders. Therefore, it is highly uncommon for patients to enter therapy seeking to change or modify their personalities. What they generally desire is symptom reduction or relief. Unfortunately, many discontinue treatment after this has been achieved but before the more challenging work leading to permanent change has begun. In a review of outcome studies, Robins (1993) found that most personality disordered patients do not respond well to standard psychotherapeutic approaches. Robins states that "research is needed to determine whether they benefit from more intensive, extensive, or integrated approaches to therapy" (p. 316). My experience has been that patients with personality disorders can achieve substantial gains with the STDP approach.

ETIOLOGY AND PATHOGENESIS

Personality disorders are a complex admixture of biogenic and psychogenic factors forming a unique matrix for each individual. Unfortunately, there is little published research on the development and pathogenesis of personality disorders. What we do know is that their roots manifest early in an individual's life, beginning with temperament. Contributing factors include genetics, biochemistry, quality of early relationships and environment. There are numerous partially supported speculations and clinical evidence such as correlations between attention-deficit/hyperactivity disorder (ADHD) and conduct disorders, chromosomal aberrations and violence, and the biological substrate for the affective spectrum of personality disorders. Watson and Clark (1994), in reviewing current research, say recent findings offer "great promise" in clarifying the underlying genetic, biological, and temperamental processes as they relate to personality and psychopathology, but they recommend caution in adopting an overly deterministic or rigidly biological view. Paris (1994) proposes a biopsychosocial model for borderline personality disorders. He states, "The most likely mechanism for this interaction of biology and environment is that in the presence of psychological risk factors—such as trauma, loss, and inadequate parenting-personality traits tend to be amplified" (p. 321). The biopsychosocial model is universally well-accepted and is useful in understanding not just the borderline disorder but all other personality disorders as well.

It is widely accepted by researchers that personality traits are highly stable over time (McCrae & Costa, 1994) although there is continuing debate regarding the validity of this evidence (Maher & Maher, 1994). Adolescents and even children may exhibit some personality disorder traits or even full-blown personality disorders, but typically, they manifest a fluid structure that incorporates varied defenses with frequently shifting constellations. During later adolescence, the adult structure begins to coalesce (Austin & Inderbitzin, 1983). Personality disorders begin to crystallize in the early 20s and then realize a more permanent form in the 30s. Most researchers and clinicians consider personality to be essentially fixed by age 30 (McCrae & Costa, 1994). For this reason, Freud believed that analysis should not be undertaken until one enters one's 30s. Since in most cases it takes many years for a personality disorder to crystallize, I next discuss the evidence that supports the possibility of rapid transformation or quantum change.

SHORT-TERM PSYCHOTHERAPY OF PERSONALITY DISORDERS: AN OXYMORON?

The idea of transforming a personality is fraught with polemics. For instance, some writers (McWilliams, 1994) hold the view that personality cannot be transformed, although it can be substantially modified. I concur with Livesley, Schroeder, Jackson, and Jang (1994), who stated, "The temporal stability of personality traits, however, does not mean that personality is immutable. Circumstances do lend to major personality change; modulation in the expression of traits across the life span is typical" (p. 14). Reich suggested this in 1933: "A compulsive character will never change into a hysteric character" (p. 117). However, he goes on to say, "the whole being of the patient becomes different . . . a change which is often more apparent to people who see the patient only occasionally, at long intervals, than to the analyst" (p. 118). Since the present-day, short-term psychotherapists have dramatically sped up the process, these changes are even more evident to those who have witnessed or conducted follow-up interviews, indicative of personality transformation. Although the patient never loses the hue or tone of his/her certain personality type, this fact does not mitigate the power of a structural transformation, where a midlevel borderline is moved to a neurotic level or an ego-syntonic obsessional character is made ego-dystonic. Although, as Reich (1945, p. 118) said, "the personal note" may never be lost, certainly the melody can change.

Most practicing clinicians have helped their patients achieve transformation in some way, though not as consistently as they might hope. In Stone's (1993) review of follow-up studies focusing on the severe personality disorders, he concludes that "beneficial changes can often occur," and that "current treatment approaches can often be instrumental in effecting positive changes" (p. 152). The potential for in-depth personality restructuring and rapid change *does* exist when the appropriate candidate is matched with the optimal approach. Under certain conditions that will be described, short-term dynamically oriented therapy can effectively transform a personality; in other cases, a gradual shift results.

Skepticism in certain doses may be healthy for science, but it can be debilitating to those trying to alleviate psychological pain. Most psychotherapists have, at some point in their careers, participated in what Miller and C'deBaca (1994) describe as "discontinuous transformational experiences"—or nonincremental change, although perhaps not as frequently as desired.[4] In fact, psychotherapy as a clinical process is predicated on the belief that with help, change *is* possible. To dismiss centuries of reported radical and quickly made character transformations denies the practitioner a unique way of understanding the phenomenon of rapid change. The following sources provide convergent evidence of the possibility of rapid and enduring personality change:

- A series of psychotherapy outcome studies showing significant change in personality disordered patients.
- Research showing naturally occurring quantum change leading to transformation of personality.
- Documented case reports by generations of clinicians showing major characterological change.
- Videotaped sessions showing the process of change.
- Outcome evaluations showing stability of change from 1 to 7 years.
- Evidence from centuries of reports on conversion experiences.
- Descriptions in the literary, autobiographical, and biographical works of personality transformations.

• Increasing consensus that severe trauma can result in major personality change.

Some of the evidence cited above can be found in various literature on
short-term dynamic therapy, as well as in the general psychological literature. An excellent summary that comprehensively reviews much of this
material can be found in the book *Can Personality Change?* (Heatherton
& Weinberger, 1995). Since so many excellent sources are available, I
emphasize the most current research and briefly summarize the clinical
literature. The remainder of the book provides evidence of outcome from
follow-up and summary of the process of change from videotaped sessions.
The reader should definitely take the opportunity to read the original case
descriptions by Davanloo, Malan, Mann, and Sifneos, as well as many of
the third-generation clinicians who have been trained by those masters.

Psychotherapy Outcome Findings: Efficacy of Brief Dynamic Psychotherapy

Although there is an ever-growing body of evidence that proves that
short-term psychodynamic psychotherapy is effective in symptom reduction
(Horowitz, Marmar, Weiss, Kaltreider, & Wilner, 1986), very little research
has been done applying the treatment model to personality disorders,
although what has been reported is promising (Monsen, Odland, Faugli,
Daae, & Eilertsen, 1995). An excellent study by Horowitz et al. (1984),
although not primarily concerned with the treatment of personality disorders, suggests that short-term dynamic therapy has a positive effect on
characterological modification. Thirty-three women and two men who
were coping with the death of a parent were treated with brief psychodynamic psychotherapy. Thirty of the subjects received an Axis II (DSM-III-R;
American Psychiatric Association, 1987) diagnosis of personality disorder.
Outcome was evaluated using multiple criteria: the patient, the evaluating
clinician, the treating clinician, and independent judges, who viewed pre-
and posttreatment videotapes. Patients with the highest severity of characterological disturbance (narcissistic and borderline) were more likely to
have poor to fair outcomes. Patients with less severe personality disorders
fared better. The researchers consistently found that the patients experienced symptom relief after STDP as measured by all four criteria. There
was also an improvement in assertiveness, level of adaptive functioning, and
in composite self-concept and interpersonal variables. Although there were
only "modest gains" in these measures of psychosocial adaptation, the
researchers believed that this was in part a function of the focus on loss in

the therapy. They suggested that short-term therapies that focus on character change might produce more powerful results.

In 1991, A. Winston et al. treated a cohort of patients with compulsive, avoidant, dependent, passive–aggressive, histrionic, and mixed personality disorders. Thirty-two patients were treated with either STDP based on Davanloo's principles or with brief adaptive psychotherapy (BAP; Pollack & Horner, 1985), based primarily on Sifneos's principles. The findings indicated that the two treatment groups demonstrated significantly greater improvement than a control group. There was not only symptomatic improvement but also a change in the level of social adjustment. The researchers were greatly encouraged by the results, particularly so because of the patients' long-standing characterological difficulties and histories of extensive prior treatment. Along similar lines of investigation, the efficacy of defense restructuring with personality disordered patients has been demonstrated over the course of brief dynamic treatment (B. Winston, Samstag, Winston, & Muran, 1994).

A. Winston et al. (1994) conducted a follow-up study 1½ years following termination of 38 personality disordered patients treated with BAP and STDP. The results showed that the improvement in target complaints seen at termination, as measured by the Symptom Checklist-90 (SCL-90),[5] held with the passage of time. The results indicate that STDP is effective with predominately Cluster C personality disorders and, furthermore, that the gains are lasting.

There was also evidence of clinically significant symptom improvement in a study that emphasized the process of change during psychotherapy (Jones, Parke, & Pulos, 1992). A sample of 30 patients diagnosed with depression, dysthymia, phobias, panic disorder, generalized anxiety, obsessive–compulsive disorder, as well as other problems were treated with STDP (16 sessions) in a private practice setting. All showed a gradual shift from an external orientation to an inner orientation. Although these patients were described by the authors of the study as suffering from neurotic disorders, the severity of the problems treated leads one to believe that some of these patients may have had coexisting Axis II diagnoses as well.

Self-concept is generally considered an enduring and pervasive measure of change reflecting personality modification (Svartberg, Seltzer, & Stiles, 1996). In their study, Svartberg and associates treated 13 clients with 20 sessions of short-term anxiety-provoking psychotherapy (STAPP). The results were significant and showed that self-concept improved at termination and continued to show improvement 2 years following termination. The researchers' assumption was that change was due to "clients' learning to solve an emotional core problem which is being evoked in the transference through anxiety-provoking techniques" (p. 45). What the authors found noteworthy in their results was the fact that, after termination, the clients developed a "self-freeing self-concept." Although the sample size was small, the results support the possibility of personality change, albeit with a higher functioning group than the population this book describes.

Although the research evidence is limited at this time, there is substantial evidence of clinically significant change using STDP with personality disorders. I briefly review this in the following section, but the interested reader should definitely review the primary sources, where case material is reported.

The Clinical Evidence

What degree of change can the clinician realistically hope for when confronted with a personality disordered patient? Some researcher/clinicians have reported *rapid characterological transformation* and symptom resolution with long-standing character disturbances (Alexander & French, 1946; Davanloo, 1980, 1990; Malan, 1963, 1976, 1979; Malan & Osimo, 1992). However, many of the pioneers of short-term psychotherapy were charismatic and possessed enormous clinical genius. The force of their personality, intellect, or attunement to the unconscious may have overshadowed technique.

What can the rest of the psychotherapeutic community hope to achieve? Many clinicians are capable of effecting major transformation with difficult patients *at times*. Most of us can remember a case in which significant change occurred and held. Many times we dismiss these results as having little to do with our psychotherapeutic acumen. If we do attribute these dramatic results to our skill or perseverance, we may not fathom what has occurred on a conceptual level or know how to do it again, though most of us strive for consistency in achieving positive results. It has been my experience, however, that what works with one patient may have the opposite outcome with another patient, even though the two appear similar diagnostically. For example, one patient with a severe obsessional character with narcissistic features responded poorly to suggestions that he undertake brief treatment. He stated that no one could understand his complexities without knowing him for years. He seemed to have a romanticized notion of his disturbance; in fact, he seemed to derive a sense of power from his recalcitrant nature and the fact that no therapist had ever succeeded in helping him. Challenging his defenses only made him feel misunderstood. Yet another patient with obsessive–compulsive personality responded positively to one of the more challenging approaches. This example serves to illustrate that although diagnostic categories are useful insofar as they alert the clinician to existing possibilities, they cannot provide a thorough reading of the structural integrity of the patient's ego system. I intend to show how systematic structural assessment and collaboration with the patient, as a partner in the process, will increase the likelihood that an appropriate restructuring method will be selected. When this match occurs, significant gains are more likely to result. In any event, treatment will be challenging, and pitfalls do exist that we discuss later.

Strangely enough, many personality disordered patients report that they are proud of their defenses. This makes treatment especially challenging. For example, I have treated some patients who have romanticized their severe detachment by adopting what I call the "Dirty Harry" persona. In the Dirty Harry movies, Clint Eastwood portrays the stereotypical emotionless male who relies on no one but himself. Many severely emotionally disconnected patients report that they made a conscious decision to be "strong" like Dirty Harry and actually take pride in this manufactured stoicism. Most of these patients are men with severe detachment predating the Dirty Harry movies, who, upon seeing these movies, strongly identify with the character. What they fail to appreciate is the cost of this style of relating, both to themselves and others. Many have left a trail of relationships they have destroyed, not unlike the bodies that Dirty Harry leaves behind him in film. Interpersonal disturbances are common in these types of cases (Frommer, Reissner, Tress, & Langenbach, 1996). It is only when the destructiveness of this manner of relating is squarely faced, and the concomitant grief is accessed, that profound and lasting transformation can occur. We refer to these character types as "ego-syntonic," and until Davanloo (1980) advanced the work carried out by Reich, little could be done for them in any type of treatment. These people simply would not tolerate long-term therapy.

I have found that some character disordered patients identify with the persona of Mr. Spock from *Star Trek*. These patients strongly resemble the alexithymic patients first described by Nemiah (1975). They have also been referred to as "submerged personalities" (Wolf & Kutash, 1991) having an "empty core" (Seinfeld, 1991). Such individuals are severely disconnected from their affect and are truly incapable of affective responses. Again, many of these patients pride themselves on their "rationalism" and fail to understand the emotional disturbance the defense masks. These severely disconnected patients require techniques that are capable of mobilizing massive amounts of anxiety such as those Sifneos used with his higher-functioning patients.

In cases where major transformation is unlikely, the clinician *can* create a positive feedback loop, addressing a single key issue. Even a small degree of change in a patient's personality is in itself significant and can have a major impact on others in the patient's life. Often, a small change will bring systemic change and alter the self-reinforcing feedback loops that are well articulated in the interpersonal model (Benjamin, 1993).

Some personality disordered patients present with fragile egos. With these patients, clinicians can work to achieve rapid *symptom resolution* and prevent further deterioration leading to a break down of defenses, which would then result in a fragmentation of the personality. The cognitive restructuring techniques are quite useful in strengthening the patient's defense system in the hope that, at a future point, derepressive work and a more comprehensive restructuring will be possible.

Millon (1981) has stated that personality is the first line of defense against stress. Stone (1993) agreed, using the metaphor of a radial tire that must withstand the stresses and shocks of the road and preserve the air (self-esteem) inside; if the system is penetrated, breakdown results. Axis I disorders such as posttraumatic stress disorder, anxiety, and anorexia often represent a failure of the personality to handle chronic stress (Stone, 1993). Stone (1993) described the process of traumatic breakdown of the defensive layer this way:

> If all other layers of the self are overwhelmed—either because the stress is truly overwhelming (concentration camp torture, public humiliation, rage, sudden rejection by a lover) or because the individual is fragile— one may witness psychological collapse. In this state we encounter the extremes of maladaptive reaction: murder, psychosis, fragmentation of the personality (as in "multiple" personality), or annihilation of the self (as seen in certain concentration camp inmates, who become robot-like or "zombies," having lost all dignity and coping ability). (p. 10)

On the other hand, as we have noted, these breakdowns, if not so severe, can lead the person into treatment.

Brief interventions can often provide a patient with a measure of *inoculation* from current and future stressors (Horowitz et al., 1984). Horowitz et al. (1984) found, for example, that brief dynamic therapy was effective in treating posttraumatic stress responses. Personality disordered patients are more prone to symptomatic reactions under conditions of stress, which, as Stone pointed out, can be catastrophic. Patients suffering the effects of significant trauma can require focused intervention not aimed at fully addressing characterological disturbances. For instance, patients with pathological grief reactions often have histories of multiple unresolved losses and present with various Axis I disturbances, such as substance abuse, clinical depression, and eating disorders. Reactivating the grief and then helping the patient to face it can strengthen adaptive or mature defenses, thereby increasing protection against future loss.

WHAT DISTINGUISHES IN-DEPTH SHORT-TERM THERAPY FROM OTHER FORMS OF TREATMENT?

There are a number of factors that distinguish in-depth short-term psycho-therapy from traditional forms of treatment. Although these have been well documented elsewhere (Bauer & Kobos, 1987), they deserve recapitulation.

1. Maintaining a strong focus on the core issues—not allowing the process to go off course.
2. High activity level of the therapist—especially during the initial phase of treatment.
3. Early use of interpretation.
4. High level of emotional arousal—as much as can be tolerated.
5. Time limitations—informing the patient that treatment is time-limited.
6. Rapid derepression of unconscious—as tolerated by ego structure.
7. Depth of treatment.

The most controversial of these factors has been the foreshortening of treatment and depth of treatment. Long-term therapy presupposes that deep reconstructive work requires a long time and that early trauma must be slowly uncovered (Hoyt, 1994). Thus, the therapeutic use of time is the cornerstone of any short-term treatment approach. The expectation of finishing treatment within a specific time frame probably acts as an accel-erant of the process for most patients.

Time Limitations

In my clinical experience, it is a common phenomenon for personality disordered patients to have a distorted sense of the passage of time. Their defensive structure often protects them from the existential anxiety caused by the passing of time. Brack, Brack, and Zucker (1992) in a literature review state "that individuals with character disorders have no past to frame the present and to give meaning to their actions, and thus are time independent" (p. 337). They also note trauma survivors often have a foreshortened perspective of the future. Patients with personality disorders often are not tuned in to the ebbs and flows of time. Prescribing a short-term treatment, in and of itself, almost always mobilizes an intrapsychic crisis, centering on attachment–separation themes. Reconnecting to the limits of time in various stages of the life cycle is often a jolt. "Short-term dynamic psychotherapy bridges the gap between two otherwise non-overlapping domains: the pragmatic, results oriented world of short-term treatment and the timeless realm of deep, comprehensive psychoanalytic understanding" (Fosha, 1995, p. 297).

The response from many has been that the significant changes that occur in STDP are not substantive and represent one of the following: transference cures, symptoms that disappear during therapy but reappear after termination, flight into health, or counterphobic responses that do not hold over time (Sifneos, 1995). Well-documented research indicates otherwise. Hoyt (1985) states, "Short-term dynamic psychotherapy can be highly intensive, exploratory, and anxiety-provoking, and can result in significant and enduring insight and personality change" (p. 98). Recent researchers have focused on the crucial element of time and how best to determine the optimal length of treatment. The maximum percentage of gain is often reached in approximately 52 weekly sessions (Howard, Kopta, Krause, & Orlinsky, 1986). At this time, we do not know the exact optimal number of sessions for treating the various personality disorders.

How Short Is Short-Term?

In a meta-analysis of 375 studies, Smith, Glass, and Miller (1980) demonstrated that the average length of psychological treatment was 17 sessions. It would seem, in effect, that *most* therapy conducted is, in practice, short-term, ranging from one to 40 sessions. I prefer to categorize short-term psychotherapy for the personality disordered patient in three groupings: crises intervention, brief treatment, and short-term psychotherapy. These distinctions become particularly important when one is working with personality disordered patients. Many of these patients are originally seen for crisis intervention and then fail to continue treatment once the crisis has subsided. In fact, we have noticed in our practice that when many potential patients initially call, they describe themselves as being in crisis and request an appointment as soon as possible. If these patients cannot be seen immediately, they cancel or fail to show up for the consultation. It is likely that many of these callers are personality disordered patients, who, as soon as their equilibrium is temporarily reestablished and their crisis has passed, feel they no longer require assistance from a mental health professional.

The categories I find most useful are described as follows:

Crisis Intervention

Crisis intervention takes from 1 to 3 sessions. The purpose is simply to assist the patient in establishing his/her equilibrium after he/she has experienced a trauma.

Brief Treatment

Brief treatment requires from 4 to 12 sessions. The goal of this type of intervention is to accomplish symptom reduction and/or trait modification. The act of setting a finite number of sessions often mobilizes the patient's core issues, especially those related to grief-laden losses and those that result from paths not taken in the past (Mann, 1973).

Short-Term Psychotherapy

Short-term therapy takes considerably longer, ranging from 12 to 40 sessions in length. For the treatment-refractory group, another course of treatment is often required, increasing the upper limit to 80 sessions. This is a more ambitious undertaking in that the goals are not only symptom resolution and trait modification but also substantial characterological change.

The descriptor "short-term" is open to multiple interpretation. Although the time-limit goal of STDP is from 12 to 40 sessions (Crits-Christoph & Barber, 1991) and the average course of STDP treatment runs 20 or so sessions, not all personality disordered patients can benefit in this period of time. With refractory patients, the number of sessions is often extended to as many as 80 sessions. Some might justifiably argue that 80 sessions is long-term. I have elected to continue using the phrase "short-term" because this treatment model is derived from and utilizes short-term principles and techniques. Also, 12 to 40 sessions *is* short compared to the number required to achieve character change with traditional psychoanalysis (600 to 1,000 sessions).

I considered various methods of tallying the number of sessions. Many patients return at a later time for another course of treatment; this situation is discussed later in the clinical chapters. Also, many patients prefer the 90-minute session as opposed to the 45-minute session. I have chosen to define "session" as a unit of 45 minutes.

Depth of Treatment

"We can define the 'depth' of a therapeutic experience by the degree to which the procedures employed emphasize unconscious experience, historical determinants, and involuntary behavior, as opposed to emphasizing conscious experience, contemporary determinants, and voluntary behavior" (Beutler & Clarkin, 1990, p. 240). Beginning with Alexander and French in 1946, clinical researchers have repeatedly established that the *depth* of focus is not related to the *length* of treatment (Bauer & Kobos, 1984). Although this was considered heresy as little as two decades ago, it is now a well-accepted clinical finding, having been published in case reports and videotape presentations of initial psychotherapy sessions. These videotape presentations are shown at conferences by various presenters throughout the world. They show that the unconscious can be accessed rapidly with active psychodynamic approaches. Even in a single extended interview of 2 to 3 hours, one can unearth buried material that would have taken months, or even years, to reach with more traditional long-term approaches.

CONCLUSION

At present, the field of psychology is faced with the following dilemma: How can we provide effective treatment to all patients who suffer from personality disorders and still meet the increasingly stringent demands placed upon us by insurance companies who demand both briefer treatment and proof of efficacy? There are no easy answers. Inherent in this book, however, is the belief that STDP can provide in-depth, growth-promoting therapy for people with personality disorders. This belief is supported by evidence clearly indicating that rapid, transformational, enduring changes *are repeatedly made.*

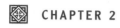 CHAPTER 2

The STRP Model: Process, Theory, and Constructs

> *Therefore, I say there is no universal method of brief psychotherapy,
> no Dante to follow for everyone. Every observing position has its
> advantages, its successes, and its dangers. Every position has a
> periphery, where important phenomena will occur and be missed,
> because of the center of interest of that position.*
>
> —GUSTAFSON (1986, p. 7)

SHORT-TERM RESTRUCTURING PSYCHOTHERAPY

The therapeutic approach explicated in this book was formulated expressly
for the treatment of personality disorders. In dynamic and existential
therapy, Singer (1971, p. 89) states that "the therapist's work is to help in
the restructuring of the total personality . . . in a shared deep and authentic
experience." The term restructuring is not new, and has been used before
by various schools of psychotherapy. Restructuring refers to an effort to
provide a new structure or organization to a personality and to resume ego
development (Loewald, 1960) and most aptly captures what clinicians view
as the central issue and ultimate treatment goal of work with the personality
disordered patient, a comprehensive restructuring of the personality (CRP).
Short-term restructuring psychotherapy (STRP) is an amalgam of existing
approaches, which represents another line in the evolutionary process of
STDP, as well as an integration of cognitive and experiential approaches. It
is a structural–integrative approach, using Freud's basic tripartite structure
(Magnavita, 1993c) of the human psyche as the foundation, to which

17

various techniques and methods are annexed. STRP assumes that no single approach or theory of psychic functioning is correct or uniformly applicable but, rather, that all provide different views of the patient. Selecting the proper treatment approach is crucial to a positive outcome (Frances, Clarkin, & Perry, 1984). Clinicians must become adept at changing lenses, especially when facing a challenging case. Very briefly, the steps of STRP, which will be elaborated in the following chapters, are as follows:

1. *Identify maladaptive trait, pattern, and style.*
   - Bring this to patient's attention. Show how it interferes with attaining goals, limits gratification, and maintains symptoms.
2. *Isolate trait.*[1]
   - Use examples from current, past, and transference relationship to highlight pattern.
3. *Select restructuring approach.*
   - Determine whether to undertake a comprehensive restructuring of the personality or a stepwise approach.
   - Select one or a combination of the following methods: [defensive]–[affective]–[cognitive] restructuring
4. *Relate patterns to core structure.*
   - Bring feelings from core difficulties to surface and assist the patient in the process of metabolizing them.
5. *Encourage more adaptive patterns.*
   - Encourage activities, challenges, and positive adaptive patterns that were previously avoided.
   - Process patient's experience and reaction.

STRP is based on the assumption that personality can be modified in a comprehensive fashion, using a mixture of three restructuring methods: defensive, cognitive, and affective restructuring. In its most simplistic sense, *defensive restructuring* is represented by the question *"What are you doing right now?"* In other words, what is going on between you and me—in the interpersonal field—or you and others, that interferes with your relationships, goals, and so on? Further, what does this indicate about intrapsychic functions?

Cognitive restructuring is represented by the question *"What are you thinking?"* That is, what is going on in your head right now that is influencing how you are behaving, feeling, and perceiving? It pinpoints the cognitive apparatus and how that apparatus is schematically organized.

Affective restructuring is represented by the question *"How are you feeling?"* It attempts to uncover the affect and its links to current problems. This entails activation of the affective schemas that are usually well protected by the patient with a personality disorder.

The clinician's ability to combine these restructuring methods in a logical and sequential fashion depends on an accurate assessment of the patient. With some patients, the goal is a *comprehensive restructuring of the personality*; with others, a more modest, *stepwise approach* is preferable. There is some overlap among the methods, and the concepts should be used heuristically to guide appropriate treatment.

At this point I briefly review the major theoretical concepts and specific approaches from which STRP draws. To do so in a truly comprehensive fashion is impossible, as I have been influenced by so many clinicians, researchers, and theoreticians. By and large, I believe that the most significant advances in this field were made by the first and second generation workers and, therefore, I draw most heavily from their work.

In order to reduce the length of treatment, pioneers in STDP continually modified existing approaches and techniques.[2] Although there is some overlap in the various techniques and theories, there remains in each much that distinguishes it from the others. All of them have at their foundation a belief in *unconscious processes* and share the conviction that, when the patient is ready, the forces of *repression* should be lifted so that nonmetabolized, affectively charged material can be worked through and put into proper perspective. This frees the patient to more actively engage the world and to pursue his/her unique developmental trajectory.

STRP does not provide a unified theory embracing drive theory, object relations, self psychology, and cognitive psychology, but rather, as Pine (1990) describes, a "multiperspective approach." And, as he points out, although there are areas of theoretical convergence, there are differences, as well. Each approach helps us understand the clinical phenomena we encounter in treating the spectrum of personality disordered patients.

In Table 2.1 I summarize the elements that are used in STRP. I then trace the natural evolution of these theories, constructs, and techniques, and the pioneers who developed them, leading to my current conceptualization (Magnavita, 1993b; Sifneos, 1981, 1984a). The reader who is not familiar with this material will need to do further reading from primary sources to assimilate these important developments. For other readers more familiar with the subject matter, this section can serve as a circumscribed review of some of the major breakthroughs that have been achieved in this century (see also *History of Psychotherapy*; Freedheim, 1992).

Theoretical Models

Specific treatment approaches derive their metapsychological concepts, theories of change, and techniques from a particular school. Each model

**TABLE 2.1. Summary of Theoretical
and Technical Components of STRP**

Theoretical models

Basic framework: structural–integrative
Drive theory
Object relations
Self psychology
Cognitive psychology

Technical components

Increasing the emotional intensity to highest level
Singling out and penetrating the character defenses
Mastering the emotional conflict in the transference
Flexibility of therapeutic stance
Flexibility of scheduling
Use of extended sessions to increase potency
Emphasis on nonverbal communication
Use of empathic mirroring
Identifying multiple core issues
Orienting treatment with triangles
Active use of techniques of defense analysis
Use of anxiety to accelerate treatment
Challenging dysfunctional beliefs/schemas
Use of time limitations to activate grief
Encouragement of extratherapeutic activities

offers a unique view of the patient and, thus, each has its own inherent limitations and advantages. The psychoanalytic models[3] that are encompassed in STRP are *structural–drive theory,* *object relations,* and *self psychology.* I also include *cognitive psychology* in this discussion because some forms of it have many similarities to psychoanalysis, and it offers a unique perspective.

Structural–Drive Theory

Structural–drive theory (Freud, 1916–1917/1953) provides the clinician with a comprehensive metapsychology, which offers an essential tool in understanding how traumatic events/conflicts and concomitant feelings are repressed and alternatively manifest in anxiety and defense. It focuses on how sexual and aggressive impulses are dealt with and managed by the defense system as well as delineates the various components and functions of the intrapsychic structure. These instinctual impulses give rise to anxiety, which then threatens to emerge into consciousness, requiring a defensive structure for containment (Fenichel, 1945). Since this is the cornerstone of the drive theory approach, I return to it in greater detail later in this chapter.

Object Relations Theory

Object relations theory offers two major contributions: It provides an understanding of early developmental tasks and how these unfold, and it also describes how pathology results when these developmental tasks remain incomplete (Johnson, 1985). Object relations theory has focused on the satisfaction that comes from positive attachments (Buckley, 1986; Fairbairn, 1954; Klein, 1948; Winnicott, 1965, 1986). The therapist's task is to form a new, positive connection with the patient in order to change fundamentally the patient's personality or "nature."

Self Psychology

Self psychology recognizes the basic human need to form a "false self" in response to a lack of attunement by parental figures to the real self (Kohut, 1971, 1977). Thus, among its major contributions is that it offers a way to understand the phenomenon of narcissism[4] and its variants. Instead of viewing anxiety as a result of fended-off libidinal and aggressive impulses alone, self psychologists believe that anxiety emanates from real or imagined injuries to self-esteem, and defenses are used as protection against this threat. Kohut (1977) has demonstrated how important a mirroring relationship is to the individual's developing self-esteem and self-cohesion. Without these relational elements, a "true self" is unable to develop, and the individual engages in an unrelenting search for affirmation.

Cognitive Psychology

Cognitive psychology emphasizes how cognitions influence emotional reactions and maintain self-defeating behavior patterns. Cognitive therapy has its roots in theories of learning and has developed along quite different lines from psychoanalytic theory. Originally, in contravention to the psychoanalytic movement, it emphasized the empirical study of human behavior. Aaron Beck (e.g., Beck, Rush, Shaw, & Emery, 1979), one of the most influential researcher/clinicians of the cognitive school, demonstrated the efficacy of this approach in the treatment of depression. He successfully used cognitive techniques, such as *challenging dysfunctional beliefs/schemas, collaborative empiricism,* and reattribution (reevaluating responsibility for outcome), on increasingly difficult cases, culminating in the publication of *Cognitive Therapy of Personality Disorders* (Beck, Freeman, & Associates, 1990). Currently, cognitive therapy concentrates on childhood themes or unconditional beliefs that represent indisputable truths about oneself and how the environment will respond to oneself (Young, 1990). "These unconscious products of early experience were incorporated into cognitive therapy under the scientifically respectable label of 'schemas' . . . which were formed early in one's experience and, once incorporated as organizing rules of behavior, forgotten" (Beutler & Clarkin, 1990, p. 8).

Essential Elements and Pioneers in the Evolution of STDP

In 1925, Ferenczi and Rank developed forms of active therapy emphasizing *increasing the emotional intensity* of the treatment by utilizing the following techniques: (1) encouraging activities avoided by the patient, (2) prohibiting stereotypical behavior patterns, (3) using forced fantasies, (4) assuming a particular transference role, and (5) setting a time limit. These technical breakthroughs were quite remarkable but were not eagerly embraced by the larger psychotherapeutic community because they were so radically different from standard analytic technique (Stanton, 1991).

In 1945, Reich advanced our understanding of character disturbances in his conceptualization of defenses crystallizing into "character armor." This armor or character defense system was recognized to be a serious impediment in standard analytic work. Access to the unconscious was sharply reduced as the patient seemed to have difficulty free associating and recalling dreams. Reich pioneered the technique of *singling out and penetrating the character defenses* so as to achieve an emotional breakthrough.[5] It was his assertion that a potent approach was required to achieve success with the characterologically disturbed patient. Horney (1937) also referred to these neurotic characters as manifesting "an invisible but impenetrable wall between the analyst and patient" (p. 157). She found that when confronted with their difficulties, these patients often broke off treatment. This *interpersonal barrier* may effectively protect against retraumatization, but it does so at the cost of further emotional growth and *intimacy* (Horney, 1939, 1950).

Alexander and French (1946) experimented with techniques similar to those used by Ferenczi and Rank. They asserted that this type of "active therapy" was deeply penetrating and that the curative factor was the ability of the patient to master the emotional conflict in the transference. This "corrective emotional experience," as it was coined, was the freedom to express emotion without the fear of punishment or censure by the therapist or the superego. They also recognized the importance of *therapeutic flexibility,* suggesting that not only should the therapist assume different therapeutic stances, but he/she should emphasize *flexibility of scheduling* and use *extended sessions.*

Balint (1969/1992), who strongly influenced Malan, felt that the more rigid techniques were effective primarily with patients with oedipal period conflicts. He states that, with patients from this more "primitive" group, clinicians deal with what he calls the "basic fault," which is not a true conflict or complex. He describes the characteristics of the basic fault as

> (a) having only events that occur exclusively in a two-person relationship—there is never a third person present; (b) having a two-person relationship of a particular nature, entirely different from the well-known human relationships of the Oedipal level; (c) having a specific dynamic force operating at this level that is not a conflict; and (d) that adult language is often useless or misleading in describing events at this level, because words have not always an agreed conventional meaning. (pp. 16–17)

Balint believes that the basic fault leads to primitive object relationships. Often, the therapeutic spotlight is on the patient's *nonverbal communication*. Patients in this group suffer from overwhelming and intense anxiety and are prone to regression under stress. It is theorized that they suffer from early disturbances in the dyadic attachment as a result of gross failures in the primary attachment. Thus, the basic ingredients necessary in laying the foundation for the development of the self are missing: trust, security, and love. *Empathy* and the patient–therapist relationship are critical elements in this reparative treatment.[6] These early developmental insults must be addressed before the personality can move ahead to a more mature level of psychic organization and a higher level of structuralization. Gustafson (1995) further delineates two categories of patients with basic faults: the malignant and benign. The malignant group consists of the more tragic patients who are in decline and for whom little can be done.

Kohut (1971) demonstrated how important a *mirroring relationship* was to an individual's development of self-esteem[7] and self-cohesion. Without these relational elements, a "true self" is unable to develop, and the individual engages in a constant search for affirmation. In a sense, these patients do not have the well-defined structural apparatus (clear differentiation between id, ego, and superego) of the higher-level, characterologically organized patients, such as one sees in the obsessional and hysteric subgroups.

Kohut observed that oedipal pathology was not evident in all patients. "The child's affectionate attitude does not have to disintegrate into fragmented sexual impulses as a result of unempathic and rejecting responses" (Rowe & Mac Isaac, 1991, p. 88). Kohut viewed the oedipal phase as a part of normal development, rather than as an "inevitable complex of problems." "The healthy child will enter the oedipal phase in a joyous manner and will experience pride in his or her developmental achievements if the parents can recognize and appreciate them" (p. 88). Disturbances in *selfobject* relations, (injuries to the self), however, can lead to rage and intense sexual impulses. The issue in determining the source of psychopathology then becomes whether or not the patient's parents had adequate self-structure to meet their child's selfobject needs, rather than whether or not the patient, as a child, experienced one or more traumatic events.

Another major advancement in the field was achieved by David Malan.[8] In 1963, Malan published a series of outcome studies to test the proposition that in-depth change could be achieved using a "focal approach" originally developed by Michael Balint, who was strongly influenced by Sandor Ferenczi.[9] The focal approach is based on *identifying one core issue,* which becomes the emphasis of selective attention and interpretation.[10]

Malan (1979) was the first to combine two essential constructs that can describe all psychodynamic treatment. The first, the "triangle of insight" (transference, current life figures, and past figures) was originally presented by Menninger (1958) and renamed the "triangle of person" by Malan, who thought this phrasing more accurately described the construct. Malan also borrowed from Ezriel (1952) in creating the second construct, the "triangle of conflict," and it consists of defense, anxiety, and hidden feeling. The "triangle of conflict" is related to the "triangle of person" in that hidden feeling can be directed toward any corner of the "triangle of person." On the importance of these triangles, Malan said:

> Each triangle stands on an apex, which represents the fact that the aim of most dynamic psychotherapy is to reach, beneath the *defense* and the *anxiety,* to the hidden feeling, and then to trace this feeling back from the present to its origins *in the past,* usually in the relation with parents. . . . The importance of these two triangles is that between them they can be used to represent almost every intervention that a therapist makes; and that much of a therapist's skill consists of knowing which parts of which triangle to include in his [her] interpretation at any given moment. (p. 80)

I feel these two constructs provide both clarity and parsimony and are testament to Malan's genius as a theorist and clinician.

About the same time, Davanloo was working in Montreal with similar methods having application to character disturbances (Della Selva, 1996). Davanloo's (1980) intensive short-term dynamic psychotherapy (IS-TDP) was heralded as a major conceptual and technical advance by Malan himself, who described it as "a twentieth century miracle." Davanloo's highly confrontational approach places heavy emphasis on *intensifying affect* (Laikin, Winston, & McCullough, 1991). Although Malan introduced the concept of "trial therapy," Davanloo also used it as a tool in determining a prospective patient's suitability for short-term treatment. Trial therapy is typically an extended 2- to 3-hour interview, during which the patient's response to the approach can be evaluated. Davanloo's brilliance is in his advancement of *techniques of defense analysis,* pioneered by Reich, but with greater technical specificity.

Meanwhile, Sifneos was working in Boston along similar lines. He developed a style of treatment called "short-term anxiety provoking psychotherapy" (STAPP; 1987), which had a primarily oedipal focus. Like Malan and Davanloo, Sifneos developed a highly focused form of treatment that, instead of actively working with the defense system, relies mostly on deep interpretation and anxiety-provoking clarifications to keep the tension level high, and thus *disrupt the defenses.* Sifneos showed how *increasing anxiety* can accelerate the psychotherapy. Unlike Davanloo's method, Sifneos (1984b) interprets material before systematically analyzing defense mechanisms.

About the same time that Davanloo and Sifneos were advancing their approaches, Mann (1973; Mann & Goldman, 1982) was also working independently on a similar accelerated dynamic approach. Mann's time-limited psychotherapy (TLP) is based on a 12-session model that *activates issues of attachment and separation.* Mann's work was influenced by Otto Rank (1929/1973) who elaborated the concept of separation–individuation emphasizing the interpersonal process in dealing with these issues. Thus, forming an attachment and then separating from the therapist mobilizes the patient's core issues. The central focus is brought up by the need to deal with termination so quickly and usually relates to unresolved losses. It differs from IS-TDP and STAPP in that it does not rely on anxiety-provoking intervention or challenge to defenses but, rather, uses a more empathic approach. In other words, the essential elements of the treatment are the nonspecific "common" therapeutic factors that were elaborated by Rogers (1957) and include genuineness, acceptance, nonjudgmentalness, empathy, and prizing.

This emphasis on the relationship encourages the therapist to be more real, vulnerable, and mutual than traditional psychoanalytic models (Jordan, 1995). In a short-term treatment model, this relational emphasis *rapidly activates unresolved grief,* as well as other affects, but primarily grief-laden feeling. Its greatest value seems to be in addressing the sectors of the personality that have experienced self-injuries or attachment disruptions existing at a preoedipal level. The use of empathy and mutuality allows the therapist to bypass the defenses (Fosha, 1995).

Given the heterogeneity and complexity of the clinical conditions subsumed under the classification personality disorder, there is no doubt that any one approach will not do justice to the clinical phenomenon. In the next section, I briefly review this need for a multiperspective approach with the personality disordered patient. I follow with a more detailed discussion of the metapsychological assumptions and important constructs of the structural model.

The Need for a Multiperspective Approach

Human beings are far too complex for us believe that any one model of treatment will work for most. Although psychotherapy integration has its critics, most clinicians who write about and treat personality disturbances value various theoretical perspectives and technical eclecticism (Beutler & Clarkin, 1990; Clarkin & Lenzenweger, 1996; Gustafson, 1986; Johnson, 1994; Millon, Everly, & Davis, 1993; Stone, 1993). Stone (1993) comments:

> One cannot prescribe *ex cathedra* which path will be the more suitable for any given therapist. Those who follow one authority closely will have the advantage of depth, but at the sacrifice of breadth in terms of the range of narcissistic subtypes with which the therapist can work efficiently. (p. 276)

> The eclectic approach that is usually necessary in treating problems in personality (single maladaptive traits as well as full-fledged disorders) consists, then, of supportive interventions (useful in fostering a therapeutic alliance), psychoanalytically informed interventions (useful in resolving negative transference at the outset), and cognitive-behavioral interventions (useful in development of new habits and attitudes). Special interventions, such as the use of medication or of group therapy, will often be necessary as well. (p. 164)

Guerette (1995),[11] after more than 12 years of observing over 160 different therapists and their work, commented, "What has struck me time and time again are the many similarities in what they were doing, yet they used different language in which to describe what they understand and what they do." At present, three routes toward psychotherapy integration are used. In addition to technical eclecticism (which emphasizes using techniques that work regardless of theoretical concerns) and common factors (which emphasizes the essential ingredients in all forms of psychotherapy), the other is theoretical integration (developing a connecting metatheory) (Norcross & Goldfried, 1992). It seems clear that a flexible approach is necessary for a positive outcome (Budman, 1981, 1994; Gustafson, 1986; Stone, 1993). This requires therapists to be familiar with and skilled in various approaches. If one approach or technique does not work, another should be tried.

STRUCTURAL FRAMEWORK AS THE CORNERSTONE

In my clinical work, I have found that the structural model provides indispensable guiding principles for assessing and treating patients with personality disorders. I agree with Lacan that "the unconscious is structured like a language" quoted in (Lemaire, 1970/1994, p. 7). Therefore, I have used this as the basic conceptual framework for STRP. Although the structural model's explanatory value is weakest with early developmental psychopathology, we can view object relations and self-validation as the initial organizing influences leading to the beginning of intrapsychic structure.

Pine (1990) emphasizes the essential nature of "structuralization, or internalization, or intrapsychic differentiation" (p. 63) in various domains. The primary goal in treating personality disordered patients is to increase the structuralization[12] of the psychic apparatus by utilizing strategies that will lead to higher levels of differentiation and balance. Increased structuralization refers to the psychotherapeutic goal of increasing differentiation of, and reorganizing the psychic structures (id, ego, and superego)[13] at increasingly higher levels of adaptation (see Figure 2.1). Such restructuring (see Chapter 6), which includes the defensive, affective, and cognitive realms, leads to enhanced emotional tolerance, more mature defense usage, increased adaptation, and clearer cognitive and perceptual fields. Each personality disordered patient manifests a different level of structuralization. For example, in some patients, the id–ego matrix has failed to lead to the development of an autonomous ego (York et al., 1989). The id–ego matrix is an unstable substitute for the ego, and the ego's lack of independent status causes distortions in thinking and acting. In other cases, however, the division between the id and ego is too strong and fixed, which

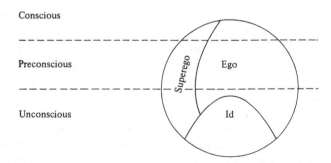

FIGURE 2.1. The relationship of the structural model of personality to levels of awareness. (Adapted from Wolman, 1968.) From Hjelle and Ziegler (1976, p. 25). Copyright 1976 by McGraw-Hill. Reprinted by permission.

causes antagonism toward the drives. Consequently, such a person cannot behave in uninhibited or creative ways.

Yet, other problems occur if the emergence of the superego is either incomplete or too complete. In the case of an overly active superego, the ego and superego can never reach agreement, and unjustified guilt feelings will constantly interfere with functioning. If the superego does not emerge, the dominant ego will support dystocial and egocentric behavior.

In clinical terms, structuralization refers to the attempt to unblock developmental fixations so that the individual can achieve higher levels of maturity and psychic integration. Blatt (1991) describes this dialectic process, alternating between the development of a consolidated self and the increased capacity to form reciprocal interpersonal relations. This is accomplished differently depending on the type of psychopathology the clinician is confronting. The "neurotic character disorders" (Shapiro, 1989; loosely translated to DSM terms are the Cluster C patients) result from internal incompatibility of the id, ego, and superego agencies and are characterized by frustration, anxiety, and repression. The intrapsychic structure is out of balance. "It seems that the person has tendencies that his own character cannot tolerate and reacts against, with remarkable consequences" (Shapiro, 1989, p. 3). Disavowed or repressed hostile impulses are the main source from which anxiety and defense spring (Horney, 1937). Horney realized that anxiety does not spring from sexual urges except when coupled with hostile impulses to humiliate or hurt another. This "introjected" group is much more likely to be struggling with aggression and self-assertion (Blatt, 1991).

In cases of "developmental psychopathology"[14] (loosely translated to DSM terms are the Cluster B patients), often referred to as preoedipal, the structural agencies have failed to clearly emerge and differentiate. There is a defect in the psychic apparatus. Blatt and Felsen (1993) term these "anaclitic" disorders primarily concerned with interpersonal relatedness. These patients often have a fragile structure (Davanloo, 1980; Pine, 1990) or unstable self.

The creation of a functioning intrapsychic world is predicated on the development of successful object relations and self–other representations. Without affection and love, basic object relatedness is flawed—the "basic fault." These disturbances usually characterize the Cluster A disorders. A satisfactory attachment is the first step in structuralization. The highest level of differentiation and fluidity of structural agencies is seen in the patient who is capable of clearly identifying feelings, anxiety, and defense (see Figure 2.2). Moving from the left to the right side of the continuum, we find the following:

1. A patient on left side lacks differentiation of psychic apparatus. The patient reports feeling strong affect states unconnected to transference or

Self disorder	Structural defects	Structural integrity
x————————	———— x ————	———————— x ——
[Undifferentiated self]	[Highly defended]	[Neurotic/oedipal]
Unstable structure	Overly fixed	Stable structure
Primitive defenses	Primitive/neurotic	Mature defenses
Profound disturbance in object relations		Positive attachment

FIGURE 2.2. Structural spectrum of personality disorders.

unconscious conflict. Anxiety is free floating and primitive, primarily related to abandonment and annihilation fears. The basic structure of the self has been impaired because of the absence of crucial developmental needs. There is a basic fault in the parent–child attachment.

2. A patient near the middle of the continuum shows structural integrity, but the system is overly rigid or fixed. This patient has the ability to repress and has a developed psychic structure (id, ego, and superego). Anxiety is aroused by impulses and feelings but is bound by character defenses and symptoms. Defenses serve to keep repressed material buried.

3. A patient on the extreme right has some access to unconscious material. Anxiety is present but tolerated; triangular relationships predominate. There has been a sufficient quantity of positive early attachment to the primary caregiver or parent(s). Difficulties arise out of the conflicts inherent in oedipal relationships, such as rivalry, and so on. The patient's personality may exhibit maladaptive traits but without a severe personality disturbance. Any preoedipal issues have colored the oedipal phase in a pathological manner (York et al., 1989).

STRP is based on the following assumptions drawn from research on personality and from analysis and integration of the various theories presented:

1. *Behavior is multidetermined.* Any system of understanding psychopathology is only one of many possible perspectives. Viewing patients only from an intrapsychic perspective misses the strong influences of the interpersonal field in maintaining and reinforcing maladaptive patterns. Being able to change lenses, that is, to view the behavior through alternative theories, multiplies our angles of comprehension.

2. *A personality disordered patient may have clear structural defects or a disorder of the self.* Treatment implications are very different for each. This distinction must be established at the outset by careful diagnostic assessment.

3. *The more evidence of self disorder present, the more emphasis should be placed on creating and nurturing the therapeutic alliance.* This

does not preclude the use of anxiety provoking defense analysis, but empathic responsiveness must be blended with these interventions or used in oscillating phases.

4. *The greater the evidence of structural defect, the more technical interventions aimed at derepression should be utilized.* Patients with structural defects have proceeded in their development to the point of repressing aggressive and sexual feeling toward the genetic figures. Anxiety-arousing interventions should be aimed toward bringing these affects to the surface so that they can be metabolized.

5. *Personality disordered patients often have combinations of pregenital (dyadic) and oedipal (triangular) conflicts/injuries.* In clinical practice, most patients have a blend of preoedipal and oedipal pathology, and for a comprehensive working-through to be achieved, both areas must be addressed.

6. *Biological, neuropsychological, and temperamental influences may contribute to the predisposition, development, and maintenance of personality disorders.* All personality disorders have their genesis in a mixture of both biological or psychogenic factors, which must be taken into consideration. For those with primarily biological loadings, medications should be used to mend neurophysiological deficits.

PRINCIPLES TO ORGANIZE COMPLEX DATA

The clinician, when processing the complex stimuli presented by the personality disordered patient, faces a daunting task indeed. This is amplified by the strenuous demands of short-term treatment wherein rapid identification of core issues needs to be achieved and then interpreted (Hoyt, 1985). Nonverbal communications, symptom constellations, character defenses, countertransference reactions, and verbal content are all expressed simultaneously, so that even highly experienced clinicians sometimes feel overwhelmed. With my first encounter, I begin to organize the various channels through which the patient communicates his/her developmental block, be it conflict or deficit. I then review the well-established metapsychological assumptions of the psychoanalytic model and then return to the two triangles that enable us to monitor the therapeutic process very precisely.

METAPSYCHOLOGICAL ASSUMPTIONS

Rapaport and Gill (1967), in a paper entitled "The Points of View and Assumptions of Metapsychology," review certain assumptions that are crucial in understanding the metapsychology of the psychoanalytic approach. These metapsychological assumptions are considered to represent the highest level of abstraction, literally beyond psychology. These assumptions serve as conceptual tools that establish the foundation for systematizing and organizing clinical data and formulations (Moore & Fine, 1990). There is a significant body of scientific research that supports these assumptions (Westen, 1986). Familiarity with these assumptions enlivens and enriches clinical formulations and provides a window into complex mental phenomena. These assumptions are well worth understanding. They include the following:

1. *Dynamic.* The dynamic viewpoint demands that any psychological phenomenon include propositions concerning the psychological forces within the psyche and interpersonally that create the phenomenon. Thus, any personality pattern or symptom constellation can be explained by these dynamic forces.

2. *Economic.* The economic viewpoint demands that the explanation of any psychological phenomenon include propositions concerning the excitation and discharge of psychic energy involved in the phenomenon. This might be observed in self-defeating behavior, where the build-up of unconscious guilt drives the penchant for self-punishment or for a patient at a lower level of structuralization, a behavioral reenactment of what is seeking expression. The more advanced the level of structural integration and development, the more economically the system works to enhance one's potential.

3. *Structural.* The structural viewpoint assumes the explanation of any psychological phenomenon will include postulations concerning the psychological configurations—ego, id, and superego (structures) involved in the phenomenon. Essentially, there is a hierarchical level of organization of the psychic apparatus for each patient. Thus, a patient who has not had a sufficient exposure to a secure dyadic relationship will structurally be organized at a psychotic or borderline level.

4. *Genetic.* The genetic viewpoint states that the explanation of any psychological phenomenon should include propositions concerning its psychological origin and development. Childhood experiences are crucial in shaping personality. Therefore, we seek to discover what caused the original injury or developmental insult. This is crucial when one is attempting to develop the core issue(s)[15] because this is the location where the deepest working through needs to occur.

5. *Adaptive.* The adaptive viewpoint postulates that the explanation of any psychological phenomenon include propositions concerning its relationship to interpersonal, environmental, and societal factors. Thus, personality is a unique adaptation to the complex biopsychosocial field. However, the adaptive value becomes lost as development proceeds. Devel-

oping an avoidant personality to cope with overwhelming parental conflict loses its adaptive value. For example, retreating to one's room as an adult to avoid conflict with one's spouse no longer has adaptive value.

6. *Topographic.* This refers to the regions of the psychic structure where conscious, preconscious, and unconscious sectors are delimited, as well as id, ego, and superego (Noy, 1977). These represent useful theoretical and metaphorical concepts (Harriman, 1947). Much of mental life, including emotional and cognitive schemas, exist at an unconscious level, especially for the personality disordered patient. From this perspective, the aim is to make the unconscious conscious and effect a full affective and cognitive restructuring.

These assumptions are used to establish conceptual understanding, formulate structural diagnosis, and plan treatment strategies. I agree with Noy (1977) that these concepts should not be reified beyond their usefulness, and yet they remain powerful organizing principles. However, with the addition of Malan's two essential constructs of the triangle of persons and the triangle of conflict, these assumptions have tremendous clinical utility.

Two Essential Psychodynamic Constructs

The main constructs that I use to orient myself and keep on track are the triangle of persons and triangle of conflict. The necessity of understanding the domain in which you are operating is crucial because of the goal of linking past patterns to current and transference patterns. Before proceeding, it would behoove you, as the clinician, to review and master these constructs. After learning them and using them to orient your treatment interventions, I am certain that you will appreciate both their elegance and Malan's genius in bringing them together.

Triangle of Persons

The triangle of persons includes *transference* (T), *current life figures* (C), and *significant past figures* (P) (see Figure 2.3). These corners are described below.

Transference. This term refers to the feelings, attitudes, and conflicts activated in relationship to the therapist. Reich (1945) found that character analysis will always intensify the hatred toward the therapist, but strong positive feelings are always generated by the therapist's continued attention and interest. Thus, there are elements of both positive and negative affect existing simultaneously in the transference. Patients may come into sessions with a build-up of transference feeling toward the therapist, or, alternatively,

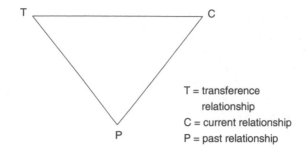

FIGURE 2.3. Triangle of persons.

it may arise slowly during the session or be indirectly expressed immediately in the character defenses. For example, one patient entered therapy for the first time taking a highly passive position in his verbal and nonverbal communications (slouched posture, low energy, quite voice, defeated demeanor) describing how unhappy he felt about his marriage. When he was asked to be specific about his complaints, he showed signs of being irritated with the therapist for disrupting his equilibrium.

Current. This term refers to the feelings, attitudes, and conflicts present in the patient's significant relationships at the time he or she enters into treatment. The current interpersonal conflicts are often part of the presenting complaint, involving spouses, friends, lovers, and colleagues. The above-mentioned patient described how, for 23 years, he was dominated and controlled by his wife but experienced overwhelming guilt whenever he tried to leave her. He declared, "I have spent my entire life unsuccessfully trying to please her." The C includes all the feelings, attitudes both conscious and unconscious, dynamics, and relational patterns that are in operation with current life figures.

Past. This term refers to the buried feeling, attitudes, and conflicts directed toward significant past figures and generally not consciously available to the patient. These are the feelings against which the patient must defend him/herself, usually because they are too painful to the conscious ego. In the above-mentioned case, the patient had been severely dominated and controlled by his mother from an early age and repressed all his negative feeling toward her, which resulted in tremendous passivity.

The use of this triangle can offer the therapist tremendous advantages. To mobilize the treatment, the therapist should be able to identify, in each interaction, on which corner of the triangle the interaction occurs. The therapist's object is to link two, or preferably three, corners of a triangle in a verbal interpretation (T–C, T–P, T–C–P interpretations). Using the case presented above, a T–C–P interpretation links the patient's anger toward the therapist (manifested in the transference communication—I won't budge, and I will prove how ineffective you are—to his "castrated" position with his wife and retaliation—I will never give her anything emotional—to his rage toward his mother that he had swallowed in the past and now expresses in his passivity.

Triangle of Conflict

The triangle of conflict refers to the interplay among defense/anxiety/impulse–feeling (see Figure 2.4). Buried feelings and impulses, especially aggressive and sexual feelings but also affectionate ones, give rise to anxiety. This anxiety is kept at bay with an assortment of symptom formations and character defenses. In the personality disordered patient, the main defenses are characterological and serve to keep anxiety within certain limits to maintain equilibrium, often at the cost of fuller functioning. These concepts are explained below.

Defense (D). This refers to intrapsychic mechanisms that involuntarily regulate nonmetabolized and highly charged affective states and instinctual impulses that are unacceptable or overwhelming to the conscious self. Defenses allow the individual to deal with sudden changes in the external world or internal surges that are activated by threats to esteem or anxiety-provoking stimuli.

To return to the case of the unhappily married man, his defenses— avoidance, withdrawal, complaining, repression, isolation of affect, and so on—culminated in a passive character. This defensive system served to keep impulses and anxiety contained.

Anxiety (A). This refers to physiological activation of the central

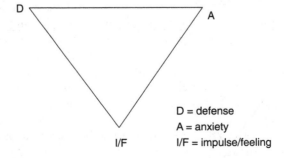

FIGURE 2.4. Triangle of conflict.

nervous system (CNS), resulting in a number of sensations, such as increased heart rate, perspiration, dry mouth, muscle tension, or need to urinate. Such CNS activation prepares the organism for the "fight or flight" response and is a reaction to perceived or unconscious threat of danger. The patient was asked to describe an incident with his wife that was troubling to him. He described an unprovoked tirade showered on him by his wife when she thought he had looked at another woman. He described his state of anxiety prior to walking out of the house: "My heart was beating faster, my mouth became dry and my hands were sweaty."

Impulse/Feeling (I/F). This refers to instinctual physiological reactions, such as sexual or aggressive urges. The aggressive impulse, for example, when fully experienced, is described by patients as a hot, "boiling" sensation that emanates from deep within the trunk and rises. This is often described as a feeling of explosiveness. The higher the intensity of felt emotion, the lower the level of anxiety. There is also a significant decrease in defensive representations or channels, such as muscle tension, in periods of felt emotion. In the case described above, the patient was asked what was underneath his anxiety, and he was able to identify an "explosive feeling that was frightening." This impulse he described by the action of its repression—wanting to punch the wall; this impulse was clearly aimed at his wife but was partially discharged by the displacement of the aggressive impulse. The anxiety is intensified by the threat of the aggressive impulse breaking though to the conscious zone.

Using the Two Triangles

The triangles of persons and conflict are used together as a method of orienting the therapist and maintaining focus (see Figure 2.5). We will refer to this in Chapter 6. Any given interaction depicting restructuring can be

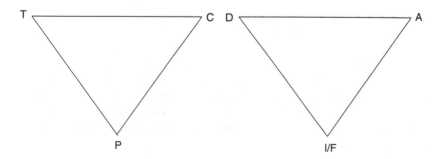

FIGURE 2.5. Triangle of persons and triangle of conflict.

understood using these templates. In this way, the therapist can have an ongoing conceptualization of the intrapsychic and interpersonal interactions. The clinician should always strive to identify in which corner of the triangle an interaction occurs or interpretation is made. Another case vignette will illustrate how the triangles are used.

PATIENT: I had a fight with my boyfriend and became angry and stormed out of the house.

> [The patient is presenting conflict in the current corner of the triangle of persons as this relates to a fight with her boyfriend.]

THERAPIST: How did you react emotionally? What did you feel?

> [The therapist is now focusing on the I/F corner of the triangle of conflict.]

PATIENT: I ran out of the house in a rage!

THERAPIST: Running out of your house is not rage. It is a defense against the rage.

> [The therapist is providing insight into the patient's defensive structure, which is focusing on the D corner of the triangle of conflict.]

PATIENT: I felt so angry inside, I could have punched him in the mouth. (*pause*) You know, my mother and I would have fights where I would run out of the house instead of punching her.

> [The patient has now shifted from her impulse to hit her boyfriend to the P on the triangle of persons.]

THERAPIST: Have you ever felt that way toward me?

> [The therapist is now focusing on the T of the triangle of persons.]

PATIENT: Yes, last week when you asked my why I was late, I wanted to run out the door.

THERAPIST: How did you feel toward me?

> [Now the therapist is attempting to link the I/F corner of the triangle of conflict to the T of the triangle of persons.]

From the brief excerpt, one can see how the therapist, using both triangles, can precisely identify the position of the patient and the interpretations can be made appropriately. An integral part of the process is educating the patient about his/her psychic structure, both cognitively and experientially, by using defensive, affective, and cognitive restructuring methods.

CONCLUSION

Although there are numerous short-term psychodynamic styles of conducting treatment (Messer & Warren, 1995), there is great theoretical diversity among them. The techniques of short-term treatment are also disparate (Magnavita, 1993a). However, they begin to make intuitive sense when one understands the structural differences in the personality disordered patient. One can see how the various approaches evolved so uniquely based on the type of patients that the clinician theoreticians encountered and were drawn to in their clinical practices. Thus, the more confrontational, anxiety-arousing approaches emanated from work with the neurotic and ego-syntonic characters where anxiety was needed to accelerate and deepen the process. In contrast, the empathic approaches derived from work with the developmentally and self-disordered patients where anxiety needed to be contained, and defenses strengthened, to keep the process from being flooded. The techniques are often diametrically opposed, so that a clinician working within a short-term framework requires a comprehensive understanding of metapsychology and developmental psychopathology, as well as the ability to conduct a rapid structural assessment. An organized model that encapsulates all the approaches will provide the clinician with a clearer conceptual understanding that leads to more efficient technical application. A patient with a disorder of the self or developmental psychopathology will clearly require a different type of treatment than a patient higher on the structural continuum. The process of making informed treatment selection decisions will become easier when the clinician embraces the full range of possibilities.

CHAPTER 3

Assessment and Treatment Planning

It is very often easier to get a clear picture of the patient's problem and life history as a whole during the first few hours of an analysis than it will be at any time later until the analysis is almost completed. It is preeminently during the period before the patient has become deeply involved emotionally in relation to the analyst that it is easiest for the analyst to gain an adequate perspective upon the patient as a whole.

—ALEXANDER AND FRENCH (1946, p. 109)

THE IMPORTANCE AND FUNCTION OF ASSESSMENT

Alexander and French (1946) first identified the need for patients to undergo a comprehensive assessment early on. This component of STDP would later be given much attention by future clinicians, and, in fact, I consider it perhaps the most crucial element of the entire process. The opportunity for a truly comprehensive evaluation is never as propitious as it is at the very beginning of treatment before transference reactions can cloud the diagnostic issues. There exists a certain clarity of vision at the very first meeting that will mutate during the later stages of therapy. Alexander believed that developing an early and comprehensive formulation was crucial to formulating a workable therapeutic plan, and I agree. Without a plan, even a tentative one, the therapy tends to drift. Clinicians of STDP need to generate a strategy rather than trust their therapeutic intuition on a "day-to-day basis," which often means dealing with the patient's difficulties as they arise. This is particularly so in STDP because of the time limitation and anxiety factors that are discussed later. Suffice it to say at this point that each session of STDP is highly important and should be used for as much effect as possible. In this chapter, I have provided a detailed overview of both the assessment process and collaborative treatment planning.

ELEMENTS OF THE ASSESSMENT PROCESS

The following represents material that must be covered and considered by the clinician during the assessment phase:

1. Presenting complaint—reason for seeking treatment
2. Descriptive phenomenology of the patient's symptoms/conflicts
3. Developmental history
4. Ego-adaptive functions assessment
5. Past history and experience of treatment
6. Diagnostic formulation
7. Genetic constellation
8. Transference reactions
9. Countertransference reactions
10. Character structure/personality
11. Dynamic formulation
12. Medical and drug and alcohol history

Presenting Complaint

The clinician can elicit the patient's view of his/her presenting complaint at the onset of the interview by asking, "What seems to be the problem?" or "What brought you here for this consultation?" The manner in which the patient frames his or her responses to these questions provides information about a number of ego functions, including psychological mindedness and insight. This is often my first clue to patient's degree of ego-syntonicity.

For example, I had a patient who responded to these basic inquiries by describing how he was referred to me by his family physician, who had been unable to determine the cause of his fatigue, gastrointestinal disturbances, and variety of vague and diffuse symptoms. He refused to discuss the nature of any other area of his life, stating repeatedly that everything is "just fine." This patient's ego-syntonicity created a barrier that made collaboration very difficult. All his feelings and conflicts were immediately expressed physically, and he had no awareness of this mechanism of somatization, which can be very difficult to restructure.

Descriptive Phenomenology

Every competent clinician works to achieve an understanding of his/her patient's experience and to assess the patient's level of distress. In order to do so, the therapist must specifically inquire about the patient's experience of his/her problems and about what it is like to look at the world through the patient's eyes. Asking the patient to describe, in specific detail, the nuances of his/her depression or anxiety and other symptoms helps build rapport and allows the therapist to get an experiential reading of the patient's suffering. I have found it helpful to have my patients rate their level of anxiety or depression on a Subjective Units of Disturbance Scale (SUDS)[1]: "From 1 to 100, how would you rate your anxiety [depression] right now?" "How would you rate it when it is at its height?"

Developmental History

The clinician should do a thorough assessment of pertinent developmental issues and conflicts in order to learn how the patient has navigated previous developmental stages. This provides insight into the adaptive capacities and struggles that the patient brings to treatment. Particular attention should be given to the patient's psychosexual development, such as onset of puberty and menstruation or history of traumatic sexual experiences. Developmental issues may also be used to guide treatment selection decisions (Burke, White, & Havens, 1979).

Assessing Ego-Adaptive Functions

Ego-adaptive capacity refers to the patient's ego strength, or the capacity to acknowledge reality, even when it is extremely unpleasant, without resorting to primitive defenses (McWilliams, 1994). A rapid but global assessment of the patient's ego-adaptive capacity will guide treatment selection decisions.

What the clinician should look for is the patient's *ability to be aware of and experience* a wide range of feelings, the *ability to stay with commitments* and keep motivated, *psychological mindedness,* the *capacity for intimacy,* the *ability to soothe oneself, stability of self-esteem,* the *ability to assert oneself,* and the *ability to tolerate being alone* (Masterson, 1988).

A detailed assessment needs to follow, taking into consideration ego functions: relation to reality, regulation and control of instinctual drives, object relations, thought processes, defenses, autonomous functions and synthetic functions (Horner, 1985) (see Table 3.1). Carefully evaluating these functions will lead to optimal treatment selection decisions. The

TABLE 3.1. Assessment of Ego Functions

Relation to reality	Reality testing
	Sense of self
	Observing self
Regulation of instinct	Capacity for delay
	Impulse control
	Adaptive expression
Object relations	Basic trust
	Level of relatedness
	Level of differentiation
	Stability
	Integration—tolerance of ambivalence
	Maturity of relationships
Thought processes	Logical and conceptual thinking
Defenses	Adequacy—tolerance of affect
	Flexibility
	Maturity of defenses
Autonomous functions	Speech, cognition, perception, motor behavior—free of conflict
	Recoverability—can be undersood in a psychological context if impaired
	Organic integrity—not impaired
Synthetic functions	Psychological mindedness
	Capacity for insight

Note. Adapted from Horner (1994, pp. 88–90). Copyright 1984 by Jason Aronson. Adapted by permission.

superego functions assessed are conscience and ego ideal (see Table 3.2). Take particular note in the assessment of the superego of the degree of punitiveness or harshness therein. Severely harsh superego functions have been associated with massive unresolved guilt over sadistic feeling. These patients have shown responsiveness to an approach that brings the aggressive/sadistic impulses to the surface and helps the patient experience his/ her

TABLE 3.2. Assessment of Superego Functions

Conscience	Standards of right and wrong
	Capacity for guilt
	Realistic standards of morality
Ego ideal	Feelings of worth
	Realistic image of self not requiring unrealistic perfection or grandiosity

Note. Adapted from Horner (1994, p. 90). Copyright 1984 by Jason Aronson. Adapted by permission.

guilt and grief over the often murderous feelings toward current and genetic figures.

Past History and Experience of Treatment

The clinician needs to explore the patient's past therapeutic relationships, especially his/her reasons for seeking treatment and the outcomes of those previous associations. There may be a history of multiple failed treatment relationships; this is often the case with personality disordered patients. The clinician should explore the reasons for ending treatment, as well as the patient's assessment of why it did or did not help. This often provides useful information about the patient's repetitive patterns and conflicts. The background of and reasons for multiple hospitalizations should also be discussed. A comprehensive review of this aspect of the patient's history can put the therapist on much firmer ground when he/she is making treatment recommendations. The work of previous therapists can and should be used to the advantage of the current evaluator. If, for example, the patient was part of a formerly positive therapeutic alliance, the current therapy may benefit by virtue of the hope and trust the patient brings. On the other hand, a past negative or damaging experience should also be discussed and dealt with early in the process so that transference resistance will be kept to a minimum.

Diagnostic Formulation

The early detection of significant character pathology is essential in guiding treatment selection. The clinician should, of course, establish a clinical diagnosis based on DSM-IV criteria, but, more importantly, he/she should complete a structural assessment (McWilliams, 1994). The ability to make differential diagnostic decisions is a skill that is essential in the effective treatment of the personality disordered patient (Beutler & Clarkin, 1990). The clinician must have a solid grounding in psychoanalytic diagnosis. Remember, personality disorders are not always evident in the patient's presentation. Therefore, before proceeding, the clinician should consider some of the following in order to determine whether or not he/she is dealing with a symptom neurosis or a personal disorder. As I stressed earlier in this chapter, how the patient formulates his/her presenting complaint and whether or not there is a clear precipitant for treatment is important in making a differential diagnosis. A symptom neurosis is typically the result of a precipitating event; a personality disorder is not.

A patient with a symptom neurosis usually has a significant increase in his/her anxiety in reaction to a specific event. The personality disordered patient, on the other hand, frequently reports generalized anxiety with no clearly precipitating events.

Also, because of the ego-syntonicity of the patient's problems, the personality disordered patient is not likely to be self-referred. These patients often have difficulty seeing how their personalities influence experience.

Personality disordered patients tend to have less-observing egos, so that they have difficulty achieving a perspective outside of themselves. Unfortunately, this hinders their ability to develop an alliance or partnership with the therapist. In other words, object relations are more primitive (McWilliams, 1994).

Genetic Constellation

In the assessment, it is important to delineate the significant figures in the patient's development and his/her relationship with them. The most obvious of these are parents and caregivers. However, it is important not to overlook other significant attachment figures, such as grandparents or members of the extended family. Sifneos (1987) gauges the patient's degree of attachment to a particular person by the level of sacrifice the person is willing to make for that other.

A preliminary attempt should be made to assess the quality of these primary relationships. Has the patient experienced a positive, affectionate relationship with one figure or two? Are the early relationships centered on one figure or are relationships triangular? Memories of traumatic events, if the patient is aware of these, should be explored.

Transference Reactions

The clinician should note and explore the meaning of any preexisting transference issues, prior to the initial encounter, and watch for those that arise very early in the interview. This should include transference feelings toward previous clinicians, as well as toward genetic figures. Especially important with personality disordered patients is unresolved transference feeling (positive and negative) toward any previous therapists, since so many have had multiple treatment experiences. The patient will most likely not spontaneously report his/her feelings in this area. Most personality disordered patients enter the treatment room with strong interpersonal expectations. The therapist should explore the thoughts, expectations, and fantasies the patient experienced prior to the session. The level of anxiety, as it relates to the patient's transference feelings, must also be assessed. Does the patient expect to be condemned, fixed, or taken care of? The therapist should note how the patient decided to see this particular therapist; that is, was it a direct referral or a fairly random choice?

Countertransference Reactions

Personality disordered patients, in particular, often engender strong countertransference reactions. The clinician is well advised to take note of them. What happens in the interpersonal field is very important, and the therapist's countertransference reactions are a measure of this (Davis, 1991). Further, gauging these reactions can be extremely valuable in assisting differential diagnosis, prognostic formulations, and treatment planning.

Kalpin (1993) aptly describes some typical reactions: "A desire to *take care* of a patient" taking the form of "urges to educate, constantly encourage, or prop up the patient. . . . [This] is an indication of *dependency* in a patient" (p. 26). Defiant patients can often stimulate the therapist to debate or to justify his/her position. *Happy agreement* can be generated by compliant patients. *Passive listening* is often a reaction to a complainer. A reaction in the therapist of *hopelessness* or *becoming entertaining* can be a response to a depressive character. "What reaction does a patient provoke in you that is different from compassion and a desire to witness, share in feelings, and facilitate change? The countertransference 'derivatives' which one can become aware of can be an important tool for understanding the patient" (Kalpin, 1993, p. 26).

Assessing Character Structure/Personality

It is crucial to the formulation of a treatment plan that a thorough evaluation of the patient's character structure—overall organization of the personality— be conducted before initiation of a course of brief treatment. Horner (1995) likens this to taking an X-ray as contrasted with a photograph. Patients who appear to fulfill the DSM-IV criteria for a particular personality disorder will have varying structural–developmental diagnoses (Cooper, Frances, & Sacks, 1986). The clinician first needs to distinguish among the neurotic, borderline, and psychotic spectrum of character structure (Kernberg, 1984; McWilliams, 1994; Stone, 1980). Important distinctions then can be made among the various character styles such as schizoid, narcissistic, and so on (Deutsch, 1965; Johnson, 1994; Wells & Glickauf-Hughes, 1993).

Stone's three-dimensional representation offers a way of illustrating three aspects of personality: genetic loadings, level of structural organization, and character type (see Figure 3.1). Patients most likely to respond to analytically oriented therapy are represented in Figure 3.2. I include the passive– aggressive, narcissistic, and schizoid personalities within this range, as well.

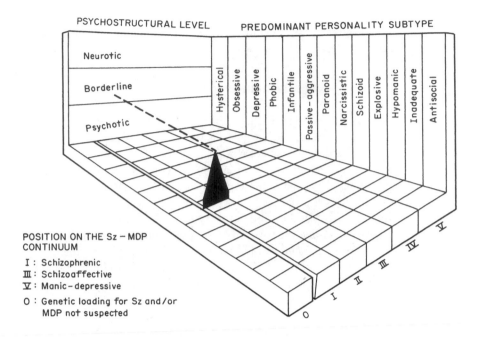

FIGURE 3.1. Stone's diagnosis cube.

Dynamic Formulation

A psychodynamic formulation or hypothesis should be established as early as possible to guide the treatment. This includes a hypothesis about the meaning of the patient's symptoms and what seems to be driving the patient's personality patterns. For example, one patient has developed an avoidant pattern to minimize strong emotions that are triggered in interpersonal relationships and, because of this pattern, has been unable to advance at work and maintain successful relationships. Such a formulation does not have to be overly complex; in fact, simplicity is desirable and will provide a framework for changing the existing patterns, that is, "The avoidant pattern and unwillingness to face your feelings has handicapped your life."

Medical and Drug and Alcohol History

The clinician should complete a medical history and consult with the patient's medical practitioner to rule out any organic pathology or other medical conditions. It is best to be on solid ground before proceeding. If

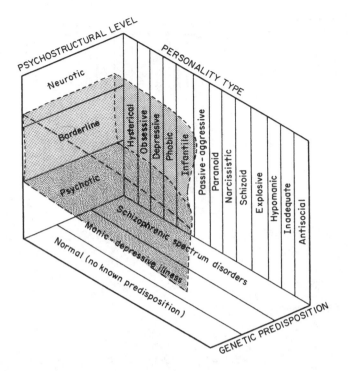

FIGURE 3.2. Stone's diagnosis cube: Region of optimal response to analytically oriented psychotherapy. *Note.* The volume outlined within the diagnosis cube delineates a territory within which "intensive" or "expressive" psychotherapy (analytically oriented psychotherapy) is generally thought to be useful.

The territory includes the borderline region, plus the lower end of the neurotic level (where certain severe phobics might be represented, for example) and the highest part of the psychotic level. The territory includes most of the "healthier" character types but begins to collapse in the region of the narcissistic and schizoid characters (the less responsive groups), vanishing altogether in the region of the nonresponsive hypomanic and antisocial characters.

concerns arise, such as questions about organic pathology, necessary consultation for neuropsychological or neurological evaluations should be completed before proceeding. A careful assessment should include a review of any psychosomatic or psychophysiological disorders such as irritable bowel, severe low-back pain, severe asthma, ulcerative colitis, Crohn's disease, and migraine headaches. If any of these is present, *the clinician should proceed with caution because anxiety-provoking techniques can precipitate a medical crisis.* If you are not trained in treating these disorders, you should not proceed with a short-term anxiety-arousing approach. If any questions arise, the patient should be medically cleared by his/her physician before treatment proceeds.

The clinician should also conduct a thorough drug and alcohol assessment, as many patients with personality disorders have comorbid substance abuse or dependency disorders. In cases where this is an active issue, treatment for this should be considered first or conjointly. Time can be lost if the patient is treated ineffectively with short-term therapy and only later it becomes apparent that there is a significant substance abuse disorder. A careful assessment will avoid many of these pitfalls.

METHODS OF ASSESSMENT

There are primarily two ways of conducting a comprehensive assessment and covering the points we have discussed. These include the clinical interview and psychodiagnostic testing, which are most effective when used in conjunction. All effective therapy with personality disordered patients follows from an accurate clinical interview, and diagnostic testing can be useful to corroborate findings.

Clinical Diagnostic Interviewing

All patients enter the first session with a complicated mix of feelings and history that, at times, may seem overwhelming to the interviewer. The clinician has multiple tasks to which he/she must attend during the initial evaluation, such as understanding the phenomenology of the patient's experience, formulating a positive working alliance, gaining sufficient background and history, and monitoring the patient's anxiety. A careful and thorough interviewer can establish rapport and keep the interview process moving along. Rapport can be established by responding empathically to any painful feeling that emerges and also by communicating an interest in understanding the patient. The interviewer must follow the patient's lead but still guide the process and prevent the patient's defenses from dominating. The therapist must attend to and validate the patient's feelings but not allow the process to bog down with too much emotion too soon. It is better for the therapist to know he/she is on solid footing before getting into anxiety-provoking material.

Balancing the Interview

Although the gathering of this information is an important part of the initial evaluation, the clinician must avoid getting too immersed in the details. If, for instance, the patient starts to obsess on one issue or go off on tangents, the interviewer should communicate to the patient that it is important that they not get bogged down by saying, "I know that the details are important and we can get back to this, but there are some other areas that we should cover today." It helps the process if the clinician is clear at the onset that the initial interview is an assessment, and, in fact, I have found that patients are often appreciative when, as interviewer, I am both meticulous and comprehensive. If resistances develop during the interview, they must be addressed, but the interviewer should try to strike a balance between gathering information and establishing a working therapeutic alliance. Information will be obtained as the interview unfolds, preferably without making it appear overly structured.

Assessing Structure Vis-à-Vis Anxiety

Kernberg (1984) uses anxiety to mobilize the defenses much the way Davanloo (1980) and Sifneos (1987) do and has set forth the detailed elements of the *structural interview*. I have found his interview quite useful. Anxiety-provoking probes and defense analysis are used to assess the patient's personality structure, that is, to determine whether it is at a psychotic, borderline, or neurotic level of organization. The structural interview also allows the therapist to make even finer distinctions in the structure and organization of the personality. This kind of psychodiagnostic assessment uses the clinician as a stimulus of the psychic system.

The "structural interview" is conducted by focusing on the patient's main conflict to increase the patient's level of tension and activate the defensive system. The therapist then monitors manifestations of the characteristic way in which the psychic apparatus functions. For example, does the patient become flooded with anxiety, typically manifested in cognitive slippage and memory loss, or does the patient characterologically defend against anxiety by becoming haughty, defiant, and sarcastic? The main focus is on patient–therapist interaction, with heavy emphasis on transference elements. Through the transference, the patient's difficulties manifest in the present through the interaction with the therapist. Clarification, confrontation, interpretation, and challenging both defenses and reality distortions are the techniques used in the evaluation, as follows:

Clarification. In clarification, the interviewer attempts to evoke conscious and preconscious material from the patient. Unclear or contradictory information is noted and explored. The Socratic method is often useful in systematically questioning and elucidating the patient's dynamics and beliefs (Overholser, 1995). Sometimes, repeating one of the patient's key words or phrases provides the patient with the comfort he/she needs to take the discussion to yet a deeper level. A typical clarifying question is, "I am puzzled by that reaction; can you tell me more?" Felix Deutsch (Deutsch & Murphy, 1955), who developed "sector therapy," used this technique and called it "associative anamnesis." When using this technique, the therapist repeats a key word or phrase that zeroes in on the patient's central conflict. "By thus speaking directly to the patient's unconscious, the therapeutic alliance is strengthened, and the patient feels understood more rapidly than by using the standard technique" (Flegenheimer, 1993, p. 34). Essentially, what the interviewer is doing is showing interest in what the patient is saying or feeling. Asking the patient to describe an example of what he/she means will also provide more specificity.

Confrontation. Using confrontation, the interviewer points out areas that are contradictory and seem to indicate conflictual preconscious and conscious material. For example, if a patient is talking about his/her anger and yet is smiling, the interviewer might say, "I'm not sure you're aware of this, but you have a smile on your face when you describe this anger."

Interpretation. This not only links conscious and preconscious material but can suggest a theory about the patient's current motivation. It takes confrontation one step further. For example, "Your anxiety seems to increase when you talk about your feelings. I wonder whether you have a fear of closeness?"

Transference interpretation. This is an unconscious reenactment of conflictual relationships from the patient's past. When it is explained to the patient and linked to the past, it becomes a transference interpretation. For example: "You smile when you discuss your anger with me. Perhaps you are concerned that I might react the way your father did when you were angry toward him."

Structural interviewing combines history taking and mental status examination while simultaneously activating the patient's defense system and object representations. This is much more anxiety provoking than taking a standard psychiatric history. If the patient's defensive system shows signs of faltering during the interview, the therapist is well-advised to revert to standard history taking, which is far less anxiety provoking. If the patient is able to tolerate the anxiety the therapist has provoked, the therapist may safely proceed with the anxiety-inducing aspects of the structural interview.

Psychological Testing

Psychological testing can be used by the evaluator in making a comprehensive assessment of the patient's cognitive, affective, intrapsychic, and interpersonal functioning but is never a substitute for a thorough clinical interview. Testing can also provide information about differential diagnostic issues, ego functions, psychodynamics, and developmental fixations. Psychodiagnostic assessment is especially valuable in short-term psychotherapy, but such assessment is often overlooked and underutilized. There are a variety of assessment instruments available that can be administered to the patient either prior to or soon after the initial consultation. These range from self-report inventories, structured clinical interviews, and personality disordered checklists to a comprehensive psychological battery including both cognitive and projective assessment. The two most widely used tests for diagnosing personality disorders are the Minnesota Multiphasic Personality Inventory (MMPI) and the Millon Clinical Multiaxial Inventory (MCMI). These can be both easily administered and computer-scored for a nominal fee. Millon and Davis (1996) describes the MCMI as an objective psychodynamic instrument "drawing on clinically established relationships among cognitive processes, interpersonal behaviors, and intrapsychic forces" (p. 157). This inventory is a highly refined clinical instrument for establishing diagnostic profiles of the personality disordered patient. Basically, self-report instruments are valuable in targeting patients who may have personality disorders so that the clinician can immediately take this into consideration before implementing a particular treatment approach. There are a variety of other assessment instruments that can be incorporated into the assessment phase or serve as treatment-monitoring devices. Millon and Davis (1996) present a comprehensive summary of these.

TREATMENT PLANNING

Rapid Transformation versus a Stepwise Approach

It is highly unlikely that your patient, upon entering treatment, will say that he/she has a personality disorder or disturbing character traits and would like to engage in a course of characterological reconstruction, no matter how difficult and painful the work might be.[2] A patient who does so would certainly demonstrate a high level of motivation to change and a *self-awareness* of the destructive nature of his/her character defenses. Instead, most personality disordered patients enter treatment with limited awareness and insight[3] into the extent of suffering they cause themselves and others. Often, they are urged into treatment by significant others or by a breakthrough of distressing symptoms.

How does a clinician assess the patient's capacity to make a rapid change, and how is the potency of treatment regulated? Personality disorders, because they are always in some way debilitating, are best treated sooner than later. Unfortunately, this is not always a viable option. When is a patient prepared for a rapid restructuring of his/her defenses and a major derepression of the unconscious?

A "rapid transformation" takes place when the patient quickly makes substantial changes in his/her personality, so that the effects are relatively clear to the patient, therapist and significant others. "Strong success cases have naturalistic outcome indexes: work and love, impossible before, now happen. There is a sense of well-being, and new dimensions open. The therapist, the patient, and questionnaires from friends agree the treatment is a success" (Gendlin, 1986, p. 131). This occurs when long-standing characterological patterns are modified so as to free the patient in all spheres of his/her life functioning. These are the "fairy tale" cases of which Gustafson (1986) speaks.

A "stepwise approach" is a more conservative intervention based on a time-limited model. It may set the stage for another, possibly more penetrating, intervention at a later time or may be part of a series of interventions over the life span of the patient. Periodic short-term interventions or "intermittent psychotherapy" (Cummings, 1991), varying in degrees of potency, can be offered to the personality disordered patient over the life span at key developmental points (Austad & Hoyt, 1992; Bennett, 1983).

The aim of the stepwise type of intervention is to accomplish some positive change, even small treatment gains, that can be expanded upon later. In these cases, as in all others, the clinician should select an approach whose potency fits with the patient's personality disorder and/or stated goals. If the patient is not interested or motivated enough to do the in-depth work needed to modify the character, he/she may be offered the opportunity to return when motivation increases or situational demands shift. At certain periods, because of increased intrapsychic demands and external stressors, the patient's defensive system may be disrupted or shifted, temporarily bringing unconscious issues to awareness. This disruption often results from a crisis in a relationship, problems at work, physical illness, external pressure from significant others to change, or increased dysphoria. The therapist should be attuned to the cues that will indicate the speed of treatment most appropriate for each case.

The Patient's Readiness for Rapid Change

In the assessment process, the therapist needs to determine the patient's suitability for short-term psychotherapy and to quickly make differential treatment selection decisions. The therapist does not experience the same degree of pressure to complete the assessment with the same rapidity when using longer-term models of psychotherapy. In a short-term approach, the therapist can utilize anxiety-increasing techniques to rapidly establish the patient's ego-adaptive capacity.

In making the determination to attempt either a rapid transformation or a stepwise treatment, the therapist must consider the following factors: (1) the patient's motivation for change, (2) the presence/absence of an optimal gestation period upon which to capitalize, (3) the degree of conscious or "felt" pain the patient is currently enduring, (4) the patient's willingness to face the external demands of character changes, (5) the patient's ego-adaptive capacity, and (6) the patient's capacity to enter into a collaborative relationship with the therapist. Each individual factor is worthy of consideration, as follows:

Motivation. The issue of motivation is a very complex one and, at this time, will be only briefly considered. It should be stated, however, that patients who appear extremely unmotivated at the beginning of an interview can later make dramatic shifts in their level of motivation. The patient who is prepared to participate in character analysis must have the motivation or the "will" (Rank, 1945, 1947) to establish closer relationships with others and risk his/her essential vulnerability, endure the pain of changing his/her life, and mourn the old self. Certainly, not all patients are prepared or presently equipped to embark upon this kind of journey; most must be systematically prepared for it.

Assessing motivation to determine whether or not a patient is a good candidate for STDP is quite straightforward. Various treatment methods are offered, including the "opportunity to as rapidly as possible get to the core of your difficulties and attempt to resolve them in a short-term approach." Thus, the patient is promptly provided with informed consent and is alerted to the fact that therapy will require very painful and hard work. The patient can also be given the option of scheduling an extended session of up to 3 hours to determine whether this approach will be acceptable and useful. A patient willing to schedule the extended session generally is indicating that his/her motivation is high. How the patient describes what he/she wants is also indicative of motivation. For example, "I really need to make some major changes, and I don't want to wait any longer." This assertion alerts the clinician that this may be an optimal gestation period. As we discuss in the clinical section, a positive extended session works both to raise hope and to enhance motivation, making subsequent sessions that much more fruitful.

Optimal Gestation Periods. There are certain phases in life when people are especially open to making changes. These often occur during a period of disequilibrium caused by a crisis. A temporary state of increased fluidity can result from the disruption caused by a crisis, which increases the patient's receptiveness to therapeutic intervention (Stierlin, 1968). "This means that the temporary state of heightened susceptibility presents an unparalleled opportunity for internal boundary realignments. It is opportunity for better—or worse" (Straker, 1980). This state of heightened susceptibility usually leads to a state of disorganization or a chaotic condition, to which Hager (1992) refers as a period of gestation. Consequently, these critical points can lead to a new synthesis. "Gestating states are usually preceded by an unusually eventful session [or event] where the client is struck by new awareness, either in the form of strong affect, a previously buried memory, and/or new self-understanding" (p. 379). During these periods, there is an increased ambivalence about the potential for making changes (Prochaska, DiClemente, & Norcross, 1992). These events may, in fact, be the precipitants for entering treatment.

Symptoms and Emotional Distress. Most patients enter treatment because they are suffering from emotional distress from which they are seeking relief; this is a powerful motivator to enter treatment. The process is no different from that caused by physical pain. The person who is suffering from dental pain will resist going to the dentist until the pain becomes unbearable and can no longer be put off. The anticipated pain caused by the dentist is eventually overshadowed by the currently experienced pain. Personality disordered patients know intuitively that opening up their inner wounds is going to be an excruciatingly painful process. In fact, the therapist must reactivate the very pain the patient is attempting to avoid, the pain that he/she will want to avoid until it becomes intolerable. The patient may have a dim awareness that old defensive structures are no longer effectively containing his/her chronically endured pain. The following is an example of a mixed narcissistic and dependent personality disordered patient who entered treatment with this reluctance.

> The patient was in his late 20s, of short stature but solid build. He reported a long history of chronic substance abuse, which he was able to give up with the help of Alcoholics Anonymous (AA) and Narcotics Anonymous (NA). The precipitant for his decision to enter psychotherapy was that he had suffered a serious leg injury while at work and needed to use a cane, which led him to a state of severe dysphoria. His image of himself as being tough and strong was completely undermined. He used to fight anyone, no matter how much bigger than himself, and he had the reputation as a "crazy man" and a vicious fighter. His narcissistic defenses no longer successfully shored up his fragile self-esteem. His massive dependency on his abusive, alcoholic father, with whom he still lived, came to the surface in the most painful manner. He continued to be fearful of his father and longed to be

accepted as being "tough" like his father. He suddenly felt that he would never win his father's acceptance now that he was crippled.

In my clinical practice, I have treated many patients with histories of chronic substance abuse who have entered AA or NA and maintained their sobriety for about a year. Because they are no longer relying on substances to dull their emotional pain and their character defenses are cracking, they enter treatment in severe emotional distress. Many of these patients have long been suffering from dependent, avoidant, narcissistic, passive–aggressive personality disorders or, more commonly, mixed types that have long been untreated.

Willingness to Face External Consequences of Character Change. Personality disordered patients are often intuitively aware of the fact that to undergo rapid transformation might entail making significant changes in their lives and lifestyles. For example, a patient who primarily has a dependent personality disorder and is married to an abusive spouse may realize that, in order to achieve a healthier life, divorce may be necessary. This can be assessed directly by asking the patient what he/she imagines would happen if he/she were to achieve the change he/she was seeking. This allows the patient's worst fear to be brought into the open and discussed. Obviously, we cannot predict what the results will be, but the patient can be assured that once he/she is more aware of his/her feelings, any decision should be clearer.

Adequate Ego-Adaptive Capacity. Personality disordered patients can be placed on an ego adaptive capacity spectrum, which is discussed in greater detail. Patients with lower levels of ego adaptive capacity are generally not good candidates for making rapid transformations. This issue is discussed later in this chapter.

Ability to Enter into a Mutually Collaborative Relationship. The patient who is capable of and motivated to undergo rapid change must also be capable of entering into a collaborative relationship with the therapist. This is one crucial aspect of the *therapeutic alliance.* "The therapeutic alliance is the emotional bond and mutual involvement between therapist and patient" (Stiles, Shapiro, & Elliott, 1986, p. 173) and may be one of the most important nonspecific factors accounting for psychotherapy efficacy (Safran, 1993). This alliance entails a sense of mutual involvement and concordance between the patient's and the clinician's treatment goals.

Although there is some blurring between the concepts of therapeutic alliance and transference, Frieswyk et al. (1986) believe the former is a relevant concept in understanding therapeutic action. They describe two kinds of therapeutic alliance, as follows: (1) The therapist is experienced as warm, supportive, and helpful; and (2) the patient has a sense that they are engaged in a joint struggle to overcome obstacles marked by a sharing of responsibility toward attaining goals.

The patient's ability to establish a collaborative relationship is one sign that the patient can tolerate an anxiety-provoking approach without causing a therapeutic fracture. I am using the word "collaborative" loosely. What I mean is that if the patient is so overwhelmed by affect resulting from primitive object relations, then, collaboration is not possible. Once this fault is mended and some trust has been established, the alliance can be shifted from a warmer, more empathic one to a more task-oriented, collaborative one. Many patients have never experienced a collaborative relationship and, yet, after an extended session, show the ability to do so.

Indications for a Stepwise Approach

There are certain factors that mitigate against the use of a rapid uncovering approach. If unwisely undertaken, iatrogenic disturbances will lead to a negative outcome. For example, patients who can be placed on the extreme left of the Structural Spectrum of Personality Disorders (see Figure 2.2) with high levels of primitive defenses such as disassociation, splitting, and projection should not be offered a rapid, in-depth restructuring approach. The reasons for this are discussed in detail in Chapter 6, in the section on the Defense Zone. A rapid restructuring approach is also unsuitable for patients with low ego-adaptive capacities, at least until effective cognitive restructuring of the defenses has been undertaken and achieved. (Assessing ego-adaptive capacity is discussed later in this chapter.) Other contraindications include parasuicidality,[4] psychotic episodes, schizophrenia, poor impulse control, and active paranoid conditions.

Setting the Stage for Short-Term Dynamic Psychotherapy

There are a number of tasks the clinician must complete in order to set the stage for successful treatment. Overlooking these can result in frustration and increased resistance on the part of the patient. When it is systematically and expertly woven into the assessment process, the patient perceives that treatment is proceeding in a collaborative, cooperative manner, and the course of treatment will benefit. Of course, there will be patients who decide not to continue or request a different approach. This is inevitable, though disappointing. Those who opt to continue, however, will be better equipped to respond to the rigorous demands of treatment.

Educating the Patient about Treatment

It is important for both the patient's well-being and for the therapy that the patient needs to understand the process, expectations, and goals of the therapy, and the therapist needs to explain the process. It is naturally incumbent upon the therapist to educate his/her patient in this. Beutler and Clarkin (1990) refer to this as "role induction," which "is a general term that describes efforts to prepare patients for treatment by educating them about treatment roles and outcomes before psychotherapy actually begins" (p. 187).

Further, the therapist cannot assume that the patient understands the process or vocabulary of psychotherapy. Although many personality disordered patients have had previous treatment experiences, some have not. In either case, the therapist must clearly articulate to the patient what the expectations and goals are for this treatment experience. For STDP in which uncovering is the goal, the following expectations[5] must be shared:

1. The patient will not censor his/her thoughts and feelings.
2. The patient will be open and honest, foremost with him/herself and then with the therapist.
3. The patient will make a commitment to change, even though it will entail hard work.
4. The patient will attend sessions on time.
5. The patient will attempt to accomplish as much as possible within the time frame.
6. The patient is willing to enter into a collaborative relationship with the therapist, with both actively participating.
7. The patient will follow through with any extratherapeutic tasks that are mutually agreed upon.

It is important to realize that the majority of personality disordered patients are not capable of fulfilling these expectations at the onset of treatment. If the patient were, he/she would not be suffering from a personality disorder. Therefore, although the situation does present a paradox, it represents the inherent developmental challenge. The patient must learn how to collaborate as a partner in his/her development. As with some forms of brief treatment, these are not used for selection criteria but, rather, as a framework to preview the patient for what will be expected. When the patient has difficulty adhering to these conditions, these resistances then become a focus of defensive analysis or cognitive restructuring and are used to deepen the therapeutic work. For example, if the patient cuts off his/her verbalizations in midsentence, the therapist might point out how censoring thoughts will sabotage the treatment process. Avoiding intimacy by blocking is invariably linked to core issues, such as trust and attachment, which will eventually come to the surface and can then be addressed.

Educating the Patient about His/Her Personality "Disorder"

Discussing your diagnostic formulation with the patient suffering from a personality disorder[6] is an issue in which timing and sensitivity to the patient's ego strengths and capacities are crucial. This topic often generates strong polemics. Some clinicians feel that providing a diagnosis is a destructive act of pejorative labeling and feel that this should never be done to any patient. They believe that any form of labeling is reductionistic and reinforces the "sick" role. I tend to disagree with this opinion. Yet, regrettably, we have all heard of mental health professionals who use diagnostic labels arrogantly and dismissively, as if labeling a patient passive–aggressive or borderline excuses us from our lack of success or allows us to feel superior. Some of us may even avoid terminology completely to spare patients the truth.

I have found that discussing my diagnostic formulations with certain patients can be a useful strategy. It can increase the patient's awareness of the entrenched nature of his/her personality traits and let that patient know that he/she is not alone in his/her condition. It can also provide the patient with a degree of comfort and hope to see descriptions of his/her behavioral patterns in print. Sometimes, I let the patient read the description of the personality disorder I have identified in DSM-IV. I have found that the typical response is a surprised, "That's me," give or take one or two of the descriptors. The patient may experience some immediate decrease in his/her feelings of alienation and take hope from the fact that the clinician is so obviously familiar with his/her particular disorder. At other times, I neither label the disorder nor give the patient the DSM-IV material to read, but, rather, I highlight orally the pertinent features in a comprehensive fashion. The cognitive schema developed for personality disorders can also serve a similar educational function.

Many clinicians (unconsciously) believe that patients are fragile and cannot tolerate the truth. The courage to face the truth with the patient communicates an important message to the patient: that he/she can be treated in an honest, straightforward manner. Even patients who appear most fragile can benefit from the knowledge that they are not alone and that researchers and clinicians are attempting to find new methods to assist them in leading fuller lives.

Other patients, particularly those who have had multiple treatment experiences and hospitalizations, may benefit from deemphasizing their diagnoses. Try to keep an open mind regarding previous diagnoses and consider pathognomonic labels. Many patients are misdiagnosed, and inappropriate prognostic statements are made from these ill-founded for-

mulations. I have treated personality disordered patients who were told that
they were manic–depressive and must be on medication for the rest of their
lives or that they have a "biochemical imbalance" and require lifelong
support of antidepressant medication. There is no question that many
disorders are indeed biologically based, but character disturbances are often
hard to diagnose. Unfortunately, patients are sometimes offered medication
when they have frustrated the clinicians working with them. Other patients
are told that they need to be in day treatment programs and are infantalized
to a degrading degree by the staff's perception that they are sick and require
expert care. Many of these patients have experienced multiple traumas and
are retraumatized by such clinicians.

Of course, there are many patients who do have primarily biochemical
disorders and require medication or structured treatment programs, but,
often, personality disordered patients unconsciously encourage their therapists to treat them the way their significant figures did. It is important to
suspend judgment and look at the patient's symptoms anew. This goes back
to how important the assessment phase of therapy is and how important
the opportunity to see the patient objectively is. One patient of mine brought
in a chart 3 inches thick documenting her previous psychiatric history to
prove how hopeless and sick she really was. Much of her behavior had been
influenced by substance abuse and a history of traumatic sexual abuse and
parental neglect. In fact, this was not the chronic patient that her chart
indicated but, rather, someone who successfully cared for a large, extended
family.

Contracting with the Patient

Patient and therapist need to collaborate and agree on the treatment goals,
anticipated length of treatment, schedule and frequency of treatment, fees
and cancellation policy. Ideally, the patient should agree to at least one final
session before prematurely terminating his/her treatment.

Treatment Goals

The ability of the patient to present a circumscribed problem has been one
of the selection criteria for determining suitability for most STDPs (Crits-
Christoph & Barber, 1991). This would certainly exclude many of the
patients I treat in my clinical practice. Few personality disordered patients
present a highly circumscribed problem. More often, the presentation
consists of a mixed description of symptoms, ego-syntonic character disturbances, and relationship problems. The therapist's task during the evaluation phase is to get a clear description of the patient's treatment goals.

These must be explicitly agreed upon as a focus for collaboration between the patient and the therapist. With personality disordered patients, this task is more complex because of the multifocal nature of their problems and their tendency at times to overwhelm the therapist with complaints, externalizations, and diffuse descriptions of general malaise. The following conversation between a therapist and a 24-year-old single male with a mixed personality disorder with both dependent and passive–aggressive traits is an example of this:

THERAPIST: What seems to be the problem?

PATIENT: I can't seem to get my life together.

THERAPIST: Yes, but it is crucial for our work together to be successful that you tell me in specific detail what you would like to accomplish here.

PATIENT: I have anger toward my mother.

THERAPIST: But still, that is vague, and if we don't get a clear picture of what you want to accomplish, then we will not know if we are successful.

PATIENT: Well, I have been feeling depressed, and I have difficulties in my relationship with my girlfriend.

THERAPIST: So what you are describing, so far, are two main issues that you would like to work on: One is depression, and the other is a disturbance in your relationship with your girlfriend.

PATIENT: Yes, that's what I'm here to work on.

In the above vignette, the therapist was attempting to undo the patient's tendency toward vagueness and generalization to get a clearer picture of the difficulties. Without doing this at the start, the process becomes muddled, and the therapist may get increasingly entangled with the patient's character defenses.

Anticipated Length of Treatment

The limitation of time in short-term therapy constitutes the cornerstone of all treatment approaches. There are two methods for handling time. The first is to set a predetermined number of sessions, such as 10 or 12, as in Mann's TLP (1973). The other is to estimate approximately how long the treatment will take, for example, 3 months. The second method permits greater flexibility. The therapist should get a reading from the patient about his/her sense of how long it will take for treatment to accomplish what they want. For example:

THERAPIST: So when you decided to come to see me and you made this appointment, how long did you anticipate it would take?

PATIENT: I don't know.

THERAPIST: But you probably had some number of sessions or period of time in your head that you thought this process would take.

PATIENT: Well, maybe but I didn't really think about it specifically.

THERAPIST: If you were to answer that right now, what number of sessions or length of time comes to your head?

PATIENT: Well I'm not sure but 3 to 6 months comes to my mind.

THERAPIST: Okay, so what you're saying is that 3 to 6 months is a time frame that we should discuss.

Some patients have totally unrealistic expectations about what can be achieved in a brief treatment model and will respond by saying, "Maybe 3 visits." But even this response provides the therapist with important information about how to proceed and how to make differential treatment selection decisions.

Frequency and Duration of Sessions

I agree with Budman (1994) who makes the point that our traditional belief about the need for once or twice a week psychotherapy is probably more the result of what he calls "lock-in" and that these "closely held beliefs about the ways that psychotherapy should be delivered have more to do with accidents of history than with clearly defensible, 'scientific' bases for treatment" (p. 2). The therapist and patient should determine what the best fit would be. For some patients, extended sessions every 2 to 3 weeks are more practical and may have a greater impact on character defenses.

A common phenomenon when one is working in traditional psychotherapy with personality disordered patients is the frustrating experience of having to start over each session. This is due to the defensive structure of the patient, which, after each session, recrystallizes. The patient then comes in with his/her unconscious blocked. This pattern will reoccur until the unconscious becomes more fluid. In such cases, extended sessions are recommended to allow greater progress at each meeting.

THERAPEUTIC FORMATS

There are numerous formats one can use as the framework for treatment (Frances, Clarkin, & Perry, 1984). I think the key here is to adapt the format to the patient's needs and the therapist's optimal working range. I use 45 minutes as the basic time interval but prefer to extend the time to 90-minute sessions for most patients. When I conduct longer sessions, appropriate breaks after each hour and a half should be taken. I attempt to be very precise about the time blocks and plan to bring up issues or derepress material when there is sufficient time to address what is brought up. In selecting the format, I consider the following factors:

1. *Physical proximity.* The distance that the patient has to travel is an important factor in determining the frequency and duration of treatment. I have often treated patients who have come from great distances, and with this model there is no problem in doing so. Obviously one would not do so with an unstable patient who does not have support where he/she lives. If the patient elects an extended session format, I schedule as many as six sessions in a day or over 2 days, if the patient is planning to stay overnight.

2. *Financial resources.* The patient's financial resources and flexibility of insurance plan should be investigated and discussed. If the patient's means are limited, this reality needs to be addressed, and sessions need to be scheduled farther apart.

3. *Desire to increase potency.* I have found that the use of extended sessions is one of the most important factors in increasing the potency of STRP. The intense therapeutic focus over the course of an extended session dramatically increases affective responding. If the patient is interested in making a rapid change, he/she will often want longer sessions.

4. *Therapist's schedule and logistics.* Using flexible scheduling may at first seem difficult logistically, but it actually maximizes one's time. It is mostly a matter of thinking in larger blocks of time. Often, patients will take a half day off from work, or if one's schedule is busy, extended sessions can be reserved for one afternoon or Saturday.

5. *Compacting the treatment process.* Frequent extended sessions are a very beneficial method of compacting the treatment process. If, for various reasons, such as relocation, a patient wants to change as quickly as possible, extending the sessions and scheduling them frequently accelerates the treatment. There does, however, have to be sufficient time between sessions so that patients can test new skills and do extratherapeutic work. The optimal between-session time should be based on each patient's level of development and available resources. For example, a patient who is married or in a significant relationship may be better able to put into practice emotional problem-solving skills than a more isolated patient.

6. *Therapist's energy level.* Conducting extended sessions may appear exhausting to therapists who have never tried this approach. Even though there is a high level of activity, the work is energizing for the most part. One does not have to wait until next week to get deeper into an issue, and the

affective involvement energizes the treatment. The patient is often surprised at how quickly time seems to pass.

Various Formats and Their Application

Weekly 45-Minute Sessions

I find this schedule most appropriate when the patient is being seen for a brief therapy and seems amenable to a stepwise approach. The weekly format is less threatening than extended sessions. Weekly sessions do not seem to have the potency of the extended session format, which many personality disordered patients require for truly in-depth work. However, if the treatment is going to emphasize attachment and separation anxiety to activate the core issues, weekly sessions over the course of 3 months have proved to be highly effective in my clinical work.

Bimonthly Double Sessions

This is often a more effective schedule for patients who are undergoing an in-depth character analysis. The every-other-week double session affords the therapist the opportunity to do extensive work on character defenses and have some time left to get to the repressed zone. The time between sessions is often quite productive for the patient in that he/she continues to work on the issues that have surfaced during treatment. Some patients elect to come weekly for a 90-minute session. During the middle phase of treatment, sessions can often be spaced farther apart—every 2 or 3 weeks but generally no longer than a month.

Extended Sessions

Extended sessions are those over 90 minutes, usually consisting of two 90-minute sessions with a 15-minute break. When possible, I almost always use an extended session of at least 3 hours with personality disordered patients at the onset of treatment. Even more sessions can be linked when appropriate, provided regular breaks are taken. As many as 10 hours of therapy have been suggested (Berenbaum, 1969). Many patients prefer this format, as it is less disruptive to their lives. Longer periods of time, such as 3 to 4 weeks, may elapse between such appointments. At times, a single extended session may suffice. Extended sessions are underutilized, and yet I find them one of the most effective treatment formats for almost all personality disordered patients. Most patients find the extended time unlike any therapy they have had in the past because of the high dosage of therapeutic contact. The main contraindication for extended sessions is a low energy level on the part of the patient, as is the case when there is a major depression, which must be treated first.

Intermittent Sessions

Scheduling sessions on an intermittent basis can be useful for patients who are not committed to a rapid in-depth approach but who can be maintained with some level of support. The therapist should be alert for signs that the patient's readiness for change has increased and then a more intensive phase can be effected. This allows the patient to regulate his/her dependency fears by scheduling the sessions when the patient feels he/she wants to and yet to establish a therapeutic alliance. The length of the session can be based on the patient's needs and ego capacity.

The Logistics of Scheduling

Most of us in clinical practice treat a heterogeneous group of patients. Therefore, we usually do not know ahead of time which patient will manifest a personality disorder. There are two methods of handling the format of the initial assessment in terms of length. The clinician can decide that all new patients will be scheduled for an extended session and declare this policy when the patient calls for an appointment. I do not think this is practical for a number of reasons. First, many patients may be put off by this policy. Second, patients with less severe disturbances usually do well with the traditional 45-minute format.

Also, the patient could be offered the opportunity to schedule an extended session, but most patients will not be interested if this alternative is suggested over the phone and they were not prepared for this, as they would be if they were referred by someone who is familiar with the model.

One must discuss the referral process in order to address this issue adequately. If the clinician is just starting to do extended sessions with personality disordered patients, it is often best to schedule a single 45-minute initial evaluation session to assess the patient. If, during this assessment, there is evidence that the patient has a personality disorder, the therapist can recommend an extended session, and the patient can then be thoroughly informed about the treatment model. I have found that this approach provides a good test of the patient's commitment and motivation. If the patient is willing, I schedule an extended session and review the approach and initial goals. I also suggest that at the end of the extended session we will have a much better estimate for the time frame.

Once the clinician has developed expertise in treating personality disorders with STRP, he or she will begin to get referrals from other professionals of patients suspected of having personality disorders or referred to as "difficult" or "resistant" patients. If the referral source is educated about the nature of the clinician's work, the referral can prep the patient by explaining that this approach is short-term and that extended sessions are often used (Magnavita, 1994a).

Informed Consent

The patient must be provided with informed consent before treatment begins, including information about potential positive and negative outcomes. For example, with the more in-depth approach, negative effects such as increased sleep disturbances, increased anxiety, panic attacks, and psychotic-like experiences may occur. In many cases, these indicate that the treatment is working, and the patient should be encouraged to report any such phenomena in session. Miller and C'deBaca (1994) also raise the ethical issue that quantum change therapies capable of producing a fundamental reorganization of values and perceptions can also induce unanticipated life changes. These issues are important to discuss.

One Final Note about Substance Use and Medication

The overreliance or abuse of prescription and nonprescription drugs and alcohol is often an issue for the personality disordered patient. Often, patients arrive for the first session having taken tranquilizers. Some patients also may have smoked marijuana or consumed alcohol, even a few days before the session. It has been my observation that the patient's use of mood-altering substances prior to or during the extended session slows the restructuring process. Many substances interfere with the metabolization of affect, thus lessening the impact of the restructuring. I encourage patients to refrain from using drugs or alcohol and any nonessential medications for *at least 48 hours but preferably longer (a week)* before the session. It is also best to have patients come off or reduce nonessential medication, especially antianxiety medication, which has a sedating effect and makes it difficult to monitor anxiety. Antidepressant medication also seems to have a slowing effect and dulls emotional responsiveness. As a result, the restructuring does not seem to have as much impact. Any medication issues should be discussed with the prescribing psychopharmacologist in advance.

CONCLUSION

The assessment phase of short-term therapy is a crucial phase of the treatment process that should influence treatment selection decisions. The amount of information that should be gleaned from the initial interview is substantial but ensures that the clinician is on firm ground before preceding with an anxiety-arousing approach. A skilled clinician can often gather this information rapidly and unobtrusively by using clinical intuition and keen observation of verbal and nonverbal communications. As we discuss in the clinical section, the assessment phase is often interwoven with defense restructuring creating a fluid process that provides the necessary information but does not let the process become too distant. In the chapter that follows, we build on this information and show how core formulations are derived.

CHAPTER 4

How to Formulate
Core Issues

*One of the approaches Alexander outlined in his technique that is
presently used in short-term psychotherapy once a "focal conflict" has
been individuated is the following. He advised his students that, once
an important conflict was localized, they should go after it to actively
interpret it and confront the patient. "Do not allow it to get cold."
"Do not wait too long to interpret it." "It will disappear. It will be
repressed, and defenses will solidify," he felt.*
—EISENSTEIN (1986, p. 183)

A successful outcome of any course of STRP is entirely dependent on the
ability of the patient and therapist to determine the central or core issues
that need to be resolved (Luborsky, Crits-Christoph, Mintz, & Auerbach,
1988). Current research has shown that interpretations congruent with core
conflicts are related to a positive therapeutic outcome (Norville, Sampson,
& Weiss, 1996). If the core issues are not established early in the process,
treatment will wander and so lose its effectiveness. If it is accurately
established, the patient will feel understood, and therapeutic rapport will
deepen. Thus, there is a great deal of pressure on the therapist in the initial
phase of treatment. Establishing the core issue(s) is one of the most complex
and challenging tasks of the short-term therapist and is especially difficult
with personality disordered patients, who often have core issues with
multiple foci. With the neurotic patient, the clinician is often able to identify
the core conflict straight away by simply inquiring into the connections that
the patient makes among symptoms, conflicts, and past history. For exam-

ple, a patient with anxiety about his impending marriage relates that he was troubled by his parents' divorce and decided that he would not repeat the same pattern of marrying, having children, and divorcing. Here, the core issue is obvious, and the therapist can proceed to the work of eliciting and helping the patient metabolize his/her feelings.

The personality disordered patient presents a much more difficult scenario. The etiology and pathogeneses of personality disorders often cloud the core issues so that they are disguised or misleading. This is largely because the defensive structure in adults with a personality disorder is so effective at keeping the content of the developmental history and associated affects out of awareness. Uncovering affect reactivates involuntary memory (Monsen et al., 1995) and leads to a clearer picture of the core issues. Therefore, the process has a certain synergy. As more affect is mobilized, repressive forces lessen, and a clearer view results. This process continues throughout therapy but is most heavily emphasized during the initial phase.

A patient may enter treatment with a declaration that he/she does not want to go into his/her past because he/she had a "good childhood" and is close to both parents. Later, after a period of defense analysis, the patient may begin to recall various previously forgotten disturbing facts and events, such as a hospitalization of a parent for mental illness, parental mistreatment, or various other traumatic experiences. One patient, whom I describe in detail later in the book, entered treatment truly believing that his childhood and family life was "typical." Later, the extent of emotional abandonment by both parental figures became apparent. The patient, because of his/her highly developed defenses and resistances, will truly believe "things weren't so bad."

DEFINITION OF CORE ISSUE

The "core issue"[1] or central conflict is the nucleus of the patient's injuries or traumas that have resulted in disturbing impulses, fantasy, and emotions; that are too overwhelming for the infantile ego; and that have never been assimilated. Instead, these unresolved feelings, against which the patient needs defense, continue to exert an organizing influence on the patient's personality. This resulted in what Horney (1937) referred to as the self-defeating patterns evident in many characterologically disturbed patients.

To illustrate, a patient with a schizoid personality will often have parents who are cold or neutral, fail to display signs of physical or emotional affection, and value objects over the patient. This severe form of emotional abandonment can create a tremendous vortex of primitive feelings and fantasies. The natural human longings for closeness may draw the patient close to others, but this patient's expectation of abandonment may lead to an unwillingness to engage. This is the patient's "genetic structure."

THE ESSENCE OF THE SHORT-TERM THERAPIST

In simple terms, I see the ability to formulate the core issues to be what makes an effective short-term therapist. The most gifted therapists, from many different schools of thought, seem to possess an extreme sensitivity and heightened intuitiveness that almost appears to be something like a sixth sense. In my years of observing many of these therapists, I have found that they work from their right brain functions, which are not driven by logical and sequential operations. My personal belief is that some people are born with this gifted extra sensitivity. For most of us, this ability is developed over years of study and clinical practice.

Part of the therapist's ability to establish accurately core issues comes from his/her familiarity with the workings of the unconscious, knowledge of metapsychological concepts, developmental psychopathology, normal development, and an experiential understanding of one's own core issues, along with an ability to synthesize these. This is not an easy proposition for STDP novices, I will admit, but it is one that is definitely attainable.

METHODS OF ESTABLISHING CORE ISSUES

Generally, patients with personality disturbances do not enter psychotherapy with a conscious awareness of their core genetic structure. This essential determination of core pathology occurs in the bipersonal field and must be established in collaboration with the therapist. Often, the patient expresses resistance in the form of not wanting to blame anyone. Patients with personality disturbances often lack psychological mindedness, so that prior to identifying the core issues, defensive, cognitive, or affective restructuring procedures must be undertaken. Restructuring, in effect, increases psychological mindedness by providing the patient with intellectual and experiential insight into his/her inner workings. This phenomenon will be more fully considered in the clinical section of the book.

In establishing the core issues, the clinician looks for the organizing theme of the material that the patient presents. Luborsky (1984) has termed this the core conflictual relationship theme (CCRT). This is derived by listening for the repetitive conflicts that emerge from three spheres: current, transference, and past relationships. These are the schemas through which all experience is filtered and processed.

During my first meeting with the patient, I begin to develop a hypothesis about the nature of the core issues. As is the case with many psychoanalytically informed therapists, this formulation is guided by theoretical constructs (Messer, 1996; Pine, 1990). In broad terms, I attempt to determine whether what the patient is communicating is best explained by *drives*, that he/she is having difficulty managing, *object* or interpersonal difficulties, or *self* disturbance. As data emerge, I modify and refine my formulation until I am ready to test its validity. My best work occurs when I am functioning from my right brain and absorb the patient's communications through all available verbal and nonverbal channels. Below, I have listed the various informational channels that, when tapped, allow the clinician to gather and synthesize data in order to formulate the core issue(s).

Multiple Informational Channels

Presenting Complaint: Symptoms

The patient's presenting complaint and symptom constellation are the most obvious derivatives of the patient's core structure, at least at the beginning. These are generally the Axis I disturbances in DSM terminology and typically what motivated the patient to enter treatment. Most commonly, these disturbances are anxiety and/or depression as well as interpersonal difficulties. The patient's symptoms and the context in which they occur provide the therapist with preliminary information concerning the area of disturbance and core structure. Take, for example, a patient with an obsessive–compulsive personality disorder, who presents that he is having frequent "blow-ups" with his wife and at work that are followed by periods of depression and anxiety. He does not feel he can ever be perfect enough to please anyone. This should cause the clinician to consider two things: (1) What is going on with this man's aggressive impulses?—*drive theory;* and (2) Who from the patient's past expected perfection?—*object relations.*

Current Conflicts

The patient's description of his/her current conflict, depicted by the triangle of persons in the C (see Figure 2.2), offers another important view of the patient's core constellation. The difficulties may be primarily interpersonal, that is, with authority figures, with members of the opposite sex, or with the social system, such as courts and institutions. For example, a patient with a passive–aggressive personality disorder may report repetitive conflicts with male authority figures. This alerts the therapist to the possibility of unresolved anger in the father–son relationship.

Areas of Strong Emotional Current

The clinician must be alert to areas in which the patient reports strong affective responses. With exploration, the clinician can determine whether or not these really are tunnels into the feeling at the core of the patient's injury. As we discuss below, this represents a step toward affective restructuring. This affective channel is depicted by the I/F corner of the triangle of conflict (see Figure 2.4). An access point to strong affect, when mobilized, will surface an association related to the core injury.

For example, a patient with a schizoid personality disorder, who is severely emotionally disconnected, mentions his fear of losing his daughter when talking about her. When he is asked, "What would happen if you lost her?" he begins to sob, showing contact with deeply painful grief-laden affect. This, his most significant attachment, wherein he experiences parental love, has acted to reactivate his grief over what was lacking in his relationship with his parents. When the waves of grief pass, he recalls an incident when he was in the hospital and his parents made only a perfunctory visit. He then begins to paint a picture of extreme emotional abandonment by both parental figures at the core of the genetic structure. Although relatively uncommon, at times this affective channeling to the unconscious does occur for even the most ego-syntonic patients.

Repetitive Maladaptive Patterns

The patient's history may contain one or more self-defeating repetitive patterns that are the sine qua non of the spectrum of personality disorders. There is frequently a masochistic element in the personality disordered patient. This is related to a repression of sadism and guilt, which drives these patterns (Reik, 1941). These patterns often provide valuable clues that will help with determining the core structure. For example, a patient with a narcissistic personalty disorder, who was employed as an executive in the insurance industry, continued to carry on affairs with female employees even though this behavior caused him considerable trouble both within his marriage and at the office. He could not explain the compulsion to repeat this self-defeating pattern. After he described a number of these incidents and his feelings of shame and humiliation when he was caught, he was asked if he had any associations and recalled an incident that characterized his relationship with his father. His father thought he was weak because he was not physically large and tough and humiliated him repeatedly "to toughen me up." His mother was emotionally unavailable. This patient's fragile self-esteem was always flagging, and his affairs were his attempts for affirmation. Thus, massive injury to the *self* was at the core of his genetic structure.

Transference Manifestations

The transference provides yet a deeper look at the patient's core issue. The manner in which the patient relates to the clinician contains all the components of the patient's original relationships, both effective and traumatic. For instance, a patient presents with a "chip on her shoulder" and is defiant of her therapist's attempts to understand her difficulties. She reports that she takes this attitude with other "authority figures," as well. She has no respect for those in authority. This is eventually linked to her history of sexual molestation and mistreatment by her father and her anger at her mother and other adults who did nothing to protect her.

Nonverbal Communication

Reik (1949), in *Listening with the Third Ear*, tells of a patient who came to therapy and mumbled inaudibly, speaking up only when requested to speak louder. All patients convey a wealth of nonverbal information, with their appearance, posture, eye contact or lack thereof, manner of dress, and so forth. These can be subtle or not-so-subtle clues about the nature of the core issue. If the patient's character armor is tight, that is, presents with tensed muscles and clipped speech, the clinician may recognize an overcontrol of impulses, as with obsessional character.

Countertransference Reactions

As we discussed earlier, the clinician's countertransference reactions provide additional information with which to formulate the core structure. Does the patient engender rescue fantasies, anger, or defensiveness in the clinician? This often represents the complementary interpersonal valence (Benjamin, 1993). The patient's communicative style recreates a force field that elicits interpersonal reactions from others, and the clinician, when attuned, can use his/her reactions as a guide. Personality can best be understood by observing the sequence of recurring events in the interpersonal field (Sullivan, 1953). The passive patient may engender an impulse in the therapist to tell him/her what to do. This may represent an aspect of the early parent–child dynamics that seek reenactment with the therapist and should be noted. In the treatment of the narcissistic patient, the therapist may find him/herself bored, angry, or unable to make sense of the material (Cooper, 1986). Recognizing and understanding these reactions can add to our intuitive understanding of the patient's core issues and their developmental context.

Issues Identified by Psychological Testing

We also touched upon the use of psychological instruments in assessing a new patient. These can be used as well in determining the core disturbance, such as attachment–loss, separation–individuation, impulse/affect regulation, and so forth. Establishing the patient's personality profile through psychological assessment can guide the process to the likely developmental disruption, alerting the clinician to object, self, or drive explanations. For example, a patient with a hysterical personality profile suggests unresolved oedipal conflicts. Testing can also provide corroboration for instinctual conclusions.

Recurrent Dreams and Earliest Memories

Another aspect of the core conflict can be observed by any recurring dreams that the patient remembers and reports. "Dream interpretation often leads directly to a person's central conflicts, even though the person previously could not articulate what was making him or her unhappy" (Hill, 1996, p. 9). These dreams often hold a metaphor for the core injury. Also, the patient's earliest memories can provide insight into the conflict and structure. One patient, for example, remembered being left alone for an extended period of time at age 3, indicative of a broader pattern of maternal abandonment.

Fantasy Material and Daydreams

The patient's fantasy productions and daydreams (Schafer, 1968) can orient the therapist to the nature of the patient's core issues. One patient had a recurring fantasy that she would wind up living the life of a "bag lady." This was later related to her identification with a schizophrenic father who was always on the edge of financial ruin. One severely self-destructive patient discussed a daydream she had prior to the first session where she was floating in a box in a pond.

Combining Informational Channels

Utilizing the informational channels described above, the therapist can begin to formulate a picture of the core genetic structure of the patient. It is best done early in the treatment process. This entails clinical deductive thinking based on sound knowledge about the roots of psychopathology and is enhanced by clinical experience.[2]

THE ROOTS OF PSYCHOPATHOLOGY

Damage from early trauma can take many forms and is not necessarily linked to a single traumatic event. Human psychopathology develops as a result of injuries received at various developmental stages, which result in the development of compensatory mechanisms, which, in turn, allow the personality disordered patient to function as effectively as possible. The most common traumas reported by patients include loss; neglect; abuse; disturbances in parent–child relationships; narcissistic injuries; family disturbances, and parental illness or hardships, such as chronic depression or schizophrenia.

Rediscovering what Horney (1937) found many years ago, Herman (1992) stated: "A secure sense of connection with caring people is the foundation of personality development" (p. 52). The roots of personality disorders are fairly well understood now, thanks to almost a century of clinical evidence. They include:

- Insufficient attachment and responsivity of early caretakers
- Incidents of sexual and or physical abuse
- Patterns of parental neglect
- Loss of object
- Injuries to the self (narcissistic exploitation)
- Unresolved oedipal issues[3]

The results of these traumatic events, which differ in severity and onset, are described in the book *Trauma and Recovery,* by Herman (1992):

> Traumatic reactions occur when action is of no avail. When neither resistance nor escape is possible, the human system of self-defense becomes overwhelmed and disorganized. Each component of the ordinary response to danger, having lost its utility, tends to persist in an altered and exaggerated state long after the actual danger is over. Traumatic events produce profound and lasting changes in physiological arousal, emotion, cognition, and memory. Moreover, traumatic events may sever these normally integrated functions from one another. The traumatized person may experience intense emotion but without clear memory of the event, or may remember everything in detail but without emotion. (p. 45)

Early attachment disruptions lead to an undifferentiated self that has not developed a clear intrapsychic organization, in other words, lack of structuralization. Later, traumatic events, injuries, and developmental insults become stratified under layers of defense, which harden and strengthen with time and become defects in structure.

Examples of Core Formulations

Core formulations, in order to be effective, must be based on an accurate and extensive understanding of the patient's essence. In formulating core issues, the clinician should strive for parsimony. If the formulations are too complex, their impact is diluted. As stated, core formulations are used by the patient and therapist to discover the patient's deepest level of injury and bring to full experience the feelings associated with these. Core formulations may emphasize or combine *drive conflict,* such as repressed aggressive or sexualized impulses toward a genetic figure; *faulty object relations,* such as early loss of a significant figure; or *self-injury,* such as a lack of parental attunement. All are associated with a complex of affects that are non-metabolized. For example:

- The loss of your mother when you were 3 resulted in painful feelings of grief, and, as a result, you have avoided close relationships so that you would not have to reexperience that pain.
- Your father's abusive actions toward you resulted in a build-up of anger that you turned into passivity in order to protect him from your wishes to murder him. You never had the closeness with him that you craved.
- Your mother's depression made her unavailable to you when you were a child, so you constantly sought other means of filling the emptiness that she left.
- The lack of a secure early attachment to either parent has left you feeling empty and chaotic, without a clearly differentiated sense of your feelings, thoughts and impulses.

Delivering the Core Formulation

One of the tasks of the initial phase of treatment is delivering the core formulation to the patient so that there is a clear understanding of the roots of the personality disturbance and symptom pattern. During the extended session, I refine the core formulation and validate this with the patient. This is a give-and-take process. At the end of the session, I usually summarize the patient's difficulties and then link this to the core formulation.

Validating the Core Formulation

Validating the hypothesis of the core formulation is a crucial step that must be done before proceeding with the working through. The core issues will evolve as therapy proceeds and new material emerges. What is important for the process is the patient's *collaboration* in formulating and acknowledging the accuracy of the formulation. There may be resistance because the feelings are painful, but the therapist needs to be sure he/she is on solid footing before proceeding.

The patient's reaction to trial formulations tests the accuracy of the theory of the patient's core issue, although this is not usually the case with highly defended patients. If a trial interpretation is accurately formulated, it will usually generate strong affect; if it is inaccurate, little disturbance in the defense–affect system will be noted. I often couch the formulation in tentative terms at first: "I'm not sure if this is correct, and if it doesn't fit, please tell me. It appears that your problems with authority figures are something you developed to protect yourself from being subjugated by your father." If an interpretation is not accepted, the therapist should not continue using it.

> *Does the core formulation surface or elicit feeling?* Often, when an accurate core formulation is presented to the patient, an increase in affect occurs. An array of feelings may be elicited. The patient will often indicate he/she feels deeply understood.
>
> *Does it shed light on character traits?* A comprehensive core formulation links, in a logical way, the core formulation to the character defense system and personality disturbance. In other words, can the core formulation explain the patient's personality disorder? There should be a connection between the theoretical constructs and resulting personality.
>
> *Is the theme apparent in dreams?* Often, the patient's dreams validate the core formulation.
>
> *Is there a shift in the defense system?* If the core formulation is valid and the associated affective material is evoked, there should be a loosening of the character defense system and greater access to the unconscious.
>
> *Does the patient report that the formulation explains the chronic pain?* Patients often report that they feel a deep affinity for themselves and

the enduring pain they have carried most of their lives. Patients often say, "I never thought of it like that, but it makes sense."

ACTIVELY MAINTAINING THE CORE FOCUS

Once the core issues are formulated and the patient is in agreement, the therapist must work to keep therapy focused so that the working through can occur. At first, patients tend to forget or minimize the relevance of the core formulation even though considerable affect has been elicited. This is especially likely to occur between sessions during the initial phase of treatment before sufficient restructuring of the defenses has taken place. This is the most crucial time for the clinician to keep the focus so that all the feeling has been elicited and metabolized. The following guidelines can serve to maintain the focus on core issues:

Starting the session by recapitulating the core issue. I have found that beginning the session by restating the core issue is helpful in maintaining the focus.

Once the core formulation is accepted, confronting resistances when they emerge. One patient came in contact with deep buried grief over the fact that her mother was a closet alcoholic and never emotionally available to her. Two weeks later, she adamantly reported that she did not want to blame her mother for her troubles. To confront this resistance, I pointed out that she wanted to protect her mother from her negative feelings and that she had done so all her life at a high psychic cost.

Reminding the patient of the therapeutic task. If the patient shows resistance to the core formulation, the clinician should remind the patient of the therapeutic task. "We are not here to blame anyone. Our goal is that we get to the truth and to the core of your difficulties so that you don't have to carry this excess baggage with you."

Using the core formulation to make interpretations relating to the patient's personality patterns. The core formulations, once established and validated, are used to interpret repetitive patterns and symptom constellations. "Interpretations" are defined as a link between the core formulation (P) and the transference (T) or current relationship (C). Thus, interpretations can be T–P, C–P, and T–C–P. Research in STDP has indicated that the best results occur when frequent T–C–P interpretations are made. That is, we demonstrate how the core genetic structure influences how the patient relates to the clinician in the transference as well as to those in the patient's current life. Two cases that follow serve to illustrate this point:

CASE A

The patient, diagnosed with an obsessive–compulsive personality, was unable to establish satisfactory relationships with men. She viewed any display of emotion in herself as weak and found herself attracted to unemotional men. The core genetic structure was as follows: (1) The patient was an only child of an attorney who was completely unaffectionate with her, expecting her to be the "perfect little girl"; (2) the patient's mother was prone to hysterical outbursts and related to her daughter as if she were a doll. She detested her mother's behavior, which seemed to be an attempt to engage her husband who was "like a rock." As soon as there was any evidence of emotion, the patient would say, "What good is emotion, it is only a display of weakness."

THERAPIST: Are you aware of how your unwillingness to contact your emotions puts a barrier between us?

PATIENT: Emotions make people behave irrationally.

THERAPIST: Yes, but we know what is at the root of that. On one side you have the rock, whom you idealized, and on the other side a hysterical woman, whom you detested. Your avoidance of your emotions makes it impossible for you to get close to anybody. You have rejected your mother's overemotionality and have become a rock.

PATIENT: Yes, but that has prevented me from getting hurt.

THERAPIST: Your unresolved feelings toward both of your parents have resulted in your erecting a wall between yourself and me, and they have destroyed your relationships.

CASE B

Another patient, diagnosed with a histrionic personality disorder, had a pattern of use and abuse relationships with men and a lack of friendships with women. She attracted men to her with seductive behavior but then could not establish any intimacy. Her endless demands for attention drove her partners away. Her core genetic structure was as follows: (1) The patient's relationship with her father was characterized by a lack of intimacy but with much sexualized affect until she entered her puberty, at which time her father greatly distanced himself; (2) her mother was chronically depressed and did not have the energy to emotionally nurture or guide the patient. In the transference, she tended toward seductiveness and identified sexual feeling but was frightened that she would be responded to by the therapist.

THERAPIST: Your lack of emotional closeness with your father resulted in your relying on your sexuality to maintain his attention, which was the only thing that he responded to. This was a substitute for emotional closeness. When that got too threatening, during adolescence, he avoided you completely.

PATIENT: But that is what happens with all men, as soon as I get sexual they leave.

THERAPIST: The same dynamic is occurring with me. You are afraid your sexual feelings are the only thing that will keep me interested, like with your father. You also seem afraid that I would respond to them.

PATIENT: Yes, but a part of me wishes you would respond.

THERAPIST: But I wonder whether the more intense craving is for an intimate caring relationship, but you're terrified to let your wall down and risk abandonment.

PATIENT: Yes, that sounds correct. It would hurt much more if I was really unlovable. At least I know men will respond to me sexually.

THERAPIST: That's right, but wouldn't it be better for you to honestly face your self-defeating behavior and work through the unresolved feelings toward both of your parents?

The patients' unresolved core issues have been recreated in current relationships and distant past relationships, as seen in the vignettes above. These core issues will also come into operation in the transference. Merely identifying the core genetic structure is not sufficient for personality transformation. Once established, the core issues must be systematically worked through by bringing the patient's feelings to surface. This is the very essence of the restructuring process. More about this will be presented in the next chapter.

CONCLUSION

The most challenging aspect of STRP with the personality disordered patient is accurately formulating the core issue(s) that are at the root of the patient's character pathology and symptoms. Although all humans are unique in their individual experience, there are surprising commonalities in developmental disturbances that affect human personality formation and psychopathology. In addition to a comprehensive assessment of the patient at the start of the process, the therapist who is attuned to the unconscious can use him/herself to develop an intuitive understanding of the patient's core issues and life struggles.

◈ CHAPTER 5

Techniques of STRP: The Use of Anxiety and Maximizing the Therapeutic Alliance

If the first transference resistance has not been preceded by sufficient production of memory material, its resolution meets with a difficulty. ... This difficulty consists in the fact that, in order to resolve the resistance, one must know the unconscious material it contains, while, on the other hand, one cannot get at this material because the resistance blocks it.

—REICH (1945, p. 28)

THE IMPORTANCE OF ANXIETY

Our inability to access the unconscious material of the highly defended patient has rendered many traditional analytic techniques useless with the spectrum of personality disorders. The use of anxiety in facilitating change and monitoring the therapeutic process is one of the most technically challenging aspects of STRP. We owe much to the pioneering work of Sifneos and Davanloo for their advancements in this regard for challenging conventional practice and carrying on the work of Reich.

Increasing the anxiety level energizes the patient's psychic system and activates defenses, causing unconscious conflicts to surface and bringing concomitant feelings and memories to the preconscious or conscious level of awareness. Increased anxiety activates the patient's defensive system, which can then be confronted, restructured, or strengthened depending on the patient's personality organization. The therapist must maintain constant vigilance to observe how the patient metabolizes his/her anxiety. Too little anxiety and the therapeutic process can become stagnant, and the process can falter because there is no access to the unconscious. Conversely, too high a level of anxiety can overwhelm the patient and lead to regressive behavior or disturbance in the patient's perceptual field. It is difficult to discuss anxiety fully without first examining defenses, which we do in Chapter 6. However, if the treatment process is to be optimized, it is necessary to understand thoroughly how anxiety is used in the therapeutic process.

MONITORING ANXIETY: THE BAROMETER OF THE PROCESS

Monitoring the patient's anxiety is equivalent to the weatherperson's use of the barometer to predict weather patterns. When the therapist is acutely sensitive to manifestations of anxiety, he/she can use this as a barometer of the treatment process. As discussed, the ability to tolerate anxiety without becoming symptomatic is a measure of ego-adaptive capacity. Fluctuations in anxiety levels inform the therapist by indicating the topics or issues to which the patient is unconsciously resonating and how the patient's defenses are organized to manage the increasing anxiety. The therapist should follow the anxiety, as it is the smoke of the emotional life, but at the same time, he/she should prepare the patient for the journey by assuring an adequate ego-adaptive capacity.

Arousal by Exposure

For some patients, especially those with borderline structures, emotional arousal is too high to allow for effective therapeutic work, and cognitive restructuring is required. This group of patients requires assistance in emotional regulation before work at a core level can begin. Patients at a higher level of structural integrity are in a sense emotionally over-regulated. These patients require sufficient emotional arousal to activate the unconscious zone. "In all models of psychotherapy, the therapist introduces arousal by *exposure*. Arousal can be created by confronting a patient with those aspects of experience, behavior, and sensation that are being avoided or by preventing the exercise of usual coping strategies" (Beutler & Clarkin, 1990). A therapist would not want to confront a fragile patient with highly emotional material, such as abuse or traumatic memories, until the patient's defensive structure has been strengthened, or psychotic reactions might occur.

Patient's Level of Anxiety

Personality disordered patients will exhibit the full range of anxiety levels and manifestations (Frommer et al., 1996), from free-floating primitive anxiety, typically present in the borderline states, to an absence of anxiety in the ego-syntonic character disturbances. Generalized anxiety and panic attacks are often apparent, but we may also have anxiety and not be aware of it even though it may be a determining factor in our life (Horney, 1937). When meeting with a patient, one of the clinician's first tasks must be to establish a baseline of the patient's level of conscious anxiety. This is extremely difficult with the personality disordered patient and requires hypervigilance on the therapist's part. It is absolutely necessary for the therapist's subsequent application of emotional arousal to determine how much anxiety the patient can tolerate before he/she will resort to regressive defenses.

Nonverbal Manifestations of Anxiety

The therapist can begin to evaluate the patient's level of anxiety before the patient has even spoken a word. The very first handshake provides clues to the patient's anxiety level, such as revealing the presence or absence of sweaty palms and warm or cold hands. Observing the patient's demeanor also provides information. The patient may be fidgety, restless, or rigid. He/she may sigh frequently, hyperventilate, or become frozen. These are all manifestations of some degree of anxiety, and they should be noted by the therapist from the start. Other anxiety release mechanisms, such as glancing away, changing posture, drumming one's fingers, and other motoric activity, serve to siphon off anxiety. By discouraging the patient from engaging in such activity, the therapist is able to escalate the patient's anxiety, thereby increasing access to the unconscious material. Often, merely pointing out the motoric activities to the patient is often sufficient to block the channel of motoric discharge.

The Importance of Nonverbal Communication
in the Interpersonal Field

The connection among unconscious conflict, relationship style, and emo-tional blockage is directly linked to physiological manifestations and character armor. Observing both the blatant and subtle nonverbal styles and responses of the patient are often as revealing, if not more so, than the patient's verbal communication (Ekman & Friesen, 1969). We discuss how to address nonverbal defenses therapeutically in the following chapter. Harper, Wiens, and Matarazzo (1978) present an excellent summary of the research to that date in nonverbal communication. Harper et al. (1978) describe the importance of the nonverbal: "Information that we may withhold verbally and fail to display in our facial expressions may be 'leaked' through movements of our hands, legs, feet, and so forth, which are less under our conscious control and more likely to reflect our emotional state at the moment" (pp. x–xi). Often, nonverbal communication is more efficient than verbal communication. The clinician should observe the following nonverbal modes of communication:

> *Paralinguistic phenomena.* These include moans and yells, as well as the tempo, range, and pitch of speech.
>
> *Kinetics.* This is defined by Harper et al. (1978) as discriminable movements of the body. "A person who moves about in intense and jerky movements would be nonverbally contradicting any concurrent verbal claim that he [she] was not upset" (p. 120). In studying psychotherapy sessions, researchers have found that micromomentary fist-like motions are associated with expressions of anger.
>
> *Facial expressions.* This may be the best indicator of the patient's feelings and can be accurately identified (Keltner, Moffitt, & Stouthamer-Loeber, 1995). Facial expressions appear to be universal, rather than culture specific. The face is able to convey emotion and a large quantity of information quickly and with force (National Advisory Mental Health Council, 1995).
>
> *Visual behavior.* Visual behavior is the information conveyed by the interpersonal gaze. Averting one's gaze or looking directly into another's eyes are basic elements in the initiation and maintenance of interpersonal communication, and they are most often related to intimacy. Prolonged looking produces flight or avoidance responses in strangers.
>
> *Proxemics.* This relates to the impact of space on interpersonal interactions. Personal space is the physical distance or boundary zone evident in various types of interpersonal interaction. For example, reporting feelings of invasion when someone gets too close is usually a manifestation of anxiety arousal.

Listening, sensing, experiencing, and observing are ways in which the therapist can monitor the anxiety in the therapeutic process. Observing the patient's nonverbal manifestations and channels of anxiety will orient the therapist by keying her/him into which topics increase the patient's nonverbal activity and provide signposts along the trail of smoke to the unconscious.

Therapists can increase their sensitivity to nonverbal communication by viewing videotapes of patients with the audio turned off to sharpen their intuitive feel for these modes of communication. During these exercises try to get a sense of what the patient is communicating and then go back and listen to the verbal communication. Trust the nonverbal!

Exploration of Anxiety

The therapist can also assess the level of anxiety by exploring the anxiety of which the patient is aware, that is, "conscious anxiety." The patient must first be educated in the proper terminology, so that both patient and therapist speak precisely and use the same language. The patient can be asked to describe his/her anxiety in specific physical terms, such as the presence of rapid heart beat, dry mouth, sweaty palms, and muscle tension, so that the phenomenon is anchored to the patient's felt experience. It is important that the therapist not unintentionally foster miscommunication by assuming that the patient knows exactly what anxiety is. Clarification and specific behavioral terminology are in order. Once a shared definition is agreed upon, subjective ratings by the patient are much easier to establish.

The Use of Anxiety to Mobilize the Unconscious Process
Activating Anxiety

As discussed in Chapter 3 in the section on (patient) Assessment, the structural interview will reveal much about how the patient metabolizes anxiety. The *triangle of conflict* depicts how mobilizing the patient's anxiety increases defensive responding. Watching the patient and listening carefully will be most important in monitoring the treatment process.

For some patients, anxiety is a sign that unconscious feeling has reached the preconscious zone, whereas for other patients, anxiety is secondary to fragmentation and loss of contact. The therapist must be knowledgeable in this area before proceeding with any of the anxiety-arousing techniques or defensive challenging approaches. As stated before, the purpose of increasing the patient's anxiety is to gain access to unconscious material; the therapist must therefore recognize when the patient is in the domain of the unconscious. Let us compare two patients:

Patient A is a 30-year-old man who, after the initial evaluation, shows that he is unable to identify any feeling and has little psychological

understanding of the events leading to his decision to try psychotherapy. From week to week, he does not recall the issues discussed. There
is little continuity; each session, by reestablishing rapport and defining
the problems, seems like starting over. He reports no memory of any
dreams or even fantasy material.

Patient B is a 46-year-old divorced woman who realizes that she is
unable to make a commitment to her current love interest and is
conflicted about this. Although she uses compartmentalization, she
shows a capacity to express her feeling. Each session seems contiguous,
as themes are followed. She reports significant dreams and shows some
ability to determine their meaning.

Patient A's unconscious is not accessible to the therapist. His defensive
system is completely closed, and there is very little collaboration between
him and his therapist. The patient appears almost wooden and one-dimen-
sional. Patient B, on the other hand, has meaningfully accessed her unconscious, and the therapist is able to guide her in exploring important areas.
It is crucial to know when the unconscious process is accessed. Once the
patient is communicating from the unconscious zone, anxiety-arousing
techniques should not be used, and affective restructuring is indicated.
    The patient's unconscious has been accessed when the following
indicators are present:

1. The patient remembers his/her dreams.
2. Themes are not forgotten from one session to the next.
3. The patient relaxes his/her defenses.
4. There is a spirit of mutual collaboration.
5. The patient recalls important early life experiences.
6. The patient can make use of psychological constructs to further
   self-understanding and awareness.
7. Painful waves of affect are accessed with minimal defense analysis.
8. Fantasy material is freely reported.
9. There is a continuity of themes within sessions and from session to
   session.

When the unconscious has been accessed, the patient's level of motivation
increases, and the patient is relating to the therapist in the way a patient at
a higher level of ego-adaptive capacity would relate. There is much less
resistance, and the therapist does not need to be as active. This process will
ebb and flow. Even though one gains an access point, this does not mean
that the defenses and resistances will not return around another aspect of
the core genetic structure.

The Question of Empathic Attunement versus Provoking Anxiety

Most clinicians are trained to provide empathic attunement, and it often comes naturally to those who are attracted to the practice of psychotherapy. We consider ourselves caring and accepting individuals and are unaccustomed to confrontational approaches and defense-challenging techniques. However, in my experience as well as many that of my peers, without defense analysis, treatment of the personality disordered patient is needlessly protracted and, in many cases, unlikely to lead to significant structural modification.

Rogers (1942) noted many years ago that *an overly supportive approach may in fact encourage repression.* The patient may begin to feel that he/she is not permitted to bring less acceptable impulses and fantasy material to the session. Although an anxiety-provoking approach may seem diametrically opposed to an empathic one, it is not dichotomous. Although few clinical theorists report mixing these approaches, in clinical practice, most therapists probably do so naturally as they gain more experience.

I would propose that the rule of thumb in STRP is to use as much defense analysis as the patient can tolerate and incorporate empathic phases when the patient responds negatively. These shifts can occur within the frame of one session. The trick is not to get too bogged down in the empathic phase unless you are clearly working at the level of the unconscious. Also, defense analysis and anxiety-provoking techniques are generally emphasized during the early phase of treatment, although one would certainly go the other way with a patient with a fragile structure.

METHODS USED TO INCREASE ANXIETY

There are a variety of technical interventions that effectively raise anxiety that are especially well-suited for use with the personality disordered patient. Remember, the purpose of intensifying anxiety is to stimulate the patient's unconscious memories and buried feelings and, thus, to activate the core structure of the patient so that it can be fully experienced and worked through systematically by metabolizing the affect and thus reducing its significance. Effective psychotherapy reactivates the emotional pain that has been avoided, and the threat of intimate exposure to the therapist will create anxiety and resistance. "Resistance refers to the customary and automatic ways clients both reveal and keep hidden aspects of themselves from the other, especially as they occur in their relationship with the therapist" (Messer, 1996, p. 26). Thus, there is a strong pull–push paradox: In order to accomplish the therapeutic goals, the patient must expose his/her deepest vulnerabilities.

Intimacy and the Approach–Avoid Paradox

The very act of entering psychotherapy will activate the patient's anxiety about intimacy, which, for most personality disordered patients, is something they crave, yet also fear. Many of these patients long to establish meaningful contact, yet their experience had been that "intimacy is dangerous, hurtful, neglectful, engulfing, sexual and so on." For many, merely employing the term "intimacy" noticeably raises anxiety. Some patients react by cringing and withdrawing, while others will assume a belligerent posture, declaring they are quite capable of attaining closeness.

This combined desire for and fear of intimacy creates a conundrum for personality disordered patients. In order for them to heal, they must allow the therapist to get close to them and establish a deep emotional attachment. Yet, most of their past relationships have been in some way injurious, and they therefore feel they have much to lose. "An intimate relationship is a separation/individuation stress in its own right because it requires self-activation and autonomy; and a patient will respond to the anxiety it creates just as she would toward any other separation or individuation stress—by utilizing the defenses" (Masterson, 1988, p. 114).

One patient described his trouble managing intimacy by saying, "I have a narrow band that is safe. If people get too close, I find it threatening because I fear exposure. On the other hand, if people get too far, I feel abandoned and strive to draw them back in." The therapist must be sensitive to this struggle. Expecting the patient to reveal him/herself in an intimate way too quickly can be extremely frightening for many patients. On the other hand, not moving closer quickly enough will trigger the patient's feelings of isolation and hopelessness.

Many personality disordered patients confuse intimacy with sexual contact. The therapist and patient should discuss the definition of intimacy. I have found that telling the patient that intimacy is "sharing your innermost personal thoughts, fantasies and feelings" clarifies the meaning of emotional versus sexual intimacy. Therapists should be alert to patients who have strong reactions to the use of the word intimacy. Patients who recoil physically or shut down may have suffered severe trauma by a genetic figure, which is closely associated with intimacy. Some patients reexperience the associated traumas in the form of flashbacks. Obviously, if this occurs, the therapist should move quickly to a less anxiety-provoking topic.

More commonly, patients report that they do, in fact, allow others to get close to them emotionally. Upon closer examination, however, it becomes clear that the patient has not really understood the question. For example, a patient who shows major resistance to opening up with the therapist says she has close friends. But what she means by this is that her friends tell her about themselves. Often, with careful use of the transference, the patient can begin to understand experientially what is meant by intimacy. This is where the concept of the false self has value. The patient often shares his/her false self with others—but never allows anyone near the real self. Another patient said that she was close to her mother because she was able to talk to her about sex. Later in therapy, she became painfully aware that her mother tolerated no emotional expression from her and only used her for vicarious gratification. Her mother's interest in her sex life was a vicarious attempt to fill the void of a sexless marriage to her father.

In-depth, short-term psychotherapy sometimes feels to the patient as though he/she has been asked to get undressed while the therapist remains clothed. The best way for the therapist to empathize with this feeling is to undergo psychotherapy him/herself.

There are various ways to directly or indirectly address resistances and thus increase anxiety. Resistances can be "realistic and unconscious" as well as "automatic or unconscious." Patients may also manifest "state resistances," resulting from the explanation of an evocative topic, or "trait resistances," wherein repetitive maladaptive patterns interfere with the therapeutic process (Van Denberg & Kiesler, 1996, p. 58). The following methods will increase anxiety and concomitant resistance and focus on lifting repressive forces.

Encouraging Intimacy

Encouraging intimacy increases anxiety. Asking a patient to reveal innermost thoughts, feelings, and fantasies is stressful. The concomitant anxiety is a treatment artifact. When pressure is placed on the patient to reveal him/herself rapidly, the anxiety can rapidly skyrocket. Focusing on how the patient is avoiding contact with the therapist can be one of the most anxiety-arousing interventions and should be used with great caution and sensitivity.

Exploring Evocative Conflictual Material

One method of increasing anxiety is to ask the patient to present conflictual material and then explore his/her affective responses. This is intense emotional evocation, wherein the patient is exposed to stimuli that are reported to be anxiety arousing. Returning to the triangle of conflict, the therapist can ask the patient to describe an incident in his/her current life (C) that is highly conflictual. The therapist can intensify the feeling by asking the patient to describe, as specifically as possible, what transpired, which has the effect of resurfacing the affect. Defenses are analyzed as they occur.

Isolating the Patient's Character–Personality Traits

"Although individual defenses are psychological processes, the propensity to use particular defenses, or *defensive style,* constitutes a personality trait" (Soldz, Budman, Demby, & Merry, 1996). The therapist can increase anxiety by pointing out the patient's character traits (Reich, 1945). Reich believed that by repeatedly identifying the trait to the patient, it would become as disturbing as a symptom. For example, "I notice that when you discuss your feelings toward your wife you sound very sarcastic," or "Every time you have reported a conflict you have reacted with avoidance."

Using Forced Fantasies

Using forced fantasies is a powerful means of increasing the patient's affective intensity. For example, if the patient is discussing a fear of losing control, the therapist can ask the patient to describe specifically what would happen under these circumstances. These questions demand that the patient consciously consider his/her unconscious fears and will quickly raise anxiety. For example, in the case of the woman with the fear of knives, we might ask, "What would have happened if you had lost control?" and "In what fashion would you have murdered your grandchild?" In a sense this is a form of desensitizing the unconscious by exposure to anxiety-provoking thoughts and fantasies. This is also an excellent technique for increasing anxiety related to buried or pathological grief, as well as other feelings, related to loss. By asking the patient to describe his/her fantasy of someone dying in as much detail as possible, the therapist can induce the patient to confront a core unconscious issue. It can also be used with patients who are suicidal to expose the nature of their suicidality. For example, a patient can be asked to portray what his/her funeral would be like. Who would attend? Who would be most upset? What would this person's good-bye be like? What would he/she say to the person's dead body at the final good-bye?

Interpreting Nonverbal Defenses

Many patients nonverbally defend against anxiety. They smile when angry, withdraw when sad, or become fidgety when anxious. Interpreting these defenses for the patient brings the patient's feelings and associated anxiety closer to the surface. For example, "I notice when I ask you how you feel, you sit back in your seat, as if to withdraw from me." Revealing the patient's nonverbal defenses increases the patient's awareness. Eventually the patient becomes ego-dystonic and, thus, raises the level of conscious anxiety. Certain groups of patients habitually smile when they are angry but are not aware of this. Bringing this to the patient's attention during various interactions increases awareness, reducing sytonicity. The patient often begins to notice a smile and declares, "I must be hiding my anger."

Focusing on Feelings

Most personality disordered patients, and neurotics as well, find discussing their feelings highly anxiety provoking. Many of them cannot specifically identify what they are feeling. Asking patients how they feel at the moment and requesting that they focus on what they notice in their bodies is one particularly effective way of demonstrating to patients the connection between what goes on in their psyche and their bodies. Exploring feelings almost always increases the patient's anxiety regarding vulnerability to, and closeness with, the therapist.

Interrupting Defenses

The therapist can intensify anxiety by interrupting the patient when he/she is in a defensive posture. For example, when the patient, during a discussion of an emotionally laden conflict, launches upon a needlessly elaborate or circumstantial explanation, the therapist can interrupt, reorient the patient, and then examine his/her reaction to the interruption. This technique must be used judiciously, as it often activates strong negative affect. Some patients will respond with irritation, for example, "You interrupted me!"

Exploring Transference Thoughts and Feelings

Transference feelings are probably the most anxiety-provoking of all feelings for the patient to acknowledge and explore. Questions such as, "How are you feeling right now toward me?" can elicit strong anxiety and concomitant defenses that can then be analyzed. This will bring intense affect closer to the surface. Encouraging the patient to report any fantasy about the therapist can also create anxiety. For example, one patient noticed another patient leaving the office and wondered who she was. She was encouraged to describe her fantasy about her. Another patient declared she "hated everyone," and the therapist indicated that this must include him, encouraging her to be honest about her hateful feelings.

Singling Out and Penetrating the Defensive Barrier

The patient's anxiety will increase if the therapist methodically singles out the patient's defenses as they appear and alerts the patient to the repetitive nature of his/her defenses in the context of relationships. When the patient's major defenses are confronted in a direct, intense way, then an increase in anxiety results, and a breakthrough to feeling can occur. Continually pointing out, for example, how a system of passive defenses interferes not only with the therapeutic task, but with the patient's full functioning, will increase anxiety and surface underlying feeling toward the therapist. "Yes, you have decided to improve your relationship with your wife, but you continue to assume a passive stance, avoiding her, becoming stubborn, coming home late, and forgetting to do what you agreed to." Each of the patient's defenses are labeled and brought to his awareness.

Anxiety-Provoking Probes and Questions

Sifneos (1987) presented a patient who spoke of the warm feelings he recalls experiencing toward his mother on wash day. Sifneos responded, "You mean 'sexual' feeling." This is a classic example of the type of anxiety-provoking intervention that will dramatically raise the patient's anxiety level. Of course, the therapist must predicate the intervention on the material the patient has revealed. These confrontations may include "paradoxical situations, illogical conclusions, ineffectual responses, irrational wishes, and maladaptive behavior patterns, all of which may not be appreciated immediately by the patient but are nevertheless true" (p. 133).

One patient discussed how he was only sexually attracted to slender women and prior to this had described his mother as slender and stated that she dresses seductively. In fact, he reported how his adolescent friends used to tell him they wanted to date her. The therapist asked about the patient's sexual feelings, which he denied. It was then pointed out how he lighted up when talking about his mother's slim body and sexy clothing and how he acknowledged his attraction to women built like his mother. His anxiety as well as his defensiveness increased: "I have never had those thoughts about my mother!"

Exhortation

The therapist can heighten emotion and increase anxiety by using vivid and intense verbal expression (Small, 1971). This technique should not be done artificially, which could damage the therapeutic alliance. "Yes, you can do something about your marriage if you don't sit back and take a passive approach!" "You must stand up for yourself and your relationship, otherwise it will be too late, and you will have lost that which you say you value!"

Shock: Toxic Metaphors

The clinician can also raise anxiety by incorporating powerful "toxic" metaphors (Fosha, 1995)in his/her speech that reflect aspects of the patient's character pathology. This, in a sense, shocks the patient and can derail defenses. For example, one patient, whenever he started to improve, would seek out a prostitute and buy cocaine, destroying the trust he built up with his family. I described this need for self-destruction with cocaine as "the cancer of his life." This labeling of the patient's patterns or defenses is meant to jolt the patient into recognizing the reality of his/her destructive pattern. It is most effective with patients who are highly syntonic characters.

Addressing Resistances

Resistance is a manifestation of the patient's defenses in the service of repression. It occurs as a reluctance to express one's thoughts and feelings interpersonally in the transference. "Close process monitoring" is acquainting the patient with his/her resistances and interpreting them (Davison, Pray, & Bristol, 1990). These resistances often manifest as silence, inappropriate affect, posture, rituals, lateness, missed appointments, not paying, and acting out. Davison and his associates suggest that, technically, the aggressive impulses should be brought to the surface first, to which I am in agreement. Once this occurs, there is greater access to the affectionate and erotic or libidinal feelings. Messer (1996) conveys an important point worth emphasizing that resistance is not the enemy of therapy but, rather, "the inevitable expression of the person's manner of relating to their [sic] inner problems and others" (p. 26).

Modulating the Anxiety to Seek the Optimal Balance

Since the therapist can never know a priori how much anxiety is necessary to maximize the treatment process, there will be occasions when too much anxiety is mobilized, and the patient cannot metabolize the underlying affects. Therefore the clinician needs to be able to intervene swiftly to reduce anxiety if the patient is beyond his/her tolerance level. This is not a static process and requires smooth shifts between interventions with careful monitoring of the nonverbal communication. Most patients can tolerate much more anxiety than is generated in most therapy. If the clinician is confident about reducing anxiety when a patient is flooded, confidence will increase, and anxiety can again be mobilized. Most clinicians are naturally more familiar with the anxiety-reducing procedures that are reviewed in the next section.

METHODS USED TO REDUCE ANXIETY

Earlier in this chapter, we touched briefly upon the fact that the therapist must be able to employ techniques rapidly to reduce the patient's level of anxiety when that anxiety threatens to flood the patient or lead to disorganization or fragmentation. Increasing the patient's anxiety to the highest level of tolerance is an affect and cognitive restructuring procedure that will, with time and use, typically increase the patient's tolerance for anxiety, as well as dysphoric affect. In the event that the patient quickly requires anxiety deescalation, the following methods can be used reliably to bring the patient's anxiety down to a manageable level. These strategies serve to increase repression and thus reduce anxiety so that it is manageable.

Moving Away from the Source of Unconscious Conflict

If the therapist senses that the patient's anxiety is becoming unmanageable, for example, the patient is showing regressive defense or is becoming disorganized, then the therapist can move away from the topic to something less anxiety laden. Shifting the focus to the patient's body awareness is often sufficient. For example: "You seem very upset." "What is happening in your body?" The therapist can also change to another subject and draw attention away from the unconscious pain.

Exploring the Phenomenology of Symptoms

Another method of reducing anxiety is to return to a discussion of the patient's symptoms and that patient's experience of current difficulties. By doing so, the therapist encourages a degree of intellectualization and distances the patient from the unconscious conflicts that have been aroused.

Intellectual Clarification

This method is related to the one described in the paragraph above, although more emphasis is placed on explanation and intellectualization, and works by offering relief to the patient in the form of distance from him/herself. The therapist may indicate causal links between precipitating events and their sequelae, for example, "Of course you walked out of the house; this is the way you learned to deal with your emotions, by watching your parents."

Providing Reassurance

The therapist may decrease the patient's level of anxiety by providing him/her with praise and encouragement. The idea is to support the patient's self-esteem and focus on comfort (Pinsker, Rosenthal, & McCullough,

1991). The therapist can bolster narcissistic defenses and provide "soothing rationalizations; and esteem-protecting generalization" (pp. 229–230). By reassuring the patient that his/her fears are not bizarre, crazy, or evil, the therapist is able to calm the patient and prevent anxiety from mushrooming beyond control.

Using a Psychoeducational Approach

By focusing on the cognitive domain, the therapist can effect a shift from anxiety-provoking interpretation and defense analysis to the more neutral topic of the patient's persistent maladaptive patterns and schema representations.

Emphasizing the Adaptive Nature of Defenses

Even the most maladaptive defense has served *some* adaptive function in the patient's life. Pointing out how and why the defense arose can serve to dampen the patient's escalating anxiety. For example, "Your ability to disassociate has protected you from unbearable feelings related to the abuse you received as a child." Fosha (1992) explains this intervention: "Even if presently counterproductive, [the defenses'] usefulness having been exhausted, their adaptive value in having been the best available means of protection for the patient in the circumstances in which they arose is explicitly acknowledged" (p. 167).

Reframing

Reframing is, in effect, the repackaging of an event or experience to make it appear benign or positive. For example, I encouraged a patient whose insomnia was a function of his preoccupation with disturbing memories to consider this time in his life as an opportunity to explore the meaning of events in his past and present in order to improve his future. Instead of confirming his insomnia as a disturbance, I reframed it as a useful and functional process, which helped reduce the patient's anxiety about the symptom.

Self-Disclosure

To reduce the patient's anxiety, the therapist can share with the patient his/her own struggles and difficulties as they relate to the issues the patient has presented. However, this technique has been the subject of heated

debate. Clearly, for some patients, the therapist's revelations can, instead of
alleviating the anxiety, actually intensify it. More commonly, self-disclosure
is appropriate when the patient notices strong feelings in the therapist and
inquires about it. For example, if a patient becomes out of control and
notices fear in the therapist and inquires, "Were you frightened?" the
therapist shares his/her fear. "When you were out of control like that, I was
frightened by your behavior."

Empathic Attunement

Empathic attunement can be used to mend the ruptures that can be caused
by anxiety-increasing techniques. In a sense, what you are doing is recognizing by acknowledging to the patient that you "pushed too hard" or were
"off track" and would like to understand what transpired. This legitimizes
the patient's expectations for accurate mirroring by communicating that the
patient's responses are appropriate, especially given the developmental
context (Patrick, 1985). This can be used to mend developmental defects
and reestablish narcissistic equilibrium (Goldberg, 1973). I illustrate this in
the following vignette:

THERAPIST: You seem upset by what I said to you.

PATIENT: Yes, I am. You are badgering me.

THERAPIST: I am sorry; it is not my intent to badger you. Let's see if we can
    understand how I approached you in the wrong way, so that we can
    work together.

PATIENT: I was feeling overwhelmed.

THERAPIST: So the approach I was taking was creating too much anxiety.
    Can you describe what it was like?

THE TECHNIQUES AND THE STANCE

Basically speaking, anxiety-arousing techniques are associated with a therapeutic stance emphasizing abstinence, and anxiety-reducing techniques are
associated with a more empathic orientation. The stance is in essence the
therapeutic attitude that the therapist conveys, ranging from an extreme of
abstinence on one end of the continuum to the other end, which emphasizes
mutuality. I realize this is a somewhat artificial contrast but nevertheless
one that has importance. Most psychotherapists are trained in providing
the core conditions of warmth, prizing, and genuineness—the common
factors that are thought to be the active ingredients in all therapy. Most of

us are comfortable with an empathic supportive approach. The reality of clinical practice requires that therapists modify their approach to suit the needs of the patient. We treat a fragile, easily injured patient with more empathic attunement than a haughty, defiant, ego-syntonic personality. This is the difference between the thin-skinned, who are sensitive to any perception of slight, and thick-skinned patients, who seem to be unaffected by anything that is said. I do not believe there is a "correct stance" but, rather, variations that will be discussed and should be considered.

The Therapeutic Stance

In STRP, the therapist modifies his/her stance to meet the developmental needs and structural level of the patient. The therapist's first goal *must* be to create the most effective and appropriate patient–therapist alliance. The stance the therapist assumes has direct bearing on the alliance. This is the predicate for all work to be done in therapy. In so doing, the therapist must decide whether to be abstinent or to reveal him/herself to the patient. If the therapist deems it appropriate to assume a less abstinent stance, he/she must then decide just how much to reveal, and when.

Finding the Correct Stance at the Right Time

Determining the correct therapeutic stance for any given moment can be extremely difficult. For example, I once treated a dependent patient with low self-esteem in her mid-30s who was married to a highly controlling partner. She had difficulty from the start in establishing a trusting therapeutic relationship. So, when she brought me a cup of coffee following one particularly productive session, I proceeded to analyze her offer as a defense. Instead of simply accepting her gesture as one of affection, which would have been a more personal and therapeutic response, I left her feeling injured and confused. Clearly, I had failed to assume the appropriate therapeutic stance. I agree with Viederman's (1991, p. 453) view that "an analytic stance dominated by strict adherence to the rules of anonymity and abstinence" can create a climate of deprivation.

Given the range of possibilities, the difficulties inherent in selecting the correct therapeutic stance at the right time are myriad. The therapist must be both vigilant and flexible. Obviously, if a therapist dogmatically adheres to one stance, some patients will not respond. The important aspect of this issue seems to be in one's ability to use empathy to strengthen a tenuous alliance, mend a narcissistic wound, or repair a rupture in the alliance but not stagnate too long, or the treatment will become long-term.

A Flexible Therapeutic Stance

The term "therapeutic stance" refers to the conditions to which the therapist adheres when conducting treatment. These conditions incorporate the basic guidelines inherent in a particular approach. Does the therapist present a "blank slate," avoid small talk, and reveal nothing of him/herself? On the other hand, does the therapist encourage the patient, provide advice, and give affirmations? Shifting one's stance may be a controversial issue among psychotherapists, but it requires careful consideration. The controversy dates back to Ferenczi's challenge of Freud's mandate of therapeutic neutrality (Ferenczi & Rank, 1925). Freud believed that responding positively to patient longings could be dangerous, whereas Ferenczi "wondered if the neutrality of the analyst might not repeat the attitudes of indifferent or neglectful parents" (Tuttman, 1982, p. 181). Therapists still argue over this issue. I believe that assuming a flexible therapeutic stance, that is, responding to the changing needs and dynamics of the patient, is by far the best way to achieve a positive outcome. Certainly, this requires that the therapist be constantly attuned to his/her patient, but the effort is well rewarded.

Naturally, the therapist's style of interaction plays a role in the therapy he/she conducts. Hammer (1990), in discussing style, stated:

> Style, however, is a function not only of one's personality, but even of one's transient mood: exuberant or dampened, playful or somber, energetic or passive, whimsical or matter-of-fact, expansive or constricted. In constructing the therapeutic relationship, the therapist inevitably draws on his own way of being and his particular method of making relationships work (even if on theoretical grounds he feels he should not); in so doing, he endows the relationship with some tone of consequence. (p. 37)

The general guidelines that I have found to be helpful in conducting STRP are as follows:

1. Allow your unique personality to emerge. Do not try to emulate someone else.
2. Highlight what is effective in your personality—being particularly sensitive, engaging, energetic, and so forth.
3. Generally assume an abstinent role, particularly during the initial phase of treatment and explain the reason for this. "I don't want to cloud what we are doing. Let's keep the focus on your difficulties." Do not rigidly adhere to this as some patients find this damaging and demeaning.

4. Assume an experimental attitude. Sometimes breaking out of an expected role is useful. Sometimes sharing how something makes you feel is immensely therapeutic.
5. Refrain from talking about yourself, except where there is a clear goal for doing so.
6. If the patient appears injured by abstinence, loosen up and emphasize the relational aspects of the transference before proceeding.

An appropriate stance that is thoughtful and respectful will enhance and strengthen the therapeutic alliance.

THE THERAPEUTIC ALLIANCE

The development and nurturing of the therapeutic alliance is especially crucial in STDP and will influence the outcome of therapy (Svartberg & Stiles, 1994; Tryon & Kane, 1995). In a panel discussion, Gatson (1994) described the professional's quandary in this way:

> If transference becomes too intense without having an alliance, the patient is going to drop out of therapy. If you don't have a good alliance with your therapist and you develop negative transference reactions, you will leave your therapist. The same thing with very positive transference. If you have a weak alliance with your therapist and you develop a very strong positive transference, there is danger you are going to be frustrated. (p. 8)

The therapeutic alliance has three important components: (1) agreement on therapeutic task; (2) agreement on treatment goals; and (3) quality of the bond (Bordin, 1979). As I have indicated, establishing a positive therapeutic alliance with the personality disordered patient is no easy task, no matter how committed the therapist. Many of these patients have become expert over the years at defeating those who have attempted to assist them in the past. The therapist's open attitude and genuine interest in helping the patient must be communicated from the start. The therapist, also, must be clear about his/her position with the patient: The therapist will bring his/her experience and training to the task, but the ultimate responsibility for change rests with the patient. Therapy must begin with a willingness by both patient and therapist to collaborate on mutually defined goals. If the therapist is invested in changing the patient for his/her own ego gratification, and the patient is able to see this, which is always the case, then patient resistance will occur and effective therapeutic work will cease.

One of the ways in which interest can be communicated is by offering the patient an opportunity to investigate his/her concerns, so that both patient and therapist have a thorough understanding of the problems and issues to be faced. The therapist also needs to communicate that he/she takes the patient's concerns seriously and that the work they are about to begin together is important and will not be taken lightly. This does not obviate the need for a sense of humor, which, if used judiciously, can be very therapeutic. Of course the therapist must communicate interest, curiosity, genuineness, positive regard, and concern for the patient.

Davanloo (1987) coined the phrase "unconscious therapeutic alliance" to describe the deepening of rapport that occurs after transference feelings have been experienced. When the patient expresses feelings directly to the therapist and the therapist can metabolize them without engaging in a countertransference maneuver, the alliance is strengthened. There is an increase in the patient's motivation, and collaboration with the therapist is characterized by "fresh memories, dreams, and fantasies; and the patient often spontaneously makes links or gives his or her own interpretations" (p. 66). Motivation increases even if the patient seemed highly reluctant to engage in therapy at the outset. When this occurs, the patient and the therapist can begin to explore the past in a meaningful way and make the connections to the patient's present problems. Once the therapeutic alliance is at a positive level and collaboration is established, the therapist can begin to mobilize the patient's anxiety and activate the defenses.

I once treated a young woman who was highly resistant to therapy but, nonetheless, chose to work on alleviating stress. She came to therapy apprehensive of being diagnosed with some serious mental illness, in part because her mother had been diagnosed as schizophrenic. She described a long history of angry, destructive outbursts wherein she would destroy her belongings. She continued to have rather extreme problems with her loss of temper, and during the course of therapy, it became clear that this issue was related to tremendous unresolved anger toward her parents. Unfortunately, the treatment prematurely focused on her anger and an exploration of her outbursts. My expectation that the patient could explore frightening feelings related to her loss of control before sufficient trust was developed created a fracture in the fragile alliance and resulted in her decision to discontinue treatment. I am convinced that if I had spent more time nurturing the therapeutic alliance, a better outcome would have resulted. Her preexisting transference feeling, that a therapist might find her disturbed like her mother, was something that could have been explored, understood, and put behind her, thus greatly reducing her anxiety about the therapeutic task ahead.

This case highlights two points: The first is that the therapeutic alliance *must* be strong enough to endure the pain of deep characterological work; the second, which will be discussed further below, is that the therapist must keep expectations realistic. Collaboration must be established by a mutual agreement on what the patient wants to accomplish and the goals that will indicate success. When collaboration is lost, it must be quickly reestablished before proceeding with treatment. The fluctuations in the level of collaboration must be monitored constantly. I had a narcissistic patient who came to treatment to work on substance abuse issues. Each time he used drugs, I brought the treatment focus back to the therapeutic contract. For many patients, the contract will have to be reexamined, in a nonpunitive fashion, throughout the early stages of treatment. Had I failed to be sensitive to the collaboration underlying the treatment of this patient, I am confident that treatment would have floundered, and the patient would have dropped out in frustration.

Using Countertransference to Monitor the Process

By frequently processing the patient's countertransference reaction, the clinician can monitor, inform, and guide the psychotherapeutic process. Since working with personality disordered patients using a short-term model is highly intensive for both patient and therapist, constantly checking the countertransference can prevent small difficulties from quickly escalating beyond manageability.

Freud (1910/1957) originally felt that countertransference impeded treatment, as it seemed to him that the therapist's own unresolved issues would corrupt the mirroring aspect of analysis. Winnicott (1949) theorized that countertransference, rather than corrupting the process, might instead enhance the course of analysis. "In its place he submitted another ideal, that of the analyst who, existing as a person in his [her] own right, *reacts* to the patient and, albeit aware of the countertransferential nature of these reactions, uses them therapeutically" (Slakter, 1987, p. 19).

There are two ways in which I use countertransference with personality disordered patients. First, I use my interpersonal reaction to guide the process (Kiesler, 1982). By taking note of my irritation toward the patient, I am able to refocus on his/her malignant defense system, which often sabotages the process. If I become frightened, it's often because the patient is accessing impulses over which he/she may have little control.

The second way that I use my countertransference reaction is to formulate preverbal needs or longings that the patient is communicating in a powerful, projective way. If, for example, I feel the urge to hold a patient, I would focus on the patient's desire for security or comfort by discussing a wish to be held physically. I would make this wish conscious without responding physically. The clinician must be very cautious when considering the use of touch (Kertay & Reviere, 1993). At other times, particularly when

I am the target of a strong projection that activates feelings in me, I describe to the patient the effect he/she has on me. Usually, when these preverbal longings are recognized and verbalized, strong affect is released, and early disruption in the patient's parent–child experience can be pinpointed and worked through.

It makes sense that the patient's characterological defenses exert a strong force on the therapist, just as they do on the people in the patient's life orbit. Tuning in to one's own reaction allows the therapist to understand many perspectives of the patient's problems and, in turn, allows the therapist the valuable opportunity to teach the patient about his/her maladaptive patterns. For example, I had a narcissistic and obsessive patient who criticized all therapists, and me in particular, for not "caring" enough and, thus, disappointing her the way everyone else in her life had done. These feelings translated into a posture of helplessness and passivity. After all, why should she bother doing anything if nothing works? In this fashion, her powerful and demanding expectations of others had driven everyone in her life away and fueled her worst fear of being unlovable.

Another aspect of the countertransference that I observe is whether or not I like the patient or develop some positive feeling toward him/her. I have found that even the most destructive person has some redeeming attribute that I can appreciate. The few patients toward whom I have had powerful negative responses were antisocial personalities or highly malignant narcissists without capacity for empathy.

The Use of Metaphors

The metaphors a therapist uses during the treatment process are central to the assumptions he/she holds about therapy and the therapeutic action of treatment. The metaphors the therapist uses in STRP should preferably be based on a comprehensive understanding of the patient's psychopathological dynamic force. At times, using "toxic" metaphoric language is effective in making the patient's defenses ego-dystonic by increasing anxiety. At other times, more "empathic" metaphors will deepen the emotional experience and avoid injury to the patient. The ideal is described by Fosha (1992) "as the evocative resonance of one's choice of words and metaphors" (p. 173).

Patient Metaphors

Patients often describe their dilemmas with powerful metaphors, of which the clinician should take note. Using the metaphors of the patient can not only deepen the therapeutic alliance, but can be powerfully evocative when highlighted. Some common metaphors used by my patients include:

"I'm on automatic pilot."
"My life is like a never-ending roller coaster."
"I have tunnel vision."
"I'm spinning my wheels."
"I feel like a robot. I'm going through the motions."
"I feel like I'm dead inside."
"I feel like a volcano."
"I feel invisible."

To illustrate working with metaphors in therapy, I have recreated below a conversation I had with one of my patients some time ago. The patient was an avoidant personality who presented herself as a "doormat" in her relationship with both her husband and her employer. One of our conversations went like this:

THERAPIST: So you present yourself as a doormat. Can you give me an example of how you are walked on?

PATIENT: Yes, I was at work the other day and my supervisor asked me to clean out the coffee pot, which I did.

THERAPIST: What did you feel when he asked you to do this?

PATIENT: Walked on!

THERAPIST: Yes, this is true, but what did you feel?

PATIENT: I don't know.

THERAPIST: As long as you avoid your feelings it is likely that you will continue to be walked on.

Therapeutic Metaphors

Most of the developers of the various STDPs have, at some time, utilized powerful metaphors in the development of their treatment approaches. It is generally agreed that powerful metaphors should not be used haphazardly during therapy but should be saved until that time when the clinician feels secure in his/her assessment of the patient's character pathology and confident in the strength of the therapeutic alliance. Generally, the more "toxic" metaphors are better suited for patients with highly cemented ego-syntonic character pathologies. Examples of commonly used therapeutic metaphors include:

The Wall. This refers to the interpersonal barrier erected between the patient and therapist. It is also described as a facade.
The False Self. This is similar to the Wall, but the barrier to be broken

through or penetrated is weaker and more ephemeral in nature than that of the Wall.

The Crippled/Paralyzed Part of You. This metaphor is used extensively by Davanloo and is an example of toxic labeling (Fosha, 1992). It is highly evocative and can even be shocking.

The Limbo State. This characterizes the ambivalence that is often present in many character disordered patients.

Mr. Spock. This term describes the patient who is totally disconnected from affect and only processes information on an intellectual basis.

Dirty Harry/Charles Bronson Persona. This often refers to detached males who shun emotional involvement.

The Caveman/Woman. This is used to describe patients who have taken refuge in extreme withdrawal and isolation.

The Injured Child. This is used to describe patients with disassociated aspects of themselves, that is, those who feel vulnerable and frightened.

Dosing Up the Therapeutic Alliance

As the therapeutic alliance strengthens, the therapist can increase the intensity of therapeutic contact and focus. Titrating the level of anxiety and shifting the therapeutic stance can make treatment more effective more rapidly. Basch (1988) discussed "potentiating a therapeutic relationship," and he concluded that with some patients, one may be taciturn and analytically reserved, and with other patients, more active by helping them organize their thoughts and actually doing most of the talking.

We have discussed the fact that most personality disordered patients enter treatment looking for symptomatic relief. If the patient enters psychotherapy and a focal issue can be established, such as treating symptoms of Axis I disorders, most commonly depression and anxiety, or interpersonal disturbance, character issues can be circumvented. However, if character disorders appear to be at the root of the patient's problems and are an impediment to treatment of those issues, the therapist can "dose-up" the relationship and address the character problems head-on or in an empathic melting of defenses.

Budman and Gurman (1988) describe the difficulty in this manner: "Most patients neither need nor want to address characterological problems. However, for one subgroup of patients, personality difficulties present such pervasive impediments in various aspects of their lives (including the ability to profit from therapy) that if any treatment intervention is to have even a chance of success, it must in part deal with personality issues" (p. 214). This, however, should not be attempted until or unless a strong positive therapeutic alliance has been established, and there are signs that the patient is willing to collaborate with the therapist. Once the therapist educates the patient about the nature of his/her self-defeating, self-limiting character patterns and how these are responsible for his/her dilemmas, the patient may see the wisdom of addressing the underlying causes and agree to undergo STRP. Timing is crucial, because if the therapist waits too long, the character defenses can become entrenched, and too much countertransference may be activated in the therapist. Naturally, the therapist should avoid pushing the patient into undergoing STRP if the patient is truly reluctant, no matter how effective the therapist knows STRP would be.

CONCLUSION

The techniques of short-term treatment are somewhat disparate, but they begin to make intuitive sense when one understands the structural differences in the personality disordered patients. One can see how the various approaches evolved so uniquely based on the type of patients that the clinician theoreticians encountered and were drawn to in their clinical practices. Thus, the more confrontational, anxiety-arousing approaches emanated from work with the neurotic and ego-syntonic characters where anxiety was needed to accelerate and deepen the process. In contrast, the empathic approaches derived from work with the developmentally and self-disordered patients in whom anxiety needed to be contained, and defenses strengthened, to keep the process from being flooded. The techniques are often diametrically opposed, so that a clinician working within a short-term framework requires a comprehensive understanding of metapsychology and developmental psychopathology as well as the ability to conduct a rapid structural assessment. An organized model that encapsulates all the approaches will provide the clinician with a clearer conceptual understanding that leads to more efficient technical application. A patient with a disorder of the self or developmental psychopathology will clearly require a different type of treatment than a patient higher on the structural continuum. Making informed treatment selection decisions will become easier when the clinician embraces the full range of possibilities.

■ **CHAPTER 6**

Comprehensive Restructuring of the Personality

By deciphering defenses, we can begin to understand the underlying pathophysiology of our patient's disorder. In contrast, by thoughtlessly challenging irritating, but partly adaptive, immature defenses, a clinician can evoke enormous anxiety and depression in a patient and rupture the alliance.

—VAILLANT (1994, p. 49)

Comprehensive restructuring of the personality (CRP) is the ultimate goal of dynamic, experiential, and cognitive psychotherapy. Although the term "restructuring" may conjure up images of overly mechanistic work, in practice, the therapist must guide treatment with a certain degree of instinctiveness. The term is used mainly to emphasize the element of precision that exists in the science of psychotherapy. In addition, I selected it because it is a recurrent technical descriptor used by various theoretical groups and seems best to capture the depth of the goals of therapy. The goals of comprehensive restructuring include (1) reorganizing the patient's defense system so that it is more mature and flexible, (2) substituting more adaptive patterns of behavior, (3) enhancing affective regulation and toler-ance, (4) changing belief systems and attitudes, (5) increasing capacity for problem solving as well as greater emotional and intellectual awareness, (6) increasing motivation, and (7) increasing capacity for intimacy. In STRP, there are three methods of restructuring. These three types of restructuring seek to effect as comprehensive a restructuring of the personality as time and patient resources permit, each with a somewhat distinct strategy.

Each of these restructuring varieties has somewhat different theoretical predicates, techniques, and aims, although there is some overlap. In simple terms, *defensive restructuring* asks, "How is the patient acting?", *affective restructuring* asks, "How is the patient feeling?", and *cognitive restructuring* asks, "What is the patient thinking?" All three methods can be utilized most effectively when considered in relation to and with an understanding of the triangle of conflict and triangle of persons. All three restructuring methods guide our strategic psychotherapeutic action in the treatment of personality disorders.

I have divided this chapter into three sections accordingly.

SECTION I: DEFENSIVE COMPONENTS

Methods of Defensive Restructuring

Defensive restructuring works by disrupting the patient's defense system by systematically eliciting and identifying maladaptive defenses in order to penetrate the affective zone and derepress the painful affect related to the patient's core genetic structure. Reich (1945) was the first to use this method of defense analysis in a systematic fashion with character disturbances, but Davanloo (1980) made the most dramatic advances in this area by developing highly specific technical maneuvers that drastically shortened the time frame. I believe it is Davanloo's work that makes it possible to apply short-term psychotherapy to a broad spectrum of personality disorders.

Defensive restructuring is typically the most rapid and anxiety provoking of the three types of restructuring. When affect follows defense analysis, outcome is enhanced (McCullough et al., 1991). For many clinicians, this method of restructuring seems to be the most foreign because it is the most confrontational. It remains the most potent of the three restructuring methods in my clinical work, and, therefore, I find it indispensable in treating the majority of personality disorders. It is most often the necessary starting point with the ego-syntonic patient, as other methods of restructuring have proved ineffective. Once sufficient work has been done to soften the defense structure, then therapy can proceed.

The focus in defense restructuring is primarily on the *current* (C) and *transference* (T) corners of the triangle of persons and the *defense* (D) corner of the triangle of conflict (see Figure 6.1).

The therapist spotlights the patient's immediate defenses by bringing these to his/her attention as the patient describes incidents in the C and then

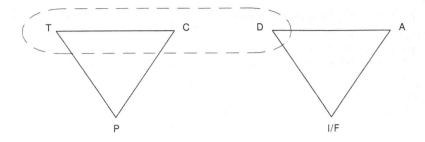

FIGURE 6.1. Defensive restructuring: Emphasis on transference and defense.

shows how the same defenses are in operation as the patient relates in the transference (T) to the therapist. This involves increasing anxiety, pointing out defenses, and explaining their maladaptive function. This persistent and unrelenting defense analysis leads to a build-up of feeling, often irritation, which the therapist hopes to evoke. When experienced, this build-up of feeling will have a link to the past (P). Once the patient expresses his/her true feeling to the therapist, the path opens for deeper unconscious communication. The potency of this method lies in the activation of the defense system, in the here and now, which is analyzed in an experiential fashion. In a sense, it is an exacerbation of the very disturbance that the patient manifests. It is particularly well suited for those with highly malignant, ego-syntonic character pathologies who are initially unresponsive to cognitive or affective restructuring. It is also the method of choice for patients with higher ego strength who nevertheless are highly defended and who prefer to undergo a rapid transformation.[1]

Goals
- Increase awareness of defenses and function
- Turn defenses ego alien
- Raise anxiety to activate underlying feeling
- Intensify feeling by persistently singling out defenses
- Capitulate defenses
- Decathect feeling over traumatic events and loss
- Increase emotional expression
- Eliminate self-defeating character patterns

Methods
- Anxiety-increasing interventions
- Establishing defense constellation
- Educating about intimacy—give examples of avoidance with therapist
- Deep interpretation

- T–C–P links creating emotional and cognitive insight
- Encourage avoided extratherapeutic activities

For example, a passive–aggressive patient who becomes defiant and stubborn, refusing to discuss the specifics of an emotionally arousing incident, must have it brought to his/her immediate awareness that these defenses will destroy the therapeutic relationship and limit the therapist's effectiveness. The following example illustrates this point.

"I notice when I ask you to be more specific about the fight with your wife you become silent and sit there defiantly, refusing to respond." The patient continues to sit silently, avoiding eye contact. "If you continue to sit silently, we will get nowhere." "You must have all the answers," the patient says sarcastically. This is a typical ploy to divert the process and provoke the therapist. The therapist must resist provocation and respond: "If you are unwilling to discuss this, then I am rendered ineffective."

In this brief vignette, we see a build-up of anger toward the therapist being defended against in the patient's characteristic style. Eventually, if the therapist maintains a focus on the defenses, the patient will experience this anger and express it in the transference. This then loosens the patient's defense system and allows enhanced unconscious communication. Once the anger is expressed, the patient can make new connections: "You know, I used to react to my father in this fashion. It was my attempt to keep him from controlling me. He always tried to squash me." Once this meaningful communication is finally expressed, the therapist is able to see the patient's core issue with far greater clarity.

The Importance of Recognizing Defenses

The clinician must be adept at systematically identifying and categorizing the array of defenses that the patient brings to therapy. This skill is vital to successful strategic psychotherapeutic planning and treatment. There are dangers in challenging defenses that are not always apparent to the novice and sometimes not even to the more experienced clinician. If defense restructuring is conducted without sufficient knowledge and experience, the patient's condition may actually worsen. If, however, the clinician is sufficiently knowledgeable about defensive functions and can quickly recognize them, there is little danger in persistently analyzing them.

Insufficient knowledge of defenses on the clinician's part can also lead to needlessly protracted psychotherapy when the patient could tolerate more intensive defense restructuring. Patients often suffer needlessly from disturbances that become crystallized in a transference neurosis, resulting in a stagnation of the process or unjustifiably long-term psychotherapy. If the therapist does not understand defenses, the patient may often be treated as if he/she has a fragile defense system, and the clinician's interventions will be too weak to support meaningful restructuring.

Pacing the revelation of disturbing material is an important corollary of understanding the nature of the defensive structure. The therapist should work to gradually increase the gradient of emotional arousal in a manner similar to systematic desensitization. When a patient seems to want to disclose too much too early, I often explain to him/her why we should not immediately get into this material. I point out the importance of establishing safety and rapport between us and then monitoring how much the patient can tolerate without flooding his/her psychic system. No matter how ripe the material seems and how tempting the opportunity to explore it, I have found that it pays to feel confident of my assessment and formulate a plan rather than to rush headlong into the patient's crisis. I also explain to my patients that they can help regulate the pace of treatment by letting me know when I am pushing too hard or not hard enough. With patients displaying more fragile defenses, I find it helpful to monitor the process frequently by asking, "Are we going at the right pace or do we need to slow down?" This systematic monitoring of the process and the patient's reaction to it should engender a feeling of collaboration in the patient.

For many patients, in addition to the therapy, a substitute for the ineffective defense is helpful. The substitutes that come to mind are 12-step programs, psychopharmacological agents, day treatment, or support groups. This is especially beneficial for patients who rely upon the more primitive defenses. I have included a brief review and explanation of defenses, but this material alone is not intended to provide, nor is it enough to provide, clinicians with a sophisticated knowledge of defensive work. In addition to understanding defenses intellectually, the clinician must also possess an experiential understanding of how defenses function. Experiential understanding comes only from clinical practice and supervision. There is no substitute for the knowledge gained the first time a clinician becomes the target of his/her patient's projective identification or witnesses a patient disassociate. This is really the only way to fully appreciate the power of defense mechanisms. Although I often mention the importance of audiovisual recording in the development and advancement of STDP, let me also say here that reviewing videotapes is particularly helpful in learning to identify defenses. I will elaborate upon the uses of videotape in Chapter 12.

The Nature and Function of Defenses

Defenses evolve throughout the course of human development and are automatically triggered when the ego is threatened. Defense reactions have numerous functions.

> They reduce emotional conflict, protect the self against its own dangerous impulses, alleviate the effects of traumatic experiences, soften failure or disappointment, eliminate clashes between attitudes and reality (cognitive dissonance), and in general help the individual maintain his [her] sense of adequacy and personal worth. (Goldenson, 1970, p. 300)

The incorporation of defenses, however, may prevent the patient from facing his/her difficulties in an honest and rational manner. Erecting a defensive barrier allows the patient to distort his/her reality and focus elsewhere. The excessive use of defenses invariably creates as many problems for the patient as it solves. Because the personality disordered patient is incapable of profiting from experience so as to be able to modify behavior, maladaptive patterns tend to repeat. Also, defenses create barriers in interpersonal relationships that prevent honest communication and aggravate extant problems.

Much of our knowledge of defenses comes from Freud's work. His daughter, Anna Freud, added considerably to our understanding of the nature and purposes of defense mechanisms (Sandler, 1985). More recently, Vaillant (1994) established an empirical methodology for the study of defenses. His longitudinal research has confirmed the hierarchical nature of defenses, which he found can even be observed in the behavior of small children. My own observations of children, those I have treated as well as my own, corroborate Vaillant's theory of defense progression. When my eldest daughter entered the phase of rapproachment, I noticed that she utilized both oppositionality and defiance in order to establish her separateness. Later, she had affective storms that resulted in temper tantrums when she did not get her way. This display of defense, although developmentally appropriate for her age, were strikingly similar to those exhibited by some of my personality disordered patients. I have found the developmental similarities comparable and have learned much by observing children.

Some controversy remains about how the therapist should view defense mechanisms—that is, whether or not they should be considered microscopically (up close) or macroscopically (as part of a whole picture). Anna Freud (Sandler, 1985) felt that the patient's gestalt was lost when the therapist focused too closely on defenses. Vaillant, on the other hand, has compared the understanding of defenses as comparable to listening to a symphony. Listening to individual instruments does not help understand symphonic complexity.

My view is that both methods have their place, especially in treating personality disturbances. I look at defenses microscopically at first and then stand back in order to experience the patient and his/her problems as a whole. While the therapist must recognize individual defenses, he/she must also attend to the patient's *constellation* and what the defenses represent for the patient.

A person's defensive style is closely related to his/her personality traits and personality pathology (Soldz, Budman, Demby, & Merry, 1995). In fact, the patient's personality type may suggest a preference for certain groups of defenses. Thus, an obsessive–compulsive personality will have a proclivity for intellectualization, isolation of affect, and repression. As I have stressed earlier in this chapter, a clinician must be well versed in defenses and their manifestation before he/she is able to conduct an accurate defense analysis. The next section provides a review and brief description of many forms of defenses.

Comprehensive Catalogue of Defense Mechanisms

Developing a truly comprehensive[2] catalogue of defenses requires that we go beyond the DSM, and so doing has proved invaluable to me in my clinical work. Defenses are like navigational aids that orient us on our therapeutic journey, just as the stars orient sailors on theirs. There is a richness in their variety and complexity that is not conveyed by the DSM. Vaillant (1994), Meissner (1981), and Perry (1990), among others, discovered that defenses can be organized hierarchically based on relative level of psychopathology. They classify defenses as psychotic, immature, neurotic (intermediate), and mature, as discussed below.

Psychotic Defenses

Patients who demonstrate defenses in this category are not suitable candidates for STDP. The incorporation of these defenses represents major disturbances in ego functions, and patients who present with these are likely to require both psychopharmacological intervention and external structure, such as day treatment or hospitalization. A patient may benefit from a short-term dynamic approach after a brief reactive psychosis, but this should be undertaken with caution. However, the fact that someone has a biochemically based affective disturbance does not preclude the presence of treatable character pathology, which can be addressed after stabilization.

Delusional projection. In delusional projection, there is a gross distortion of external reality and a feeling of being persecuted.

Denial (psychotic). With this defense, there is a gross denial of external reality.

Distortion. There is a massive reshaping of reality to better match internal need.

Immature (Primitive) Defenses

Most personality disordered patients present with a composite of immature and neurotic defenses, and, therefore, this category is commonly encountered by clinicians. The name "primitive defenses" sounds pejorative but is simply indicative of an important evolutionary stage in an individual's development. Linehan (1993) believes that the immature or primitive defenses are the patients' best attempt at taking care of themselves, even though they may have a level of self-destruction that others find frightening. When these defenses dominate over the neurotic, the patient demonstrates more psychopathology and greater severity of the personality disturbance. Overreliance on the immature defenses is typical of borderline patients. A supportive cognitive restructuring is far better suited to this patient's needs than a challenging, rapid uncovering approach. Many of these patients actually benefit from a stepwise approach, entailing supportive work first and then, when cognitive restructuring is complete, uncovering. Please note that patients with a neurotic level of organization also use defenses from this category when anxiety becomes unmanageable. I have had numerous cases of obsessive–compulsive personalities who regress and explode when their defenses falter.

   Projection. A person's undesirable impulses and feelings are perceived as belonging to another. Although projection is ubiquitous, it is only pathological when it is an unacknowledged perception.
   Schizoid fantasy. This is an overindulgence in fantasy wherein the person retreats from conflict and seeks primary satisfaction and gratification in his/her fantasy preoccupation.
   Hypochondriasis. The patient is plagued by physical symptoms that result from unmet emotional needs and unacceptable impulses/feelings. The person is often highly distressed and seeks relief from various medical specialists, to no avail.
   Passive–aggressive behavior. Unacceptable feelings of anger are expressed indirectly and through passive means.
   Acting out. Unconscious feeling and conflict are acted upon without their becoming conscious, so that affect is never experienced.
   Dissociation. With dissociation, there is a dramatic disconnection from one's identity, which serves to mitigate emotional distress.
   Blocking. This is a temporary inhibition of emotions, thoughts, or impulses.
   Introjection. A characteristic of another is internalized, the function of which is to establish closeness. Introjects can be negative, as with self-abuse, or positive. The patient often responds with a phrase or statement that does not appear to be his/her own.

Regression. This represents a return to earlier, more primitive periods of development and behavior that was surrendered. For example, some patients at the neurotic level of organization appear, on occasion, to throw temper tantrums similar to those of very young children.

Externalization. This is the tendency to see the source of one's difficulty as residing in the external world and the failure to see one's own influence in one's behavior.

Splitting. Positive and negative qualities of the self or others are separated. Things are viewed as all good or all bad; integration is not attained. There is usually oscillation between the poles.

Projective identification. Unacceptable impulses are projected onto another. The projection is often so intense that the person who is the target of the projection responds in a manner that befits the projection.

Devaluation. Negative qualities toward another person or oneself are exaggerated.

Idealization. This is the opposite of devaluation. The positive attributes of oneself or another person are unrealistically exaggerated.

Omnipotence. Acting as if oneself or others possess special powers or abilities that are not based on reality.

Withdrawal. The individual moves away from others and the external world as a means of avoiding painful affects.

Explosiveness of affect. The individual releases pent-up anxiety and affect by explosive discharge.

Weepiness. The individual becomes tearful, but there is no experience of the affect, as would occur if the patient were experiencing grief or sadness.

Depression. Many individuals use depression as defense against feeling. Often, aggressive impulses are channeled into depression, but many other feelings are also defended in this way, particularly, nonmetabolized grief.

Neurotic Defenses

This cluster of defenses is the most susceptible to modification through affective and defense restructuring. In fact, the more definitively the patient's defenses lie in this category, the better suited he/she is for an anxiety-increasing, rapid, uncovering approach.

Repression. Ideas and feelings are lost from awareness in a seemingly unexplainable loss of memory. It also encompasses those unacceptable thoughts and feelings that never reach conscious awareness.

Displacement. Feelings are shifted from one object to another, usually one that has less importance to the individual.

Reaction formation. Emotions and impulses are changed from unacceptable to acceptable by reversal.

Intellectualization. Intellectualization is, in a sense, a separation of ideas from their feelings by an abstract discussion that keeps the feeling repressed.

Somatization. The conversion of psychic energy into bodily symptoms and derivatives.

Controlling. Managing events or people in the environment excessively as a way of warding off anxiety.

Inhibition. Dampening or limiting the potential sources of ego gratification.

Isolation. Splitting the affect from the cognition and repressing or displacing either element.

Rationalization. The justification of feelings, behaviors, or thoughts that may be deemed unacceptable to the conscious ego.

Sexualization. Attributing sexual significance to people or objects that are not present, or exaggerating their presence.

Undoing. Thoughts, feelings, or actions of oneself or another are negated.

Detachment. Detachment is comparable to dissociation but is a less intensive variation. Detachment is a commonly observed defense in the spectrum of personality disorders. There is a sense that the patient is not emotionally present. Such patients appear preoccupied and emotionally distant. When these individuals emerge from a detached position, much anxiety is mobilized (Hill, 1987).

Avoidance. The individual circumvents or turns away from situations or feelings that are conflictual or anxiety provoking.

Compartmentalization. The individual is able to separate various elements of his/her life without experiencing the conflict that would inevitably result in their acknowledgment.

Complaining. Complaining is a rather insidious defense that serves to siphon off anxiety and impede true action.

Mature Defenses

Defenses in this category represent the best integration of instinct with reality constraints. Patients exhibiting defenses in this category demonstrate the healthiest adaptation to life's vicissitudes and a high tolerance for experiencing emotion.

Altruism. This represents an unselfish interest in the service to others. It provides substantial gratification with no compromise to the integrity of the self as in codependent patterns.

Humor. The capacity to express one's feelings without untoward effect on others through wit or sense of the ludicrous. Humor can also be a neurotic defense if it is used to protect oneself from genuine emotional expression.

Suppression. This reflects a capacity to keep an awareness of a conflict without repressing the emotion, reacting or becoming unduly anxious. It indicates a high tolerance for experiencing one's emotions without becoming symptomatic or using neurotic defenses.

Anticipation. The ability to plan for the future in a realistic fashion. Emotional reactions are experienced in a limited fashion and inform the ability to plan and problem solve.

Sublimation. Instincts are expressed indirectly without a loss of pleasure or negative consequences to the individual.

Ancillary Defenses

Another of Davanloo's (1980) advancements in this field is his description of a group of defenses, which he called "tactical defenses" (at Malan's suggestion). These include somewhat broader interpretations of the meaning of defenses than conceptualized by most, but I have found Davanloo's work highly informative and indispensable with the personality disordered patient. These might more aptly be considered "microdefenses": insignificant alone but in groups, quite off-putting. This array of what I term "ancillary defenses" are differentiated into three subcategories and are not listed in primary source work on defenses, and yet, they are crucial to effective CRP. These defenses are common, employed by all of us at one time or another. With almost all personality disordered patients, these defenses are a constant source of static that erodes interpersonal relationships, dampens feelings, and, if not addressed, will result in a build-up of irritation in the therapist, as it does to those in the patient's life orbit. Most therapists are familiar with these ancillary defenses but must, nonetheless, be able to respond to them appropriately.

I have subdivided these defenses to three categories: interpersonal, anxiety siphoning, and cognitive. Although these defenses are not primary, they can often be found in exaggerated forms and can be highly malignant, exerting a powerful counterforce on the psychotherapeutic process.

Interpersonal category defenses. These include smiling, sarcasm, argumentativeness, negativity, compliance, submission, blaming, poor eye contact, criticizing, defiance, stubbornness, seductiveness, complaining, provocation, teasing, and distancing. These defenses serve to put distance between the patient and therapist or significant other, as well as between the patient and his/her feelings. Some of these can become major character defenses with certain patients, for example, as with a histrionic personality who relies on seductiveness as a method of influencing others' responses.

Cognitive category defenses. These include rumination, tentativeness, vagueness, retraction, generalization, ambivalence, and equivocation. These defenses can also be major character defenses, such as with patients who suffer from major ambivalence that results in difficulty making and following through on decisions in all aspects of life. This level of defense requires major defense restructuring. On the other hand, the minor defenses in this category may be undone indirectly. For example, a patient who is showing signs of vagueness can simply be asked to be more specific.

Anxiety-siphoning defenses. These include chewing gum, cursing, fidgetiness, pacing, smoking, eating/drinking, and rocking. These defenses seem to directly reduce anxiety by acting as a siphon. Often, simply pointing out that the patient is rocking or cursing as a way of reducing anxiety will block these defenses.

Ego-Syntonicity

"Ego-syntonicity" refers to the level of identification with and petrification of the defense system. All personality disordered patients are, on some level, "ego-syntonic." That is, their defenses are so consolidated that they appear as traits. "Ego-dystonic" patients, in contrast, are capable of recognizing their defenses and suffer anxiety over them.

Patients with a highly ego-syntonic defense system are almost totally unaware of their defenses and believe their defenses are part of their "real self." Access to the unconscious is extremely unlikely without major defensive restructuring. People with high levels of ego-syntonicity are generally repellent to others. This is also often reflected in the overall physical manifestation or body armor. The passive patient appears limp, the narcissistic seems inflated, the obsessional tight, and so forth. People who attempt to come close are fended off with all manner of irritating character defenses, both verbal and nonverbal. These patients have a unique ability to bring out the most malignant traits in others. Patients who fall in the aggressive–sadistic segment often provoke hostile or passive–aggressive reactions in others and are unaware of how their interpersonal and defensive style incites these reactions (Leary, 1957). Overreliance on fewer defenses makes the system appear more cemented and less flexible. Negative response from others reinforces and justifies their style—belligerence toward others incites counterattacks. Adaptation to life is very poor, being grossly limited by the inflexible defensive structure. Emotional access is severely limited. Interpersonal relationships are generally disastrous, as defenses are of the most destructive kind: externalization, projection, and denial. Psychological mindedness is absent, and externalization makes motivation for change low. Their problems, as far as these individuals are concerned, result from the deficiencies of others or are not linked in a way that makes them understandable. If they describe their symptoms or behavior, they do so in a way that makes them incomprehensible. One patient, when asked what seemed to be the problem, responded, "My wife wrote this letter." The letter reported her concerns over his chronic exhibitionistic masturbation. The difficulties in treating patients with these highly ego-syntonic defensive structures is illustrated in the following case.

> In *The Case of the Externalizing Couple,* the couple entered treatment at the wife's urging. Both husband and wife showed signs of relying on externalization, denial, and projection as the cornerstone defenses. They had recently had a child, and the wife had given up drugs and wanted to be a good mother. Both husband and wife suffered from ego-syntonic character disturbances. The wife was primarily histrionic, and the husband was primarily passive–aggressive. The initial session was characterized by projection, blaming, arguing, sarcasm, and externalization and was quite difficult to endure. Each wanted vindication and to have the other judged guilty. As part of the evaluation protocol, each of them was seen individually, and then together.
>
> The husband, an obese man in his late 20s, seemed like an adolescent. He had recently started a job, and although he was bright and had attended excellent private schools, he was never able to hold a job for an extended period. Both husband and wife had a significant history of substance abuse. The wife had stopped when she found she was pregnant. The husband thought his wife "wasn't fun any more." Now that she was sober and with child, she found sex with him repulsive. The wife had inherited a substantial trust fund, which the couple had depleted. She spent almost all of her money buying him expensive cars, which he destroyed, and living an extravagant lifestyle. He continued to order bottles of Dom Perignon when they went out to dinner, feeling he "deserved something fun." In the individual and joint interview, he complained about what an awful "bitch" his wife was and how boring she was since the birth of their baby, whom he had not wanted them to have.
>
> The wife was considerably older than her husband and had wanted the child badly. However, it now seemed to her as if she had two children in her care. He described how exhausted he was when he came home from work and how he would lie on the sofa and drink beer to recuperate from the day. He could not understand why she nagged him so much. Occasionally, he cooked a meal but did nothing else at home. She said that every month there were 10 empty cases of beer that needed to be returned. He defended his behavior saying that he had already given up taking most drugs and that she was not going to get him to stop having a beer after work. The problem was that she

was "a control freak," which he was sure I had observed by now. He was petulant, sarcastic, and defiant in response to her attacks on him. Although her husband's motivation for treatment was nonexistent, the wife seemed somewhat more willing to work. Unfortunately, both dropped out of treatment after the evaluation. Many patients in similar situations will return when they find themselves in the midst of another severe crisis. If therapy is undertaken at the right gestation period, even difficult patients such as those described above can make substantial gains.

Aspects of Defense Analysis: Constellation Recognition

The personality disordered patient's defensive system manifests as therapeutic resistance, which is almost immediately available to the therapist for clarification and intervention. For example, a patient with a passive–aggressive personality resists the therapist's attempts to define the problem. In this manner, the patient's character defenses have entered the treatment in the form of resistance, which serves to sabotage the therapeutic alliance. The entire defensive constellation of the patient will emerge in the transference in its unique pattern, much like a fingerprint. The patient's idiosyncratic defensive style becomes clearer as the therapeutic relationship unfolds. Examining how the patient's defenses manifest in the transference can be assisted by experiencing the patient's defense system macroscopically. Does the patient present as a victim, or as helpless, defeated, exploitative, obsequious, secretive, impotent, voracious, caretaking, or self-destructive?

For example, in *The Case of the Woman with the Secret Lover,* the patient entered therapy to improve her relationship with her boyfriend but did not mention until the second session that she also was carrying on an affair with a married man. Her ability to compartmentalize her feelings for these two men was impressive. During the initial course of treatment, she would not mention her married lover, as if to keep the secret alive. Her tendency to share only portions of herself emerged as a transference resistance—if she only revealed portions of herself, she would limit my effectiveness. She did not want to discuss issues that would make her appear imperfect or flawed, believing it was best to reveal only fragments to others. Obviously, this would render me completely ineffective, like asking me to complete a jigsaw puzzle but secretly withholding many of the pieces. Once we were able to identify her resistances and establish how these defenses held her back, she began to discuss her relationship with her mother, who had narcissistically used her as a maternal object and who expected her to be perfect to affirm her as a good mother.

The therapist's ability to pinpoint the patient's constellation of defenses will guide the entire treatment process. If a high level of ego-syntonicity is apparent, this must be addressed, but whether anxiety-reducing techniques or anxiety-arousing techniques are used depends on the patient's composite of primitive and neurotic defenses, as well as on his/her ego-adaptive capacity and treatment goals.

For example, a patient with an obsessive–compulsive personality disorder may manifest a varied cluster of defenses, but the primary or cornerstone defenses are isolation of affect, repression, intellectualization, and rationalization (see Table 6.1). There will be little evidence of emotional fluidity. The patient will seem stilted, overly rational, and lacking in depth of emotion. The ancillary defenses will manifest in a tendency to ruminate in an obsessive fashion about problems. The quality of interpersonal interaction will lack a warmth and free-flow nature of more spontaneous relationships. The therapist may experience countertransference feelings of boredom or irritation. If the patient's defenses are addressed without restructuring, anxiety will build, and the patient may resort to an array of ancillary and primitive defenses, such as sarcasm, stubbornness, or defiance, or may even become explosive. Defenses are usually fluid and come in waves, changing as a function of the level of stress. Treatment would be simpler if there were homogeneity in the defense systems of various personality disorders, but as we discuss in more detail in the following section, this is not the case. In fact, it is quite rare to find clearcut DSM personality disorders. Most patients are blends of personality disorders and utilize heterogenous constellations of defenses.

Two patients diagnosed with the same personality disorder may show significant differences in how their defensive structures are organized. Each patient possesses a unique combination of defenses. Although defenses tend to cluster within diagnostic categories, one should not assume a certain defensive constellation based on diagnostic classification. As presented in

TABLE 6.1. Constellation Recognition: Obsessive–Compulsive

Primary defenses	Rating	Ancillary defenses	Countertransference
		Low anxiety	
Rationalization	4	Rumination	Boredom
Repression	4	Sarcasm	Irritation
Isolation of affect	4	Detachment	Disempowered
Intellectualization	5	Ambivalence	Stalemate
Displacement	3	Generalization	
		High anxiety	
Projection	3	Defiance	Fear
Regression	2	Stubbornness	Impotence
Explosive discharge	3		

Chapter 3, a definitive evaluation can be accomplished using a structural interview. By carefully observing fluctuations in anxiety or by increasing anxiety, the therapist can directly observe how the patient's defenses operate. Diagnostic classification will orient the clinician, but it should not be relied upon exclusively. Diagnostic categories, however, do serve to orient us. There is a high probability that a patient with a borderline personality will rely mostly on immature defenses and that an obsessive–compulsive will utilize neurotic defenses.

Cataloguing the patient's defenses, although tedious at first, becomes second nature with practice. Through the process of identifying and cataloguing defenses, the clinician increases his/her ability to predict the patient's responses in particular situations. A patient whose defensive constellation clusters mostly in the primitive category is going to have a higher probability of acting out and regressing and will require firm and consistent boundaries and limits. It is also important to remember that most defenses exist on a continuum from mild to severe. Jacobson et al. (cited in Vaillant, 1992) developed an ego defense manual that provides a global rating of patient defenses. Defenses can be individually rated: (1) minimal, (2) little, (3) moderate, (4) considerable, or (5) maximal. This scale enables the clinician to conceptualize defenses on a continuum of severity, rather than as just present or absent. A much richer clinical picture is then available.

Most defense systems have some fluidity and are dynamic. If one is blocked, another will emerge. Defensive constellations shift, depending on circumstances. Developing a feel for how the patient's defenses flow offers the clinician an opportunity to make effective interventions at the appropriate time. I have seen patients with unstable defense systems shift defense patterns from session to session and even within single sessions. This phenomenon is most commonly associated with adolescents, where frequent shifts of developmental stages and the associated defense constellations make parents continually wonder if their teen is a child or an adult.

Clinicians also use defense identification in the restructuring process to get a sense of how to time questions, particularly questions regarding emotional state. For example, asking a patient how he/she is feeling when that patient is in a regressive episode is totally counterproductive. Asking a patient what he/she is feeling when there is a sign, such as a facial signal, that emotion is close to the surface, is appropriate and productive. The patient in the regressive episode will be incapable of identifying or discussing his/her feelings because his/her defenses are in full operation. The patient whose feelings are at the preconscious level may be capable of identifying the emerging affect, and focusing on the sensations often brings the feeling into awareness and fuller experience. Generally, the greater the diversity of defenses, the better the defensive system works. This flexibility is ego-adaptive. Patients who rely on a few defenses, especially the primitive ones, are more rigid and may experience disorganization when defenses falter. Clinical reality indicates that personality disordered patients use fewer defenses than neurotics and adopt most of their defenses from the primitive and neurotic categories.

How defenses shift can been seen in the following case study:

> One patient became extremely distraught after attending an office party where her coworkers insensitively made fun of her. They "celebrated" her turning 40 by giving her morbid gifts, such as a bra for a woman with "saggy breasts" and a mass card for the dead. Her first reaction was to become "upset" (weepy and detached). When her coworkers did not relent, she left work, returned home, and retreated to her bedroom for 3 days (withdrawal and isolation). Finally, in a suicidal state, she phoned her therapist and was hospitalized (severe regression). When asked to evaluate her, I found a familial history of severe abuse, chronic alcoholism, and multiple traumatic events. This woman was deeply injured by the insensitivity of her coworkers. Their taunts reactivated her feelings and memories of profoundly traumatic events. These feelings and memories overwhelmed her ego defenses, and she shifted to primitive defenses to protect herself.

Successful defense restructuring often modifies the defense system so as to allow more effective affective restructuring, which is described in the next section.

SECTION II: AFFECTIVE COMPONENTS

Methods of Affective Restructuring

Most therapists are trained to inquire about our patient's feelings. I suspect the question "How are you feeling?" is the most commonly asked, and yet, for the personality disordered patient, the most difficult to answer. In fact, we effectively use this form of restructuring with the majority of our non-personality disordered patients. In affective restructuring, the therapist essentially bypasses the defensive system, activating emotional arousal to access core issues and pathogenic beliefs. With many personality disordered patients, this method of restructuring can be most effectively used sequentially, that is, after a course of defensive restructuring.

If we refer to Figure 6.2, we see the main emphasis is on the *impulse/feeling* (I/F) corner of the triangle, with access points primarily at the C corner of the triangle of person. As emotion is activated and experienced, links to the past will emerge in the form of associations and derepression of memories and connections. The therapist then links C to T and P.

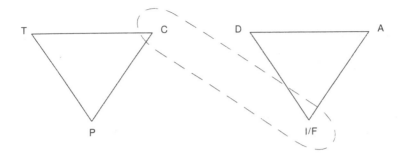

FIGURE 6.2. Affective restructuring: Emphasis on current conflicts and feeling.

Goals
- Activation of emotional schemas
- Differentiation of secondary and primary emotions
- Unblock emotional expression
- Highlight core issues/pathogenic beliefs
- Validation of feeling
- Tolerance for full emotional expression
- Metabolizing repressed emotion

Methods
- Recreate current conflictual event through detailed description
- Elicit emotions by direct focusing
- Positive affirmations
- Observe affect in facial expressions and intensify
- Emphasize empathic attunement
- Coach patient into intensifying affect
- Encourage staying with emotions
- Exaggerate physical manifestations
- After affect is experienced, explore cognition
- Educate about defenses
- Make C–P–T links

Affective restructuring is a powerful approach for many patients who are placed low on the ego-syntonic scale. This approach derives its techniques primarily from experiential psychotherapy (Greenberg, Rice, & Elliott, 1993). Exaggerating nonverbal communication can be effective in eliciting emotion. For example, asking the patient to notice a particular gesture or movement is an attempt to communicate emotionally. Using the two triangles, the therapist does not actively encourage the increase of anxiety but instead goes directly to the feeling zone. The therapist can follow a symptom or conflict to the activating event, intensify the underlying emotion by having the patient describe the incident in detail, and then focus on the felt sense. The defenses are only minimally challenged.

For example, let us reconsider the case presented in the Introduction of the patient with the obsessive–compulsive personality, who found her husband in bed with another woman and showed no reaction at the time, although she professed that she still loved him. She was asked to describe the incident in detail and focus on her internal experience and sensations. Although she described herself as always smiling and "up," there was a slight shift in her facial expression when she discussed the incident. This observation was shared, and she was asked to focus on her "bodily felt experience" (Safran & Greenberg, 1991, p. 167). She said that she felt sad but that emotions were childish. She was encouraged to stay with the emotions and see what emerged. Over the course of a few sessions, she began to describe her relationship with her father who was like a rock emotionally. I pointed out to her the link between her father and her ex-husband, which brought her deeper grief to the surface, allowing her to process this, too. Doing so usually serves to increase the positive therapeutic alliance. Cognitive restructuring techniques can then be used to strengthen the new defense system.

The Nature of Emotions

Psychotherapists have always emphasized the importance of emotions, but affective science has only recently begun to achieve the prominence that cognitive science achieved in the 1980s (Ekman & Davidson, 1994). Scientists now view emotional expression as a safeguard of survival, as well as an enriching experience. Any discussion of defenses requires an understanding of emotion, against which the patient's psyche defends. The clinician must be aware of and appreciate the dynamic interplay that exists between affect, cognition, and defenses. "It has long been an accepted tenet of psychology that the emotional life offers the best source of information about how clients think they are faring in the adaptational agendas of their lives" (Lazarus, 1991, p. 290). Adaptation entails increasing awareness and experience of emotions, as well as clearer communication of feelings. Our emotional life has a language of its own, influenced by our unconscious process.

> Granted the importance of emotions and our confusion about them, they are worth a reexamination, particularly that elusive, neglected aspect called "feelings." To do so, we must fly in the face of the experts'

advice—eschew objective analysis and return to the shadow world of the inexact, the poetic, and the subjective. (Gaylin, 1979, p. 10)

Patients with personality disorders have a particularly difficult time differentiating and accessing their emotions and are often deeply ashamed of their feelings. In fact, their feelings tend to be buried under so many stratified layers of defense that the patient often names defenses when asked how he/she feels. It is exactly this living and experiencing oneself in one's defensive layer, as opposed to the emotional level, that stultifies functioning.

Personality disordered patients have, to varying degrees, missed the early experience of having a sensitively attuned mirroring relationship, so it is often the work of therapy to provide one. In my work with these patients, I often observe affect in the patient's facial expression, which exists at a preconscious level. Observing and communicating these emotions to the patient and knowing when to begin such an intervention is possible when I allow myself to become an "emotional tuning fork."

The emotions that dominate in personality disordered patients are anger, fear, guilt, grief, shame, and sadness. Eliciting and then processing these feelings is one very important treatment goal. Many patients will avoid emotional discussions, complaining that their emotions make them "feel like a child." In fact, primary emotions are obvious in small children as well as adults and are experienced in the same way at any age.

Shame and Guilt

Shame and guilt, though similar in nature, are actually two distinct concepts (Wright, O'Leary, & Balkin, 1989). Wright (1992) defined shame as "the often sudden and painful sense of exposure for having failed to live up to one's desired self-image, or conversely, the sense of having become one's undesired or bad self."

"Guilt, on the other hand, refers to a sense of having done something wrong" (Wright, 1992, p. 7). I have found guilt is often the most tenacious and painful of emotions and has a significant place in the personality disordered patient's maintenance of self-punishment and self-defeating behavior. Why would an intelligent woman marry three alcoholic men if not, in part, to punish herself? The woman to whom I refer was enraged with her father and had repressed murderous feeling toward him, along with guilt she had never contacted. This guilt fueled her self-punishing behavior. She felt she needed to suffer for her destructive feelings toward her father. Patients like this often feel they are inherently bad and do not deserve better treatment, from themselves or from others. Many patients actually report that they believe they are "bad." The nature of the "crime," however, cannot be unearthed until the defenses have been bypassed and the core issues accessed.

Secondary Emotions

Feelings that cannot be observed, such as love, envy, jealousy, joy, disgust, humiliation, outrage, and pride are classified as secondary emotions. Personality disordered patients frequently describe their emotions as blends of defense and secondary feeling such as "feeling upset," "feeling bored," "feeling used," and "feeling hurt." In Gaylin's (1979) book *Feelings: Our Vital Signs,* the author describes *feeling upset* as an undifferentiated state of emotion where one is unaware of the specific event that has led to the feeling. "The emotion may have been isolated from it or denied and the event repressed" (p. 96). *Feeling tired* is typically a symptom of imminent or existing depression. "Tiredness as a feeling is a transient, prodromal emotion that signals a vulnerability to depression" (p. 103). It is often an indication that our psychic reserves are depleted, such as when self-esteem and self-confidence ebb and have not been replenished. Psychological strength comes from "our worth that evolves from doing, giving, loving, achieving—and the rewards inherent in love and work" (p. 110). These are the very activities that are blocked for most personality disordered patients. Thus, they often function in a state of psychic depletion, describing their internal state as "empty, hollow, or void." There is little balance. If they give, they give too much in a codependent manner, if they take, they tend toward exploitation, and if they achieve, they are driven in a compulsive way.

   Feeling bored is an anxious, restless inability to focus upon a desired goal or object. It is a passive stance that indicates a conflict not over survival but the value of survival. The *feeling of being used* "arises from the fear that the person dealing with us is not involved with us in emotional ties and affection—where there may be mutual use—but is simply using us as an instrument, a vehicle of his [her] own purposes (Gaylin, 1979, p. 157). *Feeling hurt* is a response to an injury by someone whom we believe cares about us. There is an element of unexpressed cut-off anger in feeling hurt. The personality disordered patients who are able to recognize and relate these admixtures of feeling and defense are usually closer to their emotions and less highly defended than those who cannot, as accurate identification and reflection of feelings first occurs at the nonverbal level.

Theories of Emotional Display

Nonverbal communication of feeling is typically less filtered by defensive operations and is, therefore, more clearly read by the therapist. As stated before, facial expression is the most trustworthy means of nonverbal communication available to the therapist who develops confidence and trust in her/his emotional sensitivity. Ekman's (1972) research on significant certain features of facial affect expression resulted in the following findings: (1) facial affect are universally recognized; (2) facial expression may be masked; (3) feelings coexist in blends, such as when we have a feeling about a feeling, that is, terror over contact with an angry or shameful emotion; (4) motor reactions involving the face and body manifest the activation of feeling, such as running from something frightening; (5) emotions may lead to verbal reaction; and (6) emotional arousal often has a physiological component, such as increased pulse rate, galvanic skin response, sighing, and respiration.

Sexual Differences and Emotional Development

When working with the personality disordered patient, it is important to be aware of the emotional differences between the sexes. Men and women differ in the type of personality disorders they tend to develop and how they express emotional disorder. For example, men more often develop antisocial personality disorders than do women, and women are more often labeled histrionic. Wright (1987) suggests that early developmental experiences result in the differing personality structures men and women are likely to develop: "The central experience of early life that has the greatest consequences for how children develop is that the mother is almost always the primary caregiver during infancy" (p. 242). Because of this, females are able to internalize their resemblance to the mother and benefit from this. Further, males must relinquish the maternal identification and "must repudiate femaleness and all that is associated with it, which typically includes the qualities of softness, openness, and emotional expressiveness" (p. 242). This is quite unfortunate and may have some bearing on why many men avoid the psychotherapist's office altogether. Wright comments on this terror of emotions:

> Easy expression of emotion is threatening for the male because it may expose the dependency and vulnerability he has fought so hard to master. Exposing his dependency, particularly on women, is also threatening because he experienced the radical shift from woman to man as a humiliating loss and abandonment by his first love object, mother. As a consequence, he is wary and distrustful of intimacy. It feels safer and more secure to remain cool, distant and even isolated . . . most men have a major separation-induced emotional trauma inflicted on them in early life, and carry a serious shame and humiliation based handicap with them forever. (p. 242)

Karen (1992), in his article "Shame" in the *Atlantic Monthly*, discusses the strongly masculine, scientific stance of emotional neutrality of early psychoanalysis. In contrast, the object relations theorists we discussed earlier held forth a maternal stance, relying more on empathetic relatedness than analysis of unconscious sexual and aggressive feeling. This may be the reason shame was overlooked in the past. This also sheds some light on a clinical finding that has emerged in my work. Men respond quite positively to the warlike metaphors found in Freudian psychodynamics, and women do not. Perhaps this played a part in the divergence of the empathic short-term workers. Also, men are, at first, more squeamish when I use empathic language. They see this as a shameful recognition of their vulnerability and need. Certainly, this is an area that requires some thoughtful consideration and research.

Shame can usually be dealt with effectively if it is identified and labeled for the patient early in the process. Many patients have difficulty articulating this feeling; it may manifest itself as blushing or downcast eyes. If shame is not identified, it is certain to slow the healing process. Usually, after the emotion is identified, the therapist can work through it quickly by exploring what the patient finds shameful about what has been said. The acceptance and empathy of the therapist in response to the revelation is usually all the patient needs to move on to the deeper issues.

SECTION III: COGNITIVE COMPONENTS: METHODS OF COGNITIVE RESTRUCTURING

When we ask the question "What are you thinking?" we are attempting to bring to light the cognitive schemas that influence feelings and behavior. The patient's internalized thoughts, pathogenic beliefs, and schemas are often powerful aspects of the maladaptive behavioral patterns evident in personality disorders. Cognitive schemas are enduring structures for processing and organizing information that include affect and interpersonal interactions (Blatt, 1991). Cognitive restructuring is a method for identifying and modifying these deep-seated beliefs. It is also a method for increasing the differentiation of the psychic structure and teaching emotional problem solving. This includes teaching the difference among impulses, actions, and thoughts. For example, "Wanting to kill your mother when she criticized you is an impulse and not the same as actually killing her. This was expressed in the fantasy you then had of her getting killed in a car accident." Cognitive restructuring emphasizes intellectual as opposed to emotional or experiential insight.

For example, if a patient reports self-mutilation as reaction to separation (abandonment), the therapist can help the patient recognize that the cutting is a defense against the disturbing primitive anxiety and negative cognition ("I am unlovable and will never have a relationship—I will die") that occurs when abandonment is threatened. The patient is then taught other healthier ways of coping with the anxiety and less pathogenic beliefs ("I am lovable in my own right—My father's abuse of me was *his* illness—I can reach out to a friend for support").

Cognitive restructuring occurs at the T and C corner of the triangle of persons and at the D and *anxiety* (A) corner of the triangle of conflict (see Figure 6.3). Past issues may be discussed, but there is no attempt to derepress these events by mobilizing feeling. The positive therapeutic alliance is emphasized in the transference, and the therapist acts as a teacher, collaborator, coach, and parent. The therapist teaches coping and problem-solving skills, differentiation of feeling, challenges maladaptive patterns, and attempts to substitute more adaptive beliefs. The patient is encouraged to report incidents that are upsetting, and the therapist then uses this material to examine sequentially the patient's reactions and assist the patient in developing self-awareness. The therapist repeatedly points out and labels behavior, feeling, defenses, fantasy, and cognition.

When I asked one patient how he felt when his wife was berating him, he responded, "I walked away," as if this action were indeed his feeling. Another patient in a similar situation responded, "I punched the wall." This misattribution, identifying an action as a feeling, is very common with the personality disordered patient. Even more common is describing the physiological concomitant of anxiety as the experience of emotion. That is, when asked what they feel, personality disordered patients almost always describe the physiological manifestation of their anxiety. Patients often return after our early work and report that they looked up the definition of a certain emotion, often anger, which they experienced as anxiety. This is evidence of the process of "cognitive restructuring," or, developing a conscious

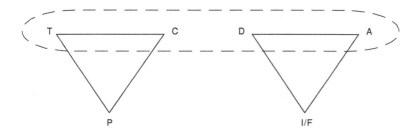

FIGURE 6.3. Cognitive restructuring: Emphasis on defense and anxiety in current relationship.

awareness and insight into one's psychic system by learning, on an intellectual level, how to differentiate among feeling, anxiety, and defense.

For extremely anxious patients or those who are severely cut off
emotionally, restructuring can be utilized to desensitize the patient to
frightening affect aroused by a breakthrough of primitive material. Discussing this frightening or overwhelming material without censure reduces the
patient's anxiety. The therapist encourages this by asking, "What are your
worst fears?" In a sense, "What would happen if you completely lost
control?" For example, one patient with a mixed obsessive and avoidant
personality had panic attacks when he visited his mother. He anxiously
reported a fantasy to stab her. By using a fantasy portrait, the patient began
to understand intellectually that repressed rage mobilized severe anxiety,
which was defended against by panic and obsessive thoughts. His fear of
murdering his mother was temporarily quelled. As with many patients, the
process of utilizing obsessional defenses (the thought of stabbing his
mother) felt as scary as actually doing it. When his anxiety diminished, the
patient was able to talk about how angry he felt.

Goals
- Develop awareness of cognitive and defensive system
- Increase capacity for collaborative relationship
- Increase psychological mindedness
- Reduce unconscious anxiety
- Build tolerance for discussing and facing disturbing material
- Increase tolerance for anxiety
- Strengthen defensive system
- Reduce acting out behavior
- Restructure, modify, or reinterpret schema
- Prepare for affective restructuring

Methods
- Ask the patient to report what he/she is thinking when he/she
  becomes blocked or diverts eye contact
- Identify sequences of reactions and beliefs by focusing on current
  conflicts or transference reactions
- Teach problem-solving skills
- Desensitize patient through imagery work
- Familiarize patient with manifestations of anxiety by focusing on
  the physiological manifestations
- Clarify the difference between anxiety and defense by repeated
  examination of incidents in the C and P providing cognitive insight
- Explain adaptive nature of defenses but emphasize more adaptive
  methods of dealing with defenses

Beginning with a cognitive restructuring approach is generally indicated for patients who are low on the continuum of structuralization or for patients with severe anxiety that threatens to flood the psychic system. Anxiety-reduction techniques are employed until the patient's psychic system is strengthened enough to begin another restructuring process. Eliciting core cognitive beliefs can be a nonthreatening way to establish a therapeutic alliance without stirring up too much anxiety. Changing schemas does have some inherent anxiety, as does any change.

Beck et al. (1990) have identified the main beliefs for the personality disorders listed in DSM-III-R (see Table 6.2).

The patient's negative cognition and core beliefs are usually not things of which he/she is aware, but which have an insidious effect on development and maintenance of self-worth. I often liken these to a cassette tape with a short loop. For example, every time one patient of mine began to reveal her feelings, she would spontaneously comment, "That's ridiculous" or "That's

TABLE 6.2. Core Beliefs Associated with Personality Disorders

Avoidant	It's terrible to be rejected, put down. If people know the real me, they will reject me. Can't tolerate unpleasant feelings.
Dependent	Need people to survive, be happy. Need for steady flow of support, encouragement.
Passive–aggressive	Others interfere with my freedom of action. Control by others is intolerable. Have to do things my own way.
Obssessive–compulsive	I know what's best. Details are crucial. People should do better, try harder.
Paranoid	Motives are suspect. Be on guard. Don't trust.
Antisocial	Entitled to break rules. Others are patsies, wimps. Others are exploitable.
Narcissistic	Since I'm special, I deserve special rules. I'm above the rules. I'm better than others.
Histrionic	People are there to serve or admire me. They have no right to deny me my just deserts. I can go by my feeling.
Schizoid	Others are unrewarding. Relationships are messy, undesirable.

Note. Adapted from Beck et al. (1990, pp. 54–55). Copyright 1990 by The Guilford Press. Adapted by permission.

childish. I shouldn't be feeling that way." Her fear of others learning her true feelings replayed internally, and repetitively, reminding her that she would be "put down" for being an "overly emotional female," just the way "my father used to humiliate me." I encourage patients to listen to these internal messages and identify whose voice they hear. Generally, the patient immediately identifies the voice of a genetic figure. Listening for the patient's internal belief systems and identifying cognitive schemas allow the therapist to lay the groundwork for cognitive restructuring.

A COMPREHENSIVE RESTRUCTURING OF THE PERSONALITY

Consolidating the Restructuring

The therapist's task is to bypass the defenses (affective restructuring) or penetrate the defenses (defensive restructuring) and contact the patient on an emotional level, which in and of itself is a corrective emotional experience with important palliative functions. Anxiety must be raised or lowered to an optimal level. "If arousal level is optimal, it will facilitate self observation, discomfirmation of pathognomic beliefs, and cognitive change . . . virtually all theories acknowledge the reciprocal nature of these processes as the therapist appropriately manages patient arousal and therapy activity" (Beutler & Clarkin, 1990, p. 272).

Many of the techniques that have been identified in Chapter 5 to increase anxiety are also techniques that will accelerate character transformation. A comprehensive restructuring can occur during the course of one treatment experience or can be completed in a stepwise fashion. The patient might, for instance, start with a cognitive restructuring step and then contract for affective restructuring. The goal of CRP is a total working through and derepression of the feeling related to the core structure of the patient, modifying the personality. The most important aspect of this process is the repetition of the cycle of eliciting emotion, encouraging the patient to experience it fully, and increasing ego-adaptive capacity. The restructuring is consolidated by linking the P with the T and C in the triangle of persons. The therapeutic action lies in the patient's and therapist's abilities to elicit repressed feeling related to trauma and then help the patient metabolize this by experiencing the pain. As layer after layer of defense and feeling over past trauma are worked through, the deeper layers will emerge, one after another. The patient's unconscious will become increasingly more fluid. Although many therapists look for major breakthroughs, which do occur on occasion, more typically, emotions are accessed and worked through in a cyclical fashion. In this way, the patient's capacity for affect tolerance is strengthened. This is the essence of the CRP.

Summary of Restructuring Indications/Contraindications

Comprehensive psychotherapy with personality disordered patients involves a blend of defense, cognitive, and affective methods of restructuring. The emphasis, however, will vary depending upon the patient's level of structural differentiation and treatment goals. The lower the level of ego adaptive capacity, the more primitive the defensive constellation, the greater the emphasis on cognitive restructuring will be. Patients at a higher level of structuralization and with higher-order defenses respond best to affective restructuring. Defensive restructuring for the high-level ego-syntonic patient entails a dismantling of the system and an increase in the emotional fluidity of the patient by successively contacting emotions at increasingly higher levels of intensity. Each time, the therapist provides the patient with encouragement and pressure to experience his/her full emotion, relying less and less on defenses.

Patients who are low on the structuralization scale can easily be overwhelmed if their defenses are eroded too quickly (Johnson, 1991). For the self-disordered patient who is prone to narcissistic injury, cognitive restructuring is enhanced by the establishment of an empathic dyadic relationship. In this fashion, primitive defenses can be replaced by fostering a positive object bond that can seed the developmental progression and increased differentiation of the psychic apparatus. The employment of defenses is supported as an adaptive response to overwhelming trauma. A patient with severe dissociation is taught to understand how the dissociation once used to protect the self is no longer effective, as it retards growth and integration.

CONCLUSION

The material covered to this point provides the background material and basic information required to understand and apply STRP to the treatment the personality disordered patient. Although we have covered a lot of material, this is a condensed version of a large body of theoretical, clinical, and research material that has been gleaned from many sources and clinical experience. Taking the time to read the original sources is truly worthwhile, as much of this work continues to be relevant. The remainder of the book focuses primarily on the clinical treatment issues and strategies with the personality disordered patient.

CHAPTER 7

Overview of the
Treatment Process

*He says a few words about the happenings of today or yesterday, but
within a few minutes they are forgotten and the past becomes as vivid
as if it were the present. Parents, long dead, come alive in his memory,
childhood scenes are re-experienced as if they were here and now and
early sorrows are felt as if today had brought them forth. Rage and
love, hate and tenderness, are expressed and thoughts that shy away
from the light of the day creep out of their hiding-places.*
—REIK (1949, p. 109)

Reawakening old wounds and bringing to life figures from the past consti-
tute an excruciatingly painful process. Psychotherapy with the personality
disordered patient rarely proceeds smoothly, although I have been surprised
on occasion. Typically, therapy with these patients is much like canoeing
down a river, in that there are likely to be periods of relative calm, where
the water is smooth, as well as turbulent stretches of rock-studded water,
where all you can do is negotiate the curves to get through intact. Expanding
on this rafting metaphor, there are also various ways of approaching and
surviving the rapids of short-term therapy involving elements of skill and a
knowledge of how the river flows. In this chapter of the book, I provide an
overview of the process of short-term therapy with personality disordered
patients and point out some of the issues that arise in the various phases of
therapy.

There are three phases or stages of the treatment process, logically
called the *initial, middle,* and *termination* stages. Each has a different set of

characteristics and tasks. Because of the compacted process and the accelerated rate of treatment, these three phases of treatment are quite distinct.

INITIAL TREATMENT PHASE

The initial phase of treatment in short-term psychotherapy of the personality disordered patient is the most complex. It is both technically and
emotionally challenging and sets the tenor for the rest of the treatment
process. If it proceeds well, the patient's motivation increases, and a sense
of hope is engendered. If this phase goes poorly, however, disappointment
results, and motivation decreases rapidly. We covered this stage of treatment
in a comprehensive fashion in previous chapters, and it has also been
highlighted in some of the clinical case presentations demonstrating the
assessment and restructuring process. Once again, the following functions
are crucial in this stage of treatment: comprehensive assessment, establishing treatment goals, educating the patient about treatment expectations,
establishing a therapeutic alliance, identifying core issues where possible,
establishing a time frame, and beginning restructuring.

Generally, all of these tasks can be completed in one extended session.
When the patient's goal is to achieve rapid character change, high levels of
defense restructuring will be required during this phase. This is especially
true for patients with high levels of ego-syntonicity. Other approaches
should be offered and, if necessary, appropriate referrals made if this type
of therapy does not seem to be what the patient wants. Some of the
characteristics of this phase are:

1. High activity level of therapist
2. High level of patient resistance
3. Mobilization of anxiety
4. Intensification of affect
5. Attachment phenomenon
6. Multiplicity of therapeutic functions
7. Greater emphasis on cognitive and defense restructuring

The Importance of the First Encounter

We have discussed the importance of the first session of therapy. The first
session of short-term psychotherapy of the personality disordered patient
is probably the most essential to the successful outcome. This typically is a
very stressful encounter for both the patient and the therapist. It holds the
promise of change and represents the realization of the patient's desire to

get help. The importance of the first session in establishing the tenor of treatment cannot be underestimated. Budman, Hoyt, and Friedman (1992) devoted an entire book, *The First Session in Brief Therapy*, to this topic:

> The brief therapist who is attempting to help his or her patients use treatment in the most productive, time-effective manner possible is advised to pay special heed to the opening phases of therapy. Although there are widely varied possibilities for the proficient practice of such treatment, the successful clinician "hits the ground running." It is unlikely that treatment that fails to quickly set a tone of active, dynamic intervention and change will lead to celertious, positive outcomes. (p. 351)

Certainly, many initial encounters fail for a variety of reasons, some obvious and others less so. The first session necessarily involves completing a psychodiagnostic interview and clinical formulation. High levels of therapist interventive activity, such as direct questioning, empathic reflections, and frequent responding facilitate engagement (Kolden & Klien, 1996). In addition to completing a comprehensive evaluation of the patient's ego functions and exploring the phenomenology of the patient's concerns, there are many other aspects of the initial consultation.[1]

Instilling Hope

During the first consultation, the patient is often very skeptical about what can occur. The therapist should communicate optimism that change is possible and that even small changes can result in quality of life improvements. At the same time, unrealistically encouraging more than is reasonable can be a grave disservice (Gustafson, 1995).

Setting Realistic Treatment Objectives

Setting realistic expectations is no easy task. If the patient's expectations are unrealistically high, damage can be done, and if they are set too low, progress can come to a standstill. In the case described below, I unrealistically set patient expectations too high.

> The patient, an accountant, entered therapy because of depression and difficulty functioning at work. A rapid approach to treating him was undertaken without due sensitivity to the nature and depth of his personality disorder. When the depression lifted, this patient showed a classic schizoid personality disorder; he could not respond to expectations that he relate in a more intimate fashion to the therapist. This was made exceptionally clear to me when he described me as a skeleton

with eyes, a hard and bony person. His depiction of me represented the primitive nature of his object relations. Human beings could not be perceived as warm or capable of empathy, and certainly not as capable of helping him in his pain.

In a subsequent evaluation, a psychiatrist decided that this patient "would not benefit from psychotherapy" and should be seen for medication management alone. Long-term psychotherapy or intermittent treatment at times of stress are alternatives that could also have been suggested. In sum, expectations should be based on a careful assessment of the patient's functioning. Otherwise, the patient will feel as if he/she is failing. If long-term treatment is deemed most appropriate, the patient should be so informed. Any therapy may produce negative effect by precipitating a psychotic episode, or increasing anxiety or depression (Strupp, Hadely, & Gomes-Schwartz, 1977), because of therapist inexperience, unpredictable patient reactions, or misapplication of an approach. On occasion, no treatment may be the appropriate recommendation, particularly in cases where the patient is being pressured by external forces to be in treatment but exhibits no desire to change. Finally, some individuals who are prone toward regression and forming severe dependency may be unsuitable candidates for psychotherapy (Beutler & Clarkin, 1990).

Creating a Spirit of Fascination

Many personality disordered patients have never experienced a significant relationship wherein an adult showed any sign of being interested in or fascinated with their development and emerging self. Many patients are severely stunted in this regard. One of my patients showed almost no capacity for self-intrigue and could not believe that I was willing to sit and show sustained interest in her. Perhaps this sensitivity to or interest in the inner workings of another human being is, as Alice Miller (1983) writes, the domain of people raised in a family in which they were prematurely used as parental objects. Whatever the reason for our occupational choice, the therapist must truly be fascinated with the complexity and healing power of the human psyche in order to derive satisfaction from and excel in this work.

The Importance of Extended Sessions

The completion of the extended session can mark the end of this phase of treatment for many patients; for others, a few more sessions are required to complete the initial therapeutic tasks. The use of extended sessions during this phase of treatment rapidly accelerates the therapeutic process and is highly recommended for patients who are amenable to this format. What might typically occur over the course of a 4-week period is experienced in the same day, keeping the intensity of affect at a high level of experience. One of the benefits of this format is that the influence of the resistance with which the personality disordered patient presents from week to week, particularly in this initial stage of treatment, can be neutralized.

The foundation upon which a self-reliant and stable personality is built is the "quality of attachments" (Bowlby, 1973). The therapist is in a natural position to become a major attachment figure for the patient. "In short, the therapist is, indeed, an object of intense affect during the formation, maintenance, disruption, renewal, and loss of the relationship, in ways consistent with early attachment relationships" (Farber, Lippert, & Nevas, 1995, p. 210). During the initial phase of treatment, the use of an extended session can serve to create a powerful bond between the patient and therapist. The detachment evident in many patients can be linked to early attachment disturbances and must be addressed, otherwise this defense will render the therapy ineffective (Della Selva, 1993). The luxury of spending four concentrated sessions with the therapist, or that amount of time with anyone, is very unusual for many personality disordered patients. The development of an attachment with the therapist engenders strong affect and is accelerated and intensified during extended sessions. Typically, at the end of this stage of treatment, a strong collaborative alliance has been forged that will provide the necessary foundation for the stresses inherent in personality transformation.

MIDDLE TREATMENT PHASE

The middle stage of treatment is often characterized as the "working-through" phase. This is where the patient and therapist have arrived at an understanding of the core difficulties and have touched upon the issues that are the source of the patient's pain. Treatment enters a period of increased collaboration and greater participation by the patient. In this phase of treatment, there are times in which the patient is doing most of the work, and the therapist is less active. In fact, it may be that the therapist has to ward off a sense of complacency at this point. The characteristics of this phase of treatment are as follows:

1. High level of collaboration—patient shares more of the load
2. Clear sense of direction—in terms of the issues that have to be resolved and work done
3. Return of resistances in less powerful forms

4. Significant evidence of patient's attempts to modify life by trying new behaviors, and so on
5. High degree of reactivated feeling that is metabolized between sessions
6. Greater access to unconscious—increased dreaming, recall of early life events, and so on
7. Greater emphasis on affective restructuring
8. High frequency of interpretations (T–C–P links)
9. Mobilization of pathological grief reactions

The therapeutic tasks shift during this phase of treatment. There is less energy expended by the clinician in developing the therapeutic alliance because successful engagement has already occurred. Less emphasis on assessment allows the therapist to turn his/her attention to encouraging and insuring the metabolization of affect and consolidation of character changes. The therapist's tasks during this period are reviewed below.

Maintain Focus on Core Issues

During the middle phase of treatment, the therapist must be vigilant about not allowing therapy to bog down and lose its focus. For the first time in their lives, patients experience the gratification of a close, nurturing relationship and may naturally want to prolong it. Although this is understandable given many of these patients' deprived backgrounds, the patient is best served when the therapist moves the process along.

The therapist should always listen for the adaptive context—"the specific reality that evokes an intrapsychic response" (Langs, 1990, p. 720) with which the patient begins the session, but he/she should not let the patient wander. If the patient initiates discussion spontaneously, the adaptive context will often set the stage for the rest of the session. If the patient is not clear about his/her focus, the therapist can recapitulate the core issues or can restate the focus of the previous session. The patient's defenses may reappear, and it may feel as if the process has begun anew. If this is the case, more defense analysis is necessary.

Identify Themes at the Beginning of Session and Plan Time Accordingly

One method to keep treatment on track is to ask the patient to list what his/her main issues are rather than to allow the patient to talk aimlessly. This provides direction for the session. After listening carefully to the patient's concerns, the therapist restates the main issues and asks which one seems the most important to begin with. This prevents the patient from bringing up an emotionally loaded issue at the last minute when it cannot be dealt with effectively. This is also a lesson in emotional problem solving that many patients have not mastered. Identifying the issues, accessing feelings, and deciding upon an appropriate course of action all strengthen ego-adaptive capacity.

One patient with a narcissistic defense system started the session with a series of philosophical ruminations. He was asked to list the issues he wanted to address in the session. He continued to wander and was again asked that he list what he wanted to talk about. This created irritation on the part of the patient toward the therapist, which was identified. The therapist then explained that the reason for listing the topics was so that the therapist can make sure enough time is allotted to address each one. The patient was grateful because he had never before learned how to identify and resolve problems in a systematic fashion. We related this to one of his core issues that his mother, who was his only parent, was depleted most of his life and unable to teach or guide him in almost every aspect of his life. He was then able to contact his grief over having been abandoned by his father.

Remind the Patient of the Time Limitations

During this middle phase of treatment, occasionally reminding the patient of time limitations and that they will "say good-bye" in a number of weeks or months keeps the process flowing. This is important in preventing the development of over dependency. The therapist should ask the patient what it will feel like to say good-bye. This also previews[2] (Trad, 1992) the next phase of treatment and surfaces issues such as unmet dependency longings and abandonment concerns, which can then be worked through.

Emphasize Affective Restructuring

When the patient's defense system is sufficiently restructured so that he/she is in touch with feelings, the therapist can work on affective restructuring techniques. The therapist must constantly monitor the patient's emotional reaction, with special attention to his/her nonverbal communication, and encourage deep experience of any emerging or preconscious feeling. Preconscious feeling often makes its first appearance in the patient's eyes or facial muscles and should be pointed out: "Are you aware that there is some painful feeling in your eyes or that you appear sad?" Patients are often not aware of this. Ask the patient, "What are you aware of in your body right now?" and "Do you notice any physical sensations or tension anywhere?"

Having the patient focus on the physical at this point can bring the affect to the conscious zone. This form of affect restructuring is usually most effective during this phase. Many patients worry that if they let their feelings out, they will lose control of their emotional state.

Provide Encouragement

The therapist must provide both support and encouragement during this phase. Some patients enter a deep state of reactivated grief and spend a good deal of time crying. This should not be cut short. The patient needs the therapist to bear witness to this deeply felt emotion. Afterward, when all the waves of feeling have passed, the patient will talk about his/her grief. If he/she does not, the therapist should acknowledge the feeling and then ask, "To what is this connected?" "What comes to your mind?" or "What are your associations?" This is the point in treatment where low therapist activity is best.

Allow Deeper Derepressions

Patients who have had multiple injuries resulting in the development of a personality disorder require multiple derepressions. This means that the same figure will be derepressed repeatedly, with the focus shifting from various incidents. Each time the patient contacts his/her deep feeling and is able to link the feeling to current and transference relationships, he/she will experience an even greater depth of feeling. As the depth of feeling increases in intensity, more memories, both positive and negative, will be accessed.

Encourage Frequent Use of Interpretations

Malan has found that interpretations that link current, transference, and past conflicts are a central curative aspect of STDP. Frequent use of interpretation is possible when the patient's defense system has been partially altered. It takes repeated use of interpretations to restructure the personality.[3] Interpretations that are followed by affect are correlated with positive outcome (McCullough et al., 1991). The patient's awareness has to be brought to the point that when something in a current relationship activates feeling, it does so on a conscious rather than unconscious level. When the patient is aware of the feeling and links it to his/her own genetic system, that patient will then have the choice of altering his/her behavioral response. The following case illustrates this.

A patient who had distanced himself from his wife, essentially cutting her off emotionally and physically, became aware of the link to his mother. She was extremely rejecting and abusive toward him. This created a severe rejection sensitivity that he defended against by adopting what he called a "stoic" defense system: "If no one gets close, they [*sic*] can't confirm that I am unwanted and unlovable." This reflects the vicious cycle in which the patient had functioned for years. "The fact that I have no close relationships is evidence of my unworthiness." Besides protecting him from any immediate pain and rejection from a current relationship, this also prevented him from having to deal with the intense negative feelings that were generated from unmet longings he had for closeness with his mother. This was amplified by his mother's treatment of his brother, whom she idealized and to whom she constantly compared him. Almost every communication from his wife for closeness triggered this system, which had led to his extreme withdrawal and hatred of her. Repeated interpretations forced this painfully to his awareness, and he realized his idealization of his mother, along with the very painful feelings he felt that were related to a lack of anything but an idealized attachment.

Encourage Limited Free Associations

Free association during this phase can further elucidate core issues. The patient can be asked to provide associations—images, thoughts, feelings, and so on, even if the patient does not understand their meaning. However, in the course of restructuring, the therapist must maintain the structure by not allowing free association to take over, turning the process into long-term dynamic treatment.

Address Guilt as Driver of Self-Defeating Cycles

When intense feelings of anger are derepressed, guilt feelings often emerge and need to be metabolized. Amplifying the behavior, thoughts, or impulses that have engendered guilt may intensify the feeling. Some patients, for example, have mistreated their genetic figures or felt unacceptable impulses toward them, such as death wishes or even mutilation fantasies. Patients often rationalize these, and when they do, their impact on the relationship is never understood. Bringing this to the patient's attention is often one of the most painful aspects of restructuring.

One patient, a highly syntonic obsessional character, reported experiencing unexplained sadness whenever a parade passed. Upon further association, it became apparent that this sadness was linked to his feeling toward his father for not having a closer relationship with him. As therapy progressed and his developmental history was filled in, the nature and force of his guilt became focal. His father had been passive and uninvolved in his life until he was a teenager. The patient had hatred toward his father because of his absence. When his father became interested during adolescence, he retaliated by stubbornly refusing to acknowledge his father's effort and by ignoring his attempts at closeness. In fact, his father died with this wall between them. He came to realize that he had denied his father the joy his father would have felt in his son's considerable success in a career he respected. This disavowed guilt fed a severe pattern of behavior that almost destroyed the patient's life. Once this was interpreted, he grieved and faced his guilt, which had led to a cycle of self-punishment.

I have observed three distinct types of guilt that often torment the unconscious of the personality disordered patient and usually become evident during this phase: *survivor's guilt, separation guilt,* and *impulse guilt.*

Survivor's Guilt

Often, when a patient fears achieving greater success in life than his/her parents or siblings have, the patient suffers a form of survivor's guilt. This guilt stems from the feeling that he/she has left his/her loved ones behind or that he/she is having a fuller life. Patients with survivor's guilt often need to work through their belief that they are responsible for the welfare of family members. This guilt is usually mixed with other feeling as well, especially grief, "I can't take them with me" and excitement, "I am free."

Separation Guilt

Separation guilt is often reactivated by moving away from parental figures, which for some is experienced unconsciously as patricide or matricide. The fear is that leaving a parent will devastate that parent, for example, "If I separate, he/she might die or go crazy." This is often evident in cases where the patient has been narcissistically used by a genetic figure and led to believe he/she is responsible for the caregiver's welfare.

Impulse Guilt

Impulse guilt is a reaction to the destructive impulse of wanting to hurt or injure someone. For example, a patient with an obsessive thought of stabbing his mother will experience strong impulse guilt. The guilt over the repressed impulse seems to have the same strength as the imagined act. This is usually evident in fantasy material. One patient in an unhappy marriage kept worrying about her spouse getting in a violent car accident.

Encourage Change in Maladaptive Patterns

During this phase of treatment, the patient may make statements about how he/she would like to do things differently or live a fuller life. Sometimes, when intense unresolved feeling has been faced with the therapist, the patient wants to face the genetic figure with his/her new self. This consolidates the gains and strengthens the ego. If the patient does not suggest these changes, the therapist may do so. Some possibilities include:

• *Patients with unresolved feelings toward genetic figures* decide, or may be encouraged, to approach the genetic figure(s) in a new and more constructive manner. In *The Case of the Man with the Skeletal View* (see Chapter 10), the patient was encouraged to spend time with his father, which he did by asking him out to lunch and talking to him in a more intimate manner than he ever had. In fact, he realized that his mother was always present, acting as a buffer between them. His father seemed pleased to be invited out and responded positively, within the spectrum that his own characterological limitations would allow. Other patients begin to assert themselves and do not experience the reaction they anticipate. Viewpoints that are often fixed or unmodified childhood perspectives shift. One patient with an abusive father said that she realized he was no longer the domineering, larger than life figure she had remembered but, rather, an aging, weak, and pathetic individual. The patient began to see her father in a new, more realistic light uncolored by the emotional reactions from the past. This increases and consolidates the mastery that the patient has experienced in solving emotional problems with the therapist.

• *Patients with unresolved grief over lost parents* may be encouraged or may decide on their own to visit the grave of the deceased figure. These are often profound experiences when, for the first time outside of the therapist's office, the patient confronts his/her grief and loss, as well as anger, toward the genetic figure. Many patients have conversations with the deceased parent where they say what they felt they could never communicate. One patient actually buried the ashes of his mother next to his father, instead of throwing them in a dumpster as he planned to do.

• *Patients who have avoided developmental milestones* may be encouraged to begin to date, take better care of themselves, or return to school as part of their commitment to themselves. The grief over what was missed has to be addressed during this process.

• *Patients who have not mastered their anger* can be encouraged to assert themselves appropriately rather than relying on old character defenses. The therapist, for example, in *The Case of the Woman who Abandoned Her Sexuality* (see Chapter 8), encouraged her to talk to her husband and express her concerns instead of withdrawing sexually and cutting him off emotionally.

• *Patients can enhance self-understanding and increase awareness of developmental issues by using psychoeducational materials.* Materials explaining cognitive schemas can be given to the patient and can alert him/her to circumstances that will trigger negative reactions. It can be explained to a patient, for example, that he/she avoids people because he/she is "rejection sensitive" and that this was an *adaptive* response, given the patient's family. The therapist can suggest readings that will increase self-acceptance. During the middle phase of treatment, I often recommend books that will help the patient understand their development and enhance compassion for themselves. Books[4] that are suggested during this phase are often digested and assimilated at deeper levels; the readings can reinforce what the patient has discovered or is experiencing in treatment.

• *Patients who need to contact missing figures* should be encouraged. This can be extremely important for patients in coming to terms with lost aspects of their lives. For example, in *The Case of the Man Who Just Heard the Words* (see Chapter 10), the patient was encouraged to follow through on his desire to contact his lost son. This does not always have a happy ending, as it did in this case. Whatever the outcome, enough time needs to be allotted to deal with the patient's reaction to these events. It is important to encourage the patient at the proper time—early enough in the treatment—and explain how it takes time to process reactions.

Identify Other Areas of Conflict

Although the therapist must be careful about enlarging the scope of treatment, at the same time he/she should watch for the emergence of other figures that have played an important role in the patient's development. For example, in *The Case of the Woman Who Abandoned Her Sexuality,* the patient's grandmother emerged as an important positive figure in her development. The patient's sense of loss and unresolved grief at her death needed to be derepressed.

Experience and Metabolize Increased Positive Feelings
toward the Therapist

During the midphase of treatment, positive feelings toward the therapist are activated that need to be elicited and linked to early positive or absent relations. The patient should be asked "How do you feel toward me?" at points where there seems to be a build-up or catharsis of feeling. For instance, after a derepression of strong grief-laden affect over a loss, there is an increased feeling of acceptance by the patient. As we shall see in *The Case of the Man Who Just Heard the Words*, the patient reported after a series of derepressions that he had never experienced any close relationships. The therapist's efforts to uncover the patient's emotions generated strong positive feeling toward the therapist. Sometimes, however, patients have as much difficulty expressing their positive feeling as they do their negative feeling. Often, when they are able to contact and identify positive feeling, they then complain that they are not able to express affection toward anyone "close" to them. This becomes another loss, that is, how the lack of close relationships early in life has handicapped relationships in the present. By focusing on the positive feeling, the therapist can follow the patient's lead and discover more about the core injury. Other patients who contact positive feeling toward the therapist remember positive feelings associated with genetic figures and come to the realization that everything was not bad. One patient recalled how her father would take her sledding and how much she savored their rare feelings of affection and love.

Help the Patient Put the Genetic Figure in a New Perspective

During the midphase of therapy, when layers of defense and repressed feeling are experienced and metabolized, the patient begins to have a greater understanding of him/herself and will most likely begin to view the genetic figure differently. Perceptions that have been fixed since childhood and have influenced the patient's relationship with the genetic figures, as well as others in his/her lives, are modified. Patients who saw their mother or father as all bad or idealized them as all good begin to have a healthier, more realistic, and balanced view of them. With this change in perspective comes an increased understanding and an acceptance of the faults of these figures. Patients also begin to understand the generational unfolding and repetition of these themes and make commitments not to have another generation suffer the way they did.

During this phase, patients often become curious about their parents' backgrounds. Many approach their parents and ask them questions that seemed taboo or forbidden but about which they are curious and seek understanding. One patient, who was told at age 14 that the man he called father was not his biological father, was shocked and felt he could not ask his mother any questions. Because he was illegitimate, he assumed his mother was deeply ashamed of the circumstances surrounding his birth. During therapy in his late 20s, he finally talked to her for the first time about his father, and she openly shared all with him. He learned some positive things about his father, whereas all he had associated with his father before therapy was shame. As a result, he felt a much greater sense of wholeness.

Use Creative Tasks

Both patient and therapist can be creative in this phase of therapy and develop tasks that allow the patient in a symbolic and literal way to experience a new character pattern. For example, patients can be encouraged to write letters to missing or dead figures. The innovative use of tasks to highlight or ritualize conflicted issues is very common in the field of family therapy. It can be helpful in STRP, as well, and it is appropriate to use whatever seems meaningful to the patient.

Examine Increase in Unconscious Activity

During the middle phase of treatment, the patient's unconscious is activated by the defense analysis and transference feeling toward the therapist. Patients generally experience a greater interest and contemplation of their unconscious process or what is often described as increased psychological mindedness. They begin to remember their dreams more vividly and often present these to the therapist at the start of the session. They also report an increased fantasy life, if this had been dormant before therapy.

Dream Interpretation

Dreams can be used to increase the depth of the treatment by permitting one to focus on the feelings they arouse, the dynamic implications of the dream, and their content. There are numerous methods of dream interpretation (Hill, 1996). One I have found useful is to relate the dream to the transference. This can be done by asking the patient how the dream relates to the therapist. In *The Case of the Woman Who Was Always a Victim*, (Chapter 9), the patient began describing a very complex dream by saying she had hit her "critical" sister in the dream. The therapist can make a transference link by asking the patient, "How does this relate to me?" In this case, the patient was experiencing a build-up of irritation toward the therapist because of the defense analysis during the previous session. She was asked if there was any irritation toward the therapist. This was brought to the surface by asking her to portray a fantasy of attacking the therapist. The therapist should make the link between the aggression toward the sister for being critical and the aggression toward the therapist for challenging her defenses. The anger can then be brought to the surface and metabolized, strengthening the defenses.

Dreams can also be related to the patient's core issue and defense constellation. The patient's desire to give up her position of victimization can be addressed, and the fact that she was always placed in the middle of her parents' conflicts can be emphasized with the intent of amplifying feeling.

Increased Fantasy

The patient often experiences an increase in fantasy productions that can be explored and brought to closure, and then related to the core issue. For example, the patient may report a sexual fantasy about the therapist or wonder what the therapist's family or personal life is like. The patient can be encouraged to elaborate on these fantasies, which will often provide a link to the core injury. For example, again in *The Case of the Woman Who Was Always a Victim*, the patient's sexual fantasy toward the therapist was related to her sexualized feeling toward her father, who related to all women as sexual objects. The patient's sexual feelings were a substitute for intimacy and closeness and represented strong unmet cravings and longings for paternal closeness. Maine (1991) so aptly describes these feelings in patients with eating disorders as "father hunger."[5] I have also found this to be so in my work with personality disordered patients. Parenthetically, the comorbidity between eating disorders and personality disorders is quite high.

Focus on Pathological Mourning: Impacted Grief

Personality disordered patients are especially vulnerable to loss and the development of pathological grief reactions. Their defensive structure has made it difficult to metabolize the feeling associated with any type of loss. The process of pathological grief has been studied by Linderman (1944) in response to the tragic fire at the Coconut Grove Night Club, which resulted in the death of 500 people. Linderman studied the reaction of family members and described the symptomatology of normal and pathological grief, reporting his findings in a landmark paper entitled "Symptomatology and Management of Acute Grief." His research indicated that the preferred method of handling grief reactions is for the therapist to help the patient experience and accept the emotional pain the loss activates. Once the patient is able to experience the grief, he/she can then be guided into examining his/her relationship with the lost figure in detail.

My clinical experience has repeatedly shown that almost all personality disordered patients have suffered numerous losses in their lives and that the second stage of the therapy usually entails substantial grief work. It is often necessary to address the surface layers of pathological grief, such as later life losses, before deeper core issues can be experientially accessed. Often, there is a complicated series of losses dating back to childhood, which the patient must face. The denial of these losses, although it provides short-term relief can leave the person functioning to outdated internal models of reality (Milbrath, Bauknight, Horowitz, Amaro, & Sugahara, 1995). The therapeutic work sometimes reactivates a full bereavement process that is very intense and has to be validated and explained by the therapist: "You have never grieved the loss of your father and are now experiencing the intense feelings over his loss." Some patients are uninformed about the course of bereavement and need an explanation about how grief is experienced and the fact that relief from grief does not happen quickly but in stages. Grief reactions vary among patients, and the therapist should be familiar with the most common types:

1. *Grief over the loss of an attachment figure.* Patients who have lost a parent or a significant attachment figure through death or abandonment will often have impacted grief, especially if the loss was early in life and there was limited cognitive structure to help mediate the loss symbolically.

2. *Grief over the lost life potential.* Many personality disordered patients have missed significant developmental opportunities because of their self-defeating patterns. Often, when they begin to face the reality of their difficulties, they are struck by their wasted potential and the things they have missed, such as establishing a career, courting, engagement, marriage, and children. This can be an extremely painful realization. One woman, a professional in her early 60s, entered into a painful grief process when she began to face how her marriage to a characterologically disturbed man with a schizophrenic disorder was a sentence to a life of misery and pain, without a fulfilling sexual relationship, children, or companionship. The recognition of her unmet longings to have a family and marriage caused intense grief and mourning.

3. *Grief over the loss of the old self.* Personality disordered patients are identified with their defenses and in many ways have survived devastating life events because of these. When the personality begins to shift, a mourning process is almost always activated. "This is the self I have known for 40 years." Saying good-bye is painful, and fear of the unknown self can be immobilizing. The therapist should view the loss

of the old self as any other significant loss and explore the process of saying good-bye to the old self.

4. *Grief over never having a meaningful affectionate attachment.* During the course of treatment, the personality disordered patient will often come to the realization that he/she never had an affectionate or effective relationship and begin to understand the meaning of this in terms of his/her developmental disruptions. This is often a painful recognition and results in grief over this deprivation. The therapeutic relationship shows the patient what an effective attachment is like, and as the void becomes obvious, the patient experiences intense pain.

5. *Grief over the loss of the therapist.* In short-term psychotherapy, the therapist and patient come together for a limited period of time and then say good-bye. For most patients, saying good-bye to the therapist is the first effective parting in their lives. The therapist must discuss this fact with the patient and explore his/her feelings so that the sadness and loss are metabolized in a different and more positive manner than were losses in the past.

6. *Grief over leaving parents and other family members behind.* At a certain point in treatment, the therapist should explore the patient's feelings about moving beyond parents and siblings in terms of resolving problems and having a more fulfilling life. In addition to the associated guilt discussed previously, many patients grieve the fact that they will not be able to get other family members to change with them and must go it alone. Some patients realize this means limited contact with family members. For others, it involves accepting the limitations of significant figures and coming to terms with the reality that the changes they have made do not necessarily lead to improvements in their relations with the important people in their lives.

7. *Grief over injuries to self.* At the core of the patient's genetic structure is the grief over the injury that has been sustained to the self. This is often the deepest layer of grief, as it relates to the way in which the patient was robbed of normal development because of abuse, abandonment, neglect, and the effects of characterological disturbances from the genetic figure.

All therapists must have a thorough understanding of the grief process and its stages in order to help patients work it through. As stated above, conducting effective short-term psychotherapy with personality disordered patients is likely to entail significant grief work. It is imperative that the therapist has faced his/her own grief and has a high tolerance for sustained contact with the reactivated pain over multiple losses. If the therapist is uncomfortable, the patient will unconsciously sense this and continue to avoid his/her grief.

When the mourning process is activated, the patient will experience waves of grief-laden feeling. The therapist should discourage verbalization until the affect has subsided. Often, the patient will want to talk to distance from the pain. Gentle reassurance and refocusing will often suffice to validate the experience and open the channel for deeper waves of affect. The therapist may first become aware that feelings are surfacing by observing changes in the patient's facial expression. Pointing this out, "You look sad," has a powerful effect on most patients and may assist them in becoming open to the experience of more feelings. More about the importance of facial affect recognition is discussed later in this chapter.

TERMINATION PHASE

The final stage of treatment is termination, which if navigated correctly, provides a first experience for many patients in appropriately facing a loss of a significant attachment figure and processing their feelings in a healthy way. When the termination phase is incomplete, the patient often misses an important learning opportunity.

Types of Termination

In my experience, the best termination is a *planned termination*, wherein the patient and I have decided to discuss ending during the same session. Often, my gut feeling that the therapy is over tracks the patient's same thought. Other kinds of termination include the following:

Premature Termination

This is an all too frequent occurrence and occurs early in the process, usually for unknown reasons. Sometimes, these patients return later for treatment. In one case, the patient was seen for an extended session, canceled his next appointment and never returned a call to reschedule. Four years later, he made an appointment and scheduled an extended session saying the first one was helpful and that he had not returned for financial reasons. After the second extended session, he again canceled and was not heard from. Cases like this are hard to explain, and they remind us of the ambiguity inherent in the life of a therapist.

Unplanned Termination

The patient, although making good progress, cancels his or her session for unspecified reasons and does not reschedule. In this situation, I usually phone the patient once and encourage him/her to make one final appointment. I respect the patient's right to terminate without notification, although this often seems unsatisfactory to me and deprives both the patient and me of a sense of closure.

Therapist-Encouraged Termination

In some cases, the patient seems to have derived maximum benefit from therapy and yet hangs on to the therapist because of strong dependency strivings. This can often be directly expressed, and a few more sessions can be taken to work out these feelings, taking particular effort to tie this to the genetic system. For example, "Of course you don't want to end, you never had a close relationship with your [mother/father/sibling], and you want to hang on to me." This often allows a deeper metabolizing of the grief to occur.

Termination by Patient before Therapist Believes He/She Is Ready

In this scenario, the patient expresses a desire to terminate before the therapist believes the therapeutic objectives have been achieved. In this case, the therapist should explore the patient's reasons for doing so and point out the benefit of continuing. The patient might expect the therapist to respond negatively, but, in most cases, the patient's reasons are valid and should be respected. The patient can be told that he/she is welcome to return if he/she feels the need to do further work. The session should be closed in the same way as any termination session.

The following are characteristics of this phase of treatment:

1. Reactivation of themes of loss
2. Struggle with meaning and importance of therapist, and feelings over loss of a positive attachment figure—"What would life have been like if I had had a parent like you?"
3. Focus on more existential issues—meaning of time, mortality, loneliness, and isolation themes
4. Discussion of commitments for new life
5. Emphasis on future hopes and plans

Tasks during Termination

The main task of termination is bringing the treatment to a conclusion and, for the patient, mourning the loss of the therapist and therapy. The importance of the termination phase is in the amplification and elucidation of themes of separation and loss and their link to the core issues. The following tasks are important elements of this phase of treatment:

Setting a Termination Date

This phase of therapy really begins when a termination date is scheduled. If the therapy is not time-limited (set number of sessions), then the patient and therapist need to determine how many more sessions will be required to accomplish the therapeutic task.

Processing the Patient's Feelings, Thoughts, and Concerns about Termination

The patient should be encouraged during the termination session to discuss how he/she feels about saying good-bye to the therapist. Previewing can be done by asking the patient to imagine the final session and what the good-bye will be like. This will inevitably surface feelings, positive, negative, or mixed in most patients. Usually, the patient is ready to get on with his/her life but feels a sadness about losing the therapist. This procedure also encourages the experience of grief over other losses as well as incomplete good-byes. These incidents should be derepressed with an affective restructuring procedure.

Saying One's Good-bye to the Patient

The therapist also needs to be aware of the impact of the good-bye and be able to express whatever is appropriate to the patient. In most cases, a strong bond has developed, and the therapist experiences sadness, especially when the patient is a more genuine and less defensive person than at the onset of treatment.

Review and Summarization of the Treatment Process

Review and summarization of therapy provide a powerful communication to the patient. This works to highlight what has been accomplished. Patients are often so involved in the process that they lose sight of the larger perspective, especially of how far they have progressed. Making final core connections and highlighting the important events and aspects of treatment are truly a gift to the patient. This shows the patient that the therapist has been attentive, careful, thoughtful, and supportive of the patient's growth.

Rating Level of Improvement

Although this is commonly used in research protocols, having the patient rate his/her progress on the issues that he/she set out to change is another way of emphasizing the patient's capacity to alter his/her life. For example, "When you entered therapy, you had a high degree of anxiety in work presentations and avoided them. On a scale of 0 to 100, how would you rate your improvement when you started as compared to now after therapy?"

Anticipating and Preplanning for Potential Problems

Pockets of potential difficulty for the patient should be anticipated and discussed. For example, a patient who has an addictive problem and is facing a situation that will place him/her at risk should be "prepped" by discussing how he/she will handle it and what preemptive steps can be taken to reduce a regression.

Making a Positive Prediction Whenever Possible

In my experience, the year after short-term treatment is one of enormous growth. I tell most patients that they can expect that things will continue to progress in ways that will enhance and consolidate the work they have done. If I think a setback is likely, I also discuss this and frame this positively by saying that sometimes a backstep is needed before a growth spurt can occur.

In Chapter 12, I present the portions of a transcript of a termination session; we now proceed to the clinical case material, covered in the next three chapters.

CONCLUSION

I am usually surprised at the passage of time during sessions. It almost always seems that time passes quickly, as if linear time has not been in operation. This is probably an artifact of working with the unconscious, where past, present, and future are often fused. The stages of therapy are not always as clearly differentiated as this chapter might suggest. Each treatment has its own rhythm and pace. Sometimes patients seem to be done, but they come back for another block of treatment. Many stop and resume, others have false starts and are not heard from again. The opportunity to "complete" the process is a privilege of being a psychotherapist. In the second part of this book, we apply what we have learned to clinical cases to see how the process unfolds.

PART II

PROCESS AND TECHNIQUE IN TREATMENT OF PERSONALITY DISORDERS

This section of the book will give the reader a better feel for how the concepts presented actually influence our clinical work. In the following three chapters, we review in depth the process of restructuring the personality with a wide spectrum of personality disturbances. Certainly the best way to integrate or master the techniques and learn the process is to observe audiovisually recorded sessions under supervision and study the process in detail. The next best method for learning the approach is to follow the actual transcripts of patients who have experienced both massive change, and have enduring outcomes, and cases where the outcomes were poor. In fact, I have learned many important lessons from my cases where the outcome was poor. These stand out in my memory as vividly as the cases where the results seemed miraculous.

Although the next three chapters are organized around DSM-IV personality clusters, I do not present a case of each personality disorder as identified in DSM. Rather, I attempt to present a variety of cases from each cluster that are encountered in clinical practice and that are illustrative of this approach. In clinical practice, patients tend to present with blends of personality types; distinct categories are hard to find.

The majority of the cases presented are based on transcripts from audiovisually recorded sessions. In one case, *The Case of the Man Who Feared He Would Be Violent,* where the patient was not audiovisually recorded, the transcript has been reproduced to as close to the original dialogue as possible, and this is so noted. Most patients willingly agree to be recorded, but for others, it is experienced as burdensome. I was surprised by the number of patients who allowed their work to be published: Almost all of those asked agreed, without hesitation. I am grateful and indebted to these patients for their trust and courage. I believe that the best way to advance our science and art is to expose our work to self scrutiny and review by others. We often expect as much or more from those who have entrusted their treatment to us.

CHAPTER 8

Cluster C Disorders: The Treatment-Responsive Group

Do you continually curtail your effort till there be nothing of it left?
. . . By non-action there is nothing which cannot be effected.
—LAO-TZE

Patients with personality disorders in Cluster C have the best outcomes with every type of short-term psychotherapy. This does not mean that we can consistently achieve rapidly induced, in-depth change and enduring outcome with all patients, but we can consistently achieve positive outcomes with most patients. Even within diagnostic categories, two patients who have avoidant personality disorders may have very different results with the same therapist, using the same approach. Diagnostic classification only depicts one aspect of the patients complexity.[1] As we have seen in previous chapters, a comprehensive evaluation takes many other factors into consideration.

QUANTUM CHANGE EXPERIENCES

Quantum change experiences occur both naturally (Miller & C'deBaca, 1994) and as a result of psychotherapeutic experiences. Psychology has been loath to recognize and investigate these experiences until recently. Most of our understanding of these events comes from studies of religious conversions, which for most scientists and psychotherapists have a dubious reputation. We know very little about what precipitates these rapid transformations, but when they occur, there is no question for the patient, significant others, and the therapist that a major shift in the patient's personality has occurred. Our job as therapists is to maximize these opportunities and to be sensitive to converging forces in the patients' lives that trigger a disruption in their characteristic patterns and induce a scanning for new solutions. A patient's decision to enter psychotherapy does not always signify that the patient is at an optimal gestation or change period, although for some it does. When we are fortunate enough to have a patient enter treatment during an optimal change period, the results can be rapid and the transformation enduring. Participating in this type of change is a rare privilege. To reiterate a point made in Chapter 3, if the patient is not ready or willing to undergo the painful work required of a rapid transformation, then a more modest, stepwise approach should be selected. We must avoid precipitating an intrapsychic crisis with a patient, who, for example, is suffering from external challenges, such as financial difficulties, an abusive relationship, or other environmental demands. The therapist must make sure that the patient understands that a rapid transformation will entail metabolizing significant emotional pain and that between sessions, there will be emotional turmoil as grief reactions are reactivated and the facts of the patient's life come to the surface.

THE OTHER SIDE OF THE COIN

Most of my patients know that I specialize in short-term reconstructive psychotherapy. In fact, I generally attempt short-term therapy as the treatment of choice unless it is obviously contraindicated. The patients who do not respond to a short-term approach and instead carry on with longer-term treatment often report that they feel like failures. In the past, I think mental health professionals have had a tendency to blame their patients for not improving. This has been a very destructive trend that is being counteracted by clinicians such as Marsha Linehan, among others, who abhor our tendency to blame the patient and not look at our inadequate approaches and mistakes. I hope that those reading this book will come away with increased knowledge and skill in identifying and participating in rapid character transformations but, more importantly, will be open to learning from our less brilliant outcomes without resorting to blaming the patient for "not wanting to change." There are patients who are not motivated to make changes but most patients seek us out because they realize they need to grow and develop. For those patients whose improvements are almost imperceptible over long periods of time but who continue to suffer unbearable emotional disturbances, I let them know that new developments are emerging in psychotherapy and psychopharmacology all the time, and I will be alert to anything that might benefit them. I stress that it is *not their fault* that they are not "getting better faster" but that we have not yet developed the approach that might be effective.

REVIEW OF THE CLUSTER C DISORDERS: THE ANXIOUS OR FEARFUL GROUP

Cluster C includes the avoidant, dependent, and obsessive–compulsive personality disorders. Passive–aggressive personality disorder, now termed negativistic personality disorder, has been moved to the Appendix of DSM-IV for further research corroboration. A new addition to Cluster C is the depressive personality disorder, which has also been added to the Appendix for further confirmation. The Cluster C personality disorders are the most responsive to anxiety-increasing, rapid uncovering approaches, particularly suited to those patients above the borderline position on structural organization.

This Cluster is characterized by difficulty experiencing and expressing anger or irritation. There are often difficulties in the sphere of sexual functioning. Of the three clusters of personality disorders, Cluster C is the lowest on the ego-dystonic scale, in that these patients experience the highest level of suffering, which causes them to seek treatment more readily than the other clusters. We often find comorbid anxiety and depressive disorders diagnosed on Axis I. Much of their frustration with life and others is internalized, and there is a high degree of self-blame (Stone, 1993). They lack assertiveness because of their emotional inhibition and fear of catastrophic reactions. Many of the patients from this group respond to and identify with the Jekyll and Hyde personality; because of their inhibition and repressed anger, they are fearful of losing control and becoming a monster.

THE PROCESS AND TECHNIQUE

As opposed to Clusters A and B, Cluster C patients almost always require direct defensive restructuring early in the process. With patients who are able to rapidly form a collaborative therapeutic alliance, the therapist can quickly begin restructuring the defenses. As with any patient, the therapist must monitor the therapeutic alliance, so that ruptures are not created. One must be ever alert for ego fragility—collapsing of ego functions, major regressive behavior, major clinical depression, psychophysiological disruptions, such as irritable bowel, migraine, and severe suicidal states. The therapist's aim is always directed at the defenses and should never contain any attack on the self. There is a certain level of confrontation that may be uncomfortable for those who are not familiar with defense analysis. Anxiety-provoking techniques are used to penetrate defenses and create an emotional breakthrough, which allows for a derepression and decathexis. This will reduce the stimulus–response connection between the traumatic event and affective reaction.

RAPID RESTRUCTURING: A QUANTUM CHANGE EXPERIENCE—THE CASE OF THE MAN WHO TOOK THE HEAT

The first case presented highlights elements of a rapid restructuring approach with a patient suffering from an obsessional character who was 42 years old when he entered treatment. Although this case was rare in that it was completed in a very brief period of time (five 45-minute sessions including assessment), it is an excellent case to highlight the sequence of events and change movements in detail. Highlights of the case are used to illustrate the restructuring and derepression of unconscious material. Each successful phase of derepression and restructuring deepens the process. Although much of the actual transcripts have been included, the reader will realize that much has been left out.

Assessment

The patient entered treatment after breaking off a 3½-year, live-in relationship. He had no previous history of mental health treatment of any type. He felt very sad and depressed about the loss of the relationship. He realized that he had a pattern of repeatedly sabotaging relationships with women. He frequently started a new relationship while still in an existing one, causing much turmoil and conflict. He reported suffering from a long-standing, low-grade depression and mild anxiety. He was moderately ego-syntonic with no major ego deficits. The patient's ability to develop a collaborative relationship seemed good. The patient wanted to be able to commit to a woman, marry, and start a family and was aware of the fact that something was preventing him from doing this; he realized that time was running out. This seemed to be a critical juncture in his life. Either he would continue his pattern, sabotaging his relationships, or come to terms with his difficulties. He seemed prepared to come to try to do the latter. He was initially seen for a 45-minute consultation, and the following presenting complaints were identified:

1. History of relationship difficulties wherein he has been unable to fully commit himself to the woman and winds up seeing another woman and getting caught in a stormy situation.
2. Trouble maintaining his sexual interest after the initial stage of the relationship and so looks to other women.
3. Mild anxiety and depression.
4. Difficulty expressing his emotions, which have exacerbated relationship difficulties.
5. Characterological disturbance, including passivity, perfectionism, obsessive devotion to work, and severe isolation of affect.

The patient agreed to be seen for an extended session, the purpose of which was described as an attempt to get a full understanding of his difficulties and get to the core of them. He seemed motivated enough to withstand a rapid derepression of his unconscious and make changes in his personality. One week later, an extended session (four 45-minute sessions back to back with one 15-minute break) was scheduled. It is important to inform patients that the treatment can be emotionally disruptive and that they might want to plan the remainder of the day accordingly. Also, if the therapist is audiovisually recording the treatment, the patient should be informed of the purposes for this and sign any necessary releases. This is discussed in greater detail in Chapter 12.

Extended Session

At the onset of the extended session, it is important for the therapist to recapitulate the therapeutic task: "Our goal today is to get to the core of your difficulties and face your feelings honestly." Also, the specific areas of change that the patient wants to attain should be listed as clearly in behavioral terms as possible. This is explained as follows: "In order for us to know when we have met the goals that you have set out for us, it is important that you be specific about how you will know that you have attained them." In this case, one goal was for the patient to be able to overcome his difficulty with commitment and be able to maintain a long-term, monogamous relationship. We begin with the opening of the extended session:

THERAPIST: The purpose of today's session is for you and me to get to the core of your difficulties, get to the root of the problem so that at the end of our time together you can live a less self-defeating, less self-sabatoging[2] life for yourself. So what do you want to start with today?

The patient's response to the opening is to be rather vague and passive as he waits for the therapist to "ask me some questions." His *noncommittal style* immediately emerges as a transference issue and is part of his character resistances. Since we have reviewed his problems and established the treatment goals, this ambivalence is viewed as character resistance and needs to be made ego-dystonic.

THERAPIST: Being on the fence is going to sabotage this relationship, because if you and I are going to get to the bottom of this, so that you can really get your freedom, sitting on the fence is never going to allow your self to be fully present with me.

[Now we are in the T at the defense corner of the triangle.]

PATIENT: I guess I just don't know where to start.

THERAPIST: There are certain difficulties that you came to me with, certain kinds of patterns that you talked about with women seemed to be important.

It is crucial that when the therapist is elucidating defenses he/she does not allow a power struggle to emerge, which frequently occurs if the collaborative nature of the alliance has not been sufficiently nurtured. The therapist must be very alert for the emergence of stubbornness and defiance and to head off a power struggle by emphasizing that the purpose of the session is first for the therapist and patient to get an understanding of the difficulties. Without agreement on the problems, collaboration to solve the disturbance is impossible. Emphasizing the joint nature of the therapeutic endeavor, and that it can only work with collaboration, is crucial.

PATIENT: Yes, there are, it seems like I don't let our relationship [with girlfriend] get to any degree of intimacy. Part of it is that—One of my things is that I tend to be passive. That's been a complaint. Shelly has been complaining for some time that it is just like being with no one.

THERAPIST: So you remain uninvolved or emotionally detached. I have a sense that there is a part of you that is really terrified of letting anybody get close to you.

[Now we are in the C at the defense corner of the triangle.]

PATIENT: I don't think I was always aware that was an issue. At least not consciously. But it has become apparent that it is an issue. I can open up from time to time, but that is not my natural mode. My actual mode is to be closed, to be aloof, is to be noncommittal. Noncommital is a big thing for me.

All signs are now positive to proceed with active defensive analysis. The patient acknowledges that there are unconscious factors that influence his behavior. When the defenses are pointed out, he recognizes what is being communicated. The session continues with identification of his constellation of defenses as they emerge. These include his detachment, avoidance of eye contact, lack of emotional involvement, ambivalence, and passivity, all of which create a wall keeping the therapist, as well as others, at a distance. The therapist proceeds with the defense analysis because it is clear the patient is accepting what is being identified. As you recall, the purpose of the defense analysis is first, *to make the defenses ego-dystonic,* and second, to *stimulate affective responding.*

PATIENT: I am kind of confused right now. Maybe that's another thing.

THERAPIST: Confusion is another way that you have of walling off other people.

PATIENT: It is really not easy for me to talk about my feelings because again I am not sure I understand what my feelings are. Well I don't know, I guess I don't know how to talk with someone on an intimate level, and I'm not sure why that is. I thought about various reasons why. You hear about things, your parents being a key factor in your life, and I always felt that's perhaps one of the things. I don't know; I've never really connected to my father.

[The patient is using tentativeness as a defense, but this is not challenged because it is minor.]

THERAPIST: You've never felt a connection with your Dad?

PATIENT: No, I never did. I really wanted to, but I remember early on what I felt. He wasn't around a lot and I never really knew him well.

At this point, quite early in the session, moderate defense analysis begins to mobilize affect. There are two reasons this occurs. First, bringing the defenses to the patient's attention starts restructuring the defense system because the patient will see their function and rely on them less. Second, the therapist's genuine interest in the patient's life begins to activate early unmet longings and feelings toward attachment figures. We also get a glimpse of the first core issues, a disturbance in the father–son relationship, which we can then use as a guide and as a focus for interventions. At this point the therapist can use affect restructuring. This should be done when there is evidence that the affect has reached the preconscious zone. Often the patient is not aware of this, and the therapist must mirror the reaction. One can observe the affect in the facial expression and eyes.

THERAPIST: I sense right now that there is some painful feeling that is coming to the surface.

PATIENT: About that? Yes.

THERAPIST: And right now there is a part of you that doesn't want to experience the intensity of that feeling right now. Why is it that you don't want to really experience the full impact of your emotional life?

PATIENT: It's too painful.

THERAPIST: But if we avoid the pain, we go around it, and then we never really get to the core of why a guy who has your potential has sabotaged so many relationships. What you have brought here is this need to destroy, kill off your relationships with women. I'm not sure I have that right. There is a lot of feeling coming to the surface now.

PATIENT: (affect very sad) Yes, there is. I mean, I guess that my father is someone I really wanted to connect with, and I'm not sure he knew how.

THERAPIST: So you wanted to have a connection with him. There was something about him that made it difficult. What was there about your father that made it difficult?

PATIENT: I'm really not sure, but it seems that—He seemed like he was a very frustrated person. Frustrated with his life. I always had a sense that he did not want to get married. I had a sense that he was not genuinely happy. He was frustrated about a lot of things.

If the patient is responding to the defense and affect restructuring, there will be increased clarity about early experience in the form of previously repressed traumatic memories, dreams, affect, and fresh associations. This offers a widening channel into the unconscious. On the other hand, if the defensive restructuring is not occurring, the patient will become more passive, depressed, defiant, and stubborn or develop psychophysiological reactions such as migraine or GI tract disruptions. At this point, it is very important to test the unconscious opening by asking for an incident concerning the genetic figure (in this case the father). If the patient cannot recall or be more specific, the repressive forces are still too high, and more restructuring must be completed.

THERAPIST: Can you give me an example, was there an incident or something we could talk about specifically that kind of gave you the sense that your dad really didn't want to be married to your mom?

PATIENT: Well, I remember when I was very little, maybe 4 or so, he came home when we were having supper, and he was upset about something. Something to do with his job or something; he just exploded.

[Now we are in the triangle at the past corner.]

THERAPIST: He exploded? You were about 4 years you say?

PATIENT: Something like that. He came home from work; he sat down at the dinner table and just exploded.

THERAPIST: What was the explosion like?

PATIENT: He was screaming, and my mother was saying something like, "not in front of the kids," and he was saying something like, "I don't care," and he started picking up plates and throwing them against the wall.

THERAPIST: Did anyone get hit?

PATIENT: No, no.

THERAPIST: How did your mother react?

PATIENT: She was pretty upset.

THERAPIST: Can you remember what she did or said?

PATIENT: Not really, but I know she was just upset. I really don't remember. She was crying and hollering at him to stop.

THERAPIST: So he came home raging?

PATIENT: I'm not sure he came home raging, but when he sat down at the table that's when he—it's kind of fuzzy, but that's what it seemed. That it just came to the surface.

The therapist should try to get as much detail about the traumatic incident, which brings more life to the scene and intensifies the derepression. The therapist might also ask the patient to describe the room and where people were situated or any sounds or smells he/she can recall.

THERAPIST: Then you must have had a lot of feeling about having that occur?

[Now we are reaching for impulse/feeling.]

PATIENT: I guess I did. I guess I felt . . . I guess I was upset and what seemed to happen was . . . at least the recollection I have is that I just kind of tightened up and stepped back from the situation.

[Now we are identifying defense.]

THERAPIST: You detached?

We can now observe the onset, although there may have been earlier incidents, wherein detachment and passivity and isolation of affect were used to protect the patient from traumatic events.

PATIENT: Yes.

THERAPIST: Because you had a lot of feeling.

PATIENT: Well, it was extremely upsetting.

Even though the patient is showing evidence of emotional pain, it has not reached high intensity. Therapists might be tempted to stop at this point, but for a comprehensive restructuring to occur, it is crucial that the most intense feeling associated with the traumatic be *experienced* and *metabolized* in the session, in the safety of the therapeutic alliance.

THERAPIST: When you say upsetting, what were the feelings toward your dad at that time, to see him throwing the dishes and seeming like he didn't want to be married to your mother?

PATIENT: It was upsetting because it's your whole world. Your parents are your whole world.

THERAPIST: So it was like your whole world was going to collapse on you.

PATIENT: Definitely.

THERAPIST: Then you had a lot of feelings to see—at 4 years old this whole world as you knew it just collapsed. And then you detached from all that feeling.

PATIENT: Yes. I can remember, I believe it was after that, standing in the bathroom and my mother was standing at the door. My father was there also, and they were talking about something, and I'm not sure whether they were arguing or not, but the thought I had was I cannot wait until I am old enough to take care of myself because I don't need this. They can't help me. They can't give me what I need.

THERAPIST: At 4 years old you felt that your mom and dad weren't capable of giving you the security you needed. And what feeling did that mobilize inside you toward your parents? And if you really were to look at that feeling inside of you?

PATIENT: I would say probably one of detachment. One of "I guess it could work."

THERAPIST: Do you notice your fists right now?

[Nonverbal indices of affect are usually noted before the patient gets fully in touch with the feeling and should be pointed out.]

PATIENT: Yes.

THERAPIST: Because detachment is not a feeling. It's the mechanism that you have been using to deal with your emotional life, but it has been crippling you.

There are many shifts that can be observed when the patient begins a round of derepression. As the feelings and memories come close to the conscious experience, the patient often starts talking in the present tense, *as if the experience is being relived in the here and now.*

The focus of this session has become the patient's fear that he would not be taken care of but that his mother would make up for that by saying that his father did not care but *she* loved him. We now have an inkling that the second core issue has to do with feeling toward his mother.

The patient then described an incident, when he was 15, where his father took him to work, and they went to visit the father's mistress, leaving him with her daughter while they went off. His father then told him not to tell his mother. The patient said, "I just felt like it's another nail in his coffin." When asked about his feelings, the patient described them in a somewhat intellectualized fashion saying he felt "inferior" and "hurt"—secondary emotional blends.[3] When the patient's defense system loosens its hold and there is activation of the emotional schema, the patient shows signs of habitual or reflex emotional reactions. The therapist must be particularly alert to important unconscious communications such as these. *The therapist can then use these communications to make "deep interpretations" that will mobilize more anxiety–defense, as well as underlying affect.* In the next vignette, we can see how this is used to deepen the process and bring the feeling closer to the conscious experience.

THERAPIST: As you said, " . . . another nail in his coffin."

PATIENT: Because I was hurt by him many times.

THERAPIST: So whose coffin did you want to put the nail in? I mean what about the anger that you had toward him? Where is that now?

PATIENT: I definitely felt anger toward him.

THERAPIST: You felt the anger? Where is that anger right now? Do you realize how rapid your breathing is? (*The patient's respiration has become more rapid, indicating a rise in anxiety.*)

PATIENT: There is a lot of rage[4] inside of you.

The patient then brings up the issue of his father abandoning the family and the loss of their house as a result. Sometimes when the affect starts to become intense, the patient may wish to move to another incident to depressurize the psychic system. The therapist must acknowledge the importance of the issue but keep the focus on the emotionally "hot" issue.

THERAPIST: I notice that when we get close to something you want to move to another topic. . . . But you touch on each topic for a brief minute, and then you want to move to another one. There is a lot of feeling inside of you, because you said that you actually found out that your father was being unfaithful to your mother. You were actually there! And then you must have a lot of feeling toward him about that. And not only that he lied to your mother. And then you said, " . . . another nail in his coffin." What's the feeling toward him that you had?

PATIENT: I think I just hated him more.

THERAPIST: How did you experience the rage?

PATIENT: I'm not sure I experienced it at the time. I think I just buried it.

THERAPIST: Have you been burying your rage all your life?

PATIENT: Probably.

THERAPIST: Because it seems to me that a part of you is terrified of that rage inside of you. Terrified of what would really happen if you became in touch with that rage toward him.

The patient then describes an incident that occurred when he was 16. His father had provoked the patient by pushing him and calling him names. The patient then reported that he could not remember what happened after that. He stated, "Right now I just want to kill him." His defenses are pointed out as he discusses this emotionally laden incident. *With each derepression, further defense analysis may be required to loosen the defensive structure.* As the therapist proceeds with the restructuring, incidents with more disturbing and intense affect are derepressed.

THERAPIST: Do you realize right now that you are frozen?

PATIENT: I guess I do. I think that's what happened.

THERAPIST: You take a very defeated position with regard to your rage.

PATIENT: When you say defeated you mean?

THERAPIST: That you don't put it out there. You don't experience it. You cut it off. And you don't allow us to get to the rage that you experience toward him.

PATIENT: If I felt I could have—I would have beat the fucking shit out of him.

THERAPIST: And how do you feel the anger inside? Can you describe that anger?

PATIENT: It's like a boiling.

THERAPIST: Boiling, there is a boiling inside. You want to beat the shit out of him? And if the rage had come out?

PATIENT: I mean if that rage came out I don't know what I would have done to him. (*The patient is clearly in touch with his anger, his body posture is upright, and there is force in his voice and hands.*)

The therapist does not want to stop at this juncture even though the patient is in touch with his rage. Fantasizing what would have happened allows the feelings to be experienced and metabolized at the deepest level of consciousness, and it opens up channels to other positive feeling that has also been repressed. The patient often develops an awareness of the mixed nature of his/her feelings that were not previously noticed. It should be noted that, if the fantasy portrait comes after the patient is in touch with his/her feeling, this comprises a "comprehensive restructuring" at the deepest affective, cognitive, and defensive level. However, if the portrait occurs before the affect is experienced at the highest level, this is a "cognitive restructuring" procedure. *When a patient is in contact with his/her feeling, there is a noticeable reduction in defenses, more signs of animation, congruence among facial signs, nonverbal communication, and expressed affect, and a marked decrease in anxiety.* In treating patients from Cluster C, the therapist should whenever possible attempt to access the buried rage that is always a central treatment task. Non-metabolized sadistic feeling leads to overwhelming guilt and an avoidance of intimacy.

THERAPIST: If that rage had come, what would you have done to him, in your fantasy?

PATIENT: Just jump out and punch him. And with my hands just punch him in the face. Punched him more and more.

THERAPIST: And what if the rage kept coming? How would you kill him?

[The therapist makes this leap based on the reference to " . . . another nail in his coffin."]

PATIENT: I'd pick up a rock and hit him in his fucking head.

THERAPIST: Just take the rock and smash his head?

PATIENT: Yes, I guess. But that wouldn't have made me very happy because I loved him. And I would have been very sorry afterward.

THERAPIST: So there are mixed feelings toward him.

Now the therapist's task is to help the patient identify all of his feelings, but the process should be slowed down to allow for the feelings to be fully metabolized. The activity level of the therapist sharply declines. This means that the therapist should wait until all the waves of affect, both positive and negative, have been processed, labeled, and understood within the context of the patient's personality organization and current disturbances. Thus, when the patient starts to sob, the therapist can make empathic comments such as, "It is very painful," but usually a minimal amount of words is needed. The emotion will continue to be processed by the patient in dreams and waves of affect after the session, but the most intense derepression usually occurs in the safety of the therapeutic relationship.

THERAPIST: The rage was overwhelming to you. And then I noticed as soon as you got in touch with the rage, your grief started to come out about the loss of the relationship with him. That you never had a close, affectionate, supportive, loving relationship with your father. You missed that as a kid. And all these feelings are mixed up in a ball for you.

As one traumatic event is derepressed and metabolized, other incidents will be reported and will be identified and worked with in the same manner.

The therapist must be vigilant about time constraints. In an extended interview, many traumatic events can be addressed, with each cycle taking 15 to 20 minutes and more for the highly ego-syntonic. Each patient will have a different rhythm in how the memories unfold and how the waves of affect emerge. The therapist should check with the patient to see if he/she is becoming exhausted. If the therapist senses that the patient is starting to tire, no new trauma should be derepressed. However, I have rarely found that the patient cannot tolerate four 45-minute sessions with a break, and many can do longer blocks. In fact, most patients are surprised at how quickly the time passes.

It is critical to remember that it is the therapist's role to pace the session and monitor the time. If the patient does recover a traumatic incident near the end of a session, the therapist should say that this is certainly an important event, but, because of time constraints, the therapist does not want to proceed. It is important to emphasize that enough time needs to be alloted to process all the information and feelings related to the incident. Often there may be multiple traumatic incidents with significant figures that need to be derepressed. Each derepression strengthens the patient's defense system and allows the natural healing process to occur. Emotions will be allowed to emerge without defenses to block them or anxiety channels to divert them. Change in the patient can usually be noted during the course of a single session with each derepression.

The therapist should not expect one derepression to complete the restructuring. Depending on the level of trauma, it may take repeated derepressions for each pathogenic figure. A good rule of thumb is that the first figure derepressed is usually the less pathogenic figure. Deeper unresolved feelings are usually saved for the more damaging relationship. This is because greater ego strength is required to face the more primitive impulse/feeling directed toward the more abusive or conflicted figure. We now return to the case as the focus shifts to the maternal figure.

THERAPIST: So you never felt as though your father valued or wanted you?

PATIENT: No, I never felt that he wanted or valued me. On the other hand my mother tried to make up for it by pouring all this emotion on us, like this love. I felt very stifled by her. I thought—well, I can get all the love I need from my mother, and maybe she felt that she had to fill this void. Kind of gooped all this—

THERAPIST: Can you give me an example of how she "gooped" all this love on you? An incident that comes to your mind where she gooped all this love on you?

The patient then brought up the relationship with his mother, but he quickly shifted back to his father. *We now have an indication that the second core issue is an overly seductive relationship with his mother.* He described an incident where his father severely beat him and his mother stood and watched and wet her pants. He described how his mother would come to his room after the beatings in scanty nightclothes and soothe him in a highly seductive fashion.

It is not uncommon to see such evidence of narcissistic exploitation by one of the parents in Cluster C patients. In this cluster, patients generally have oedipal issues that are complicated by disturbed relationships with both genetic figures. In these cases, abuse is often present, but there is also evidence of some positive object relations that have mitigated more extreme structural damage that will be evident in the patients presented from Clusters B and A. We return to the session.

THERAPIST: Do you remember your feelings toward her?

PATIENT: Just that she was some neurotic woman who didn't know what the hell was going on. That she was out of control.

THERAPIST: What feeling is that? That she doesn't know what's going on but her son is getting beaten by her husband, and she stands there crippled and paralyzed. Do you see when we get to your anger you move away? The anger inside you has been the cancer of your life. And you have been messing up your life because of all this feeling you have cut off.

PATIENT: I felt just as angry at her . . .

As often as possible, the therapist should try to have the patient describe a specific incident that illustrates what he/she is communicating. This provides an anchor for the sequence of interventions. There is now enough information to make a comprehensive core formulation. This is presented to the patient and we will see if it is validated.

THERAPIST: So she would soothe you when you were feeling . . . The more your father abused you and the more you felt defeated with him and hopeless, the more she would come and give you these goodies, shower love on you. Like she was reinforcing the defeated position that you had with your father. There must have been a lot of feeling toward her. Why would the mother let a boy get beaten, abused, intimidated, and then shower him with love, and then tell him his father is bad?

PATIENT: I don't know why she would do that. What I want to say, that's the only thing she knew how to do . . .

[He goes on intellectualizing his mother's behavior.]

THERAPIST: So you were firmly in her camp. Then your father would get resentful and angry and take it out on you. So you were really caught in the middle. Because what you said in the scenario that you just talked about was that the fight started out between your mom and dad, and it got focused on you, and she stood by and watched. It was like you took the heat off of her.

PATIENT: Yes, as a matter of fact, I did take the heat off of her. In the one instance where she had wet her pants and I was getting beat up, I did feel like I was taking the heat for whatever was wrong in his business, whatever was wrong between them. I felt that in that one particular episode, like I was the scapegoat. I was the sacrificial lamb. I mean now that I look back.

THERAPIST: I think that the real tragedy is that there is a part of you that is still sacrificing your life and sabotaging your own happiness and, in a way, always being caught in the middle of two women. [The patient had a history of starting a relationship with another woman while already living with someone in a committed relationship.] There's a connection with the need to be in the middle of something brutal and intense.

PATIENT: Either in the middle or nothing at all.

THERAPIST: But I guess being in nothing at all for you is worse for you than being in the middle because at least it is something.

PATIENT: Definitely. Yes, I don't know whether I want to laugh because, BOOM! you struck something that makes sense to me, or cry because it makes sense to me, and I have been going through all this shit because of that.

When an important connection is made that provides insight on both an emotional and intellectual level, the event is undeniable, as observed by this patient's reaction. This validates the core formulation, and we can now proceed with the "process decathexis." *We also want to provide cognitive insight into the patient's character defenses, which were an adaptive response to nonmetabolized affect generated by the genetic disturbance.* Linking the past disturbance in intimacy to the current disturbance can be underscored (C–P interpretation).

THERAPIST: There are strong feelings about what effect this has had on your life.

PATIENT: Yes, this goes back to when I told you I was 4 years old and said I didn't need them. There's the detachment. I want to get out of the middle of this. Who wants to be in the middle of this? But when you're 4 years old, you can't get out of the middle of anything . . .

THERAPIST: Then you never allowed yourself to get involved with anybody on an intimate level for a long period of time. And every time you allowed someone to get into your intimate life, you disappeared on them. And I think this is a sad thing for you.

PATIENT: Yes. I can remember having a dream, and I can remember in the dream when I was around 4, 5, 6 years old. I had it more than once. I believe I had it two or three times. The dream was I'm standing in my grandparents house, and at that time we were temporarily living there because my father was building another house for us, and he had sold the one we were in . . . I remember looking out the screened door, concrete steps, and at the bottom of the steps was my father who was wearing, like, a tennis shirt, and in one arm he was holding a 4- or 5-year-old boy who had all rags on and was dirty, and I was the boy.

THERAPIST: What is the feeling you have right now? Can you tell me about that? The father is smiling, building a new house, and then he puts his son in rags . . . What does that produce inside of you?

At this point, the patient has another derepression of feeling toward the father. He accesses more powerful rage and remorse. He then contacts powerful waves of grief, as he describes how his father's motionless body looks. He then tells how his father died, an isolated alcoholic. This ended the first hour-and-a-half of the extended session. A 15-minute break was taken.

The unconscious process has been mobilized, and the patient should be asked to report on what he was thinking and feeling over the break. This often provides a preview of the issues that need to be focused on during the remander of the session. The patient should also be asked how he/she feels toward the therapist to monitor a build-up of transference feeling. Often at this point there is much positive feeling that should be elicited and metabolized. Usually this is followed by waves of grief that the genetic figure was long ago lost and the longings for a positive attachment unmet.

During the remainder of the session, the patient focused on the seductive relationship with his mother and his sexualized attachment toward her. He was able to access his feelings toward her and grieve her death. Again, a series of derepressions were experienced.

This patient was treated in a total of five 45-minute sessions including the intake. The patient felt that at the end of the session he had met his treatment goals. He did not feel that more therapy was indicated. A follow-up phone interview was done at 5 years. The patient reported that "the therapy had totally changed his life." He had married and had a son. He tremendously enjoyed fatherhood and marriage. He was running a very successful business. He expressed his gratitude for the therapist's involvement. This was an unusually rapid transformation of a patient with life-long character pathology in five sessions. This patient came to therapy during a period of high readiness for change. These kind of quantum transformations do not occur often, but when they do, it is amazing to be a part of the process. With most patients, a follow-up session to consolidate the gains should be conducted. The restructuring of the character can be observed in such a compacted version that there is no question that a dramatic change is underway.

COMPREHENSIVE RESTRUCTURING OF AVOIDANT PERSONALITY DISORDER WITH MIXED DISTURBANCES—THE CASE OF THE WOMAN WHO ABANDONED HER SEXUALITY

The patient, a school psychologist[5] in her late 40s, entered treatment with complaints of depression, which was a chronic dysthmia. She reported difficulties at work in that she was very anxious and did not feel that she was doing an adequate job. She had difficulty at staff meetings where she would often become anxious and allow herself to be dominated by other team members. During the initial session, she seemed very shy and blushed easily. She had had a previous course of psychotherapy but did not feel that this was successful. She suffered from generalized anxiety that was most prominent in social situations. She was married, had two children, and would have liked to have more but could not due to a hysterectomy. Although clearly of above-average intelligence, she was not clear about the cause of her malaise. A pattern of long-standing characterological disturbance was noted in her history, as follows.

Originally seen for a 45-minute consultation, she was assessed to be toward the neurotic level of the structural continuum, with moderate ego-syntonicity. The option of scheduling a four-session extended interview to determine whether she was a suitable candidate for a rapid uncovering approach was explained. This was agreed to, as was audiovisually recording the treatment for research and training purposes.

Assessment

The main focus of the initial session was on the patient's depression. This was explored and found to relate to two main areas in her current life: (1) marital disturbance, and (2) anxiety and insecurity about her functioning at work. These then became the foci of the initial session. The patient was then asked to provide specific examples of the difficulties in her marital relationship and produced a vignette wherein she asked her husband to take care of some household tasks, and he agreed but never attended to the situation. This was a pattern that was longstanding, and she would then complete the task and build up negative feeling. The focus then became the way she felt when her husband ignored her requests.

The patient fulfilled the necessary requirements for a rapid uncovering approach and comprehensive restructuring. Most importantly, she responded to defense analysis with increased anxiety but with no signs of ego collapse. She displayed a high degree of motivation, she had a solid ego structure, and she was aware of the long-standing nature of her characterological difficulties. There was, however, a moderate degree of ego-syntonicity. The option of entering into STDP was discussed, and she agreed to schedule an extended session. The first assessment session was not audiovisually recorded, although subsequent sessions were.

Extended Session

The patient was seen for an extended session (four 45-minute sessions with a 15-minute break in the middle) during which the foci involved establishing the goals of treatment, making a fuller assessment, formulating the core genetic issues, and beginning the restructuring process.

Strengthening the Therapeutic Alliance

The initial portion of the extended session was devoted to assessing the level of collaboration and to *strengthening the therapeutic alliance.* This is important with all personality disordered patients. However, as we will observe in the following chapters, with the more disturbed patients in Clusters B and A, the effort is aimed at *establishing a collaborative relationship,* so treatment can proceed. The more disturbed the patient, the greater the challenge establishing a collaborative relationship. The therapist must be confident that the patient is ready to proceed, or damage to the alliance can occur. If the therapeutic alliance seems strong at this point, it usually indicates that defense work can begin. On the other hand, if the patient reports a negative, nonspecific reaction, the therapist must continue to use more empathic interventions.

THERAPIST: How did you react to the first session we had?

PATIENT: I felt very good about it. I felt hopeful, that kind of thing. It felt like we were going in the right direction.

THERAPIST: So you felt hopeful that this process might be an effective one for you.

PATIENT: Yes.

THERAPIST: And what made you feel hopeful about that?

PATIENT: The idea of really trying to make some sort of personality changes. I feel like I've been doing little "Band-Aid" changes. I would really like to try to come to grips with some stuff.

THERAPIST: What other reactions to the first session did you have?

PATIENT: I felt you really zeroed in on some things and that was stressful, but it was good.

THERAPIST: When you say stressful you mean?

PATIENT: I don't know. I just felt—

THERAPIST: Anxiety.

PATIENT: Yes.

THERAPIST: Zeroing in on some of these issues created some anxiety within you.

PATIENT: Yes. It was like WOW! But that felt good at the same time. I just feel like I'm so defended. It would be good for me to get through that. I felt a lot of anticipation in a positive sense, but anxiety, too.

THERAPIST: So there's a mixture of anxiety and hope.

PATIENT: This morning, especially, I was aware of being very, very anxious.

THERAPIST: And how were you aware of your anxiety this morning.

PATIENT: My stomach. I've been more tuned in to when I feel anxious since I was here and what I experience, and a lot of times it's in my head. It's like, not a headache, but a constricted kind of feeling.

THERAPIST: So what were you thinking this morning?

PATIENT: (*sighs*)

THERAPIST: Did you notice you made a sigh when I asked you that?

PATIENT: (*laughs*) That was one of the things that I was telling my husband, that you pick up on that kind of stuff. That's good, but it's anxiety producing too; I'm not aware of all that [referring to her defense system].

This patient discusses her fear of letting down her guard and falling apart. We may recapitulate her problems as follows:

1. Sense of being an imposter at work. Does not feel she performs adequately even though this is not evident in feedback.
2. Problem with intimacy in close relationships. Tendency to be irritable with husband and son.
3. Sexual issues in relationship with husband.
4. Chronic low-grade depression in adult life.
5. Social avoidance: "I hold back from everything."

Step 1: Identify maladaptive trait, pattern, and style. Bring this to patient's attention. Show how it limits gratification, maintains symptoms, and interferes with attaining goals.

THERAPIST: Which issue should we start with?

PATIENT: The intimacy comes to mind.

The patient discusses the fact that with acquaintances she is more willing to be open and intimate. "With my own family I'm less likely to really talk."

THERAPIST: So there is more avoidance with people you are in ongoing committed relationships with?

The therapist inquires about her sexual functioning.[6] She reports that she has suffered from painful intercourse and that intercourse has been severely curtailed by her vaginismus. She also discloses that she has been inorgasmic all her life but has avoided discussing or acknowledging this problem with her husband. She discusses how detached she was during the birth of her first child and how her milk never came.

Step 2: Isolate trait. Use examples from current, past, and transference relationships to highlight pattern.

PATIENT: What I see in my everyday life is this need to please everybody.

The above clinical vignette is the beginning phase of the defense restructuring leading to a further strengthening of the therapeutic alliance and a disclosure of a major pattern of avoidance and sexual disturbance that was not previously mentioned. The therapist's focus was on the C, the patient's relationship with her husband and also on the T, her interpersonal avoidance with the therapist.

Step 3: Select restructuring approach. (a) Determine whether to undertake a comprehensive restructuring of the personality or a stepwise approach. (b) Select one or a combination of the following methods: defensive, affective, or cognitive restructuring.

Restructuring

The patient is detached and not in touch with her feelings. The first portion of the session is devoted to establishing the constellation of defenses and familiarizing the patient with her defense system by emphasizing the transference manifestation and resistances. This builds up irritation that increases defensive responding. The patient acknowledges irritation toward the therapist saying, "What do you expect? I've been like this all my life!"

This is a common reaction with patients suffering from long-standing character pathology. Many of them believe the popular notion that you cannot change personality and certainly not in a brief time frame. The therapist should pose the question: "Why not?" The patient then describes an incident in which she was angry toward her son because he responded in an avoidant fashion. Again, to recapitulate a crucial point with the Cluster C patient: *The therapist should attempt to access the anger* whenever there is an incident that warrants this. However, *if, during the process, other emotions come to the surface first, they should be metabolized by affective and cognitive restructuring methods.*

PATIENT: I went into a big speech about—

THERAPIST: So you lectured him. How did you experience your anger toward him? Physically, you said you were angry with him; how did you experience that? Do you notice as soon as I say the word anger, you freeze?

PATIENT: When you say physically, I'm not used to really tuning into that, I guess. I don't remember what I felt. I remember more of what I thought than what I felt.

THERAPIST: But if you keep this on an intellectual level then you're not going to get the most out of this.

PATIENT: (*clearly angry, with raised hand, and increased volume*) I don't remember! I feel tense.

THERAPIST: What else besides tension?

PATIENT: Frustration (*hitting leg with fist*).

THERAPIST: Let's see how you experience the frustration?

PATIENT: (*laughs*)

THERAPIST: Because as soon as your anger comes you want to either avoid it, intellectualize it, rationalize it, or detach yourself from it, go around it in some way and not really face your feelings.

The patient reports experiencing anxiety. Cognitive restructuring is done helping the patient understand the difference between anxiety and anger. She then reports that there was an incident a month ago when she was in a rage and directed a tirade toward her husband but cannot remember the incident. She says that she cannot ever recall these incidents. More defense restructuring is undertaken because the patient's repressive forces are in operation, and her resistance is high.

PATIENT: I feel like I'm being pushed up against a wall.

THERAPIST: When your feelings come up, you have a need to put up a facade, and it creates a barrier between us.

PATIENT: I don't feel that it's within my control.

THERAPIST: You portray yourself as being helpless, which is yet another mechanism to divert us from your feelings. You took a sigh and looked away again.

The therapist brings the focus back to the incident with the patient's husband, but the resistance continues.

PATIENT: "I don't know how to feel my feelings." I feel a lump right here (*holds chest*).

She declares that she feels angry toward the therapist but smiles. Then she says what she experiences even more strongly is a sad feeling. An affect restructuring intervention—asking her to focus on the sensations—is attempted, but the defenses are too entrenched.

THERAPIST: How deep does it go?

PATIENT: I feel like there is this (*gesticulates with hands*) that wants to come out.

[The focus is on the patient's sadness and her defense against this painful affect. The defenses emerge again, are pointed out again, and a build up of anger is noted.]

PATIENT: Then it [anger] goes away, and it becomes a helplessness.

THERAPIST: You see, that is a defense. Turning helpless and then getting weepy. These are defenses that cut off your anger. (*Patient sighs.*) And that sigh, so we know there is a lot of feeling inside there.

PATIENT: That's angry. That's angry. Oh shit! [Patient's emotional schemas are activated.] (*She has clenched fists, and she pounds on her legs.*)

THERAPIST: How do you experience it physically?

PATIENT: Like I want to pound something.

THERAPIST: A feeling to pound? So there is a rage inside?

PATIENT: I guess so.

THERAPIST: So an impulse to pound. Pound whom?

PATIENT: I suppose you at the moment.

THERAPIST: In fantasy, if that impulse to pound came out how would you pound me?

PATIENT: Like this (*pounds air*).

THERAPIST: What part of me?

PATIENT: Your shoulders. Yelling and screaming and kicking in the shins.

THERAPIST: How long would it last if it emerged?

[The focus is kept to the impulse in the transference. The patient tries to divert by wanting to talk about her anger toward her husband, but the transference focus is maintained.]

PATIENT: I just picture flailing my arms and yelling, "Leave me alone!"

THERAPIST: And what would happen if that happened?

PATIENT: I'm feeling something sexual—I feel warmth and sexual tension in that part of my body.

THERAPIST: Which part?

PATIENT: In the vaginal area.

THERAPIST: So there's a sexual arousal in your genitals. Is that positive?

PATIENT: It's scary. That's embarrassing.

THERAPIST: What else are you aware of?

PATIENT: Like a tremendous constriction, a shortness of breath. That seemed to be related to when I was feeling angry.

THERAPIST: But if that kind of attack came through to me, what would happen? There is a lot of energy still left in your hand. What would happen if that—

PATIENT: I think I picture myself at 12. I'm associating to my parents. My mother, suffocating.

THERAPIST: What's the image?

PATIENT: Very overprotective, very suffocating. Instilling all kinds of prohibitions about sexuality. You'll be taken advantage of. Nice girls don't do this. I sure ended hung up as a result of it. I was terrified of boys, terrified they would do this awful stuff to me. I can remember being really frightened of what they would do and of intercourse. Getting pregnant would be the ultimate horror in my mother's eyes.

Step 4: Relate patterns to core structure. Bring feelings from core difficulties to surface and assist the patient in the process of metabolizing them.

PATIENT: The thing is so many people grew up with that. That was the thing at that age.

THERAPIST: But if we start to generalize though, we are going to get away from your feelings again. What you're describing is a relationship with your mother that was very suffocating, and this has had a tremendous impact on your life.

PATIENT: And I know that I had negative feelings about her, and I didn't want to be like her, but that's how I am now. Now I see how aloof my father was. She glommed onto me because he didn't talk about emotions.

The patient then discusses how she admired her father, although he had an awful temper, and she would blame her mother for nagging him and making him angry. She then remembers an incident at age 12 when her father threw a cup because her mother was nagging him but then says that she cannot actually picture him angry. She then reports that her father is living and that she has always worked hard to please him. She discusses hating her mother who died 8 years ago. The focus then returns to analyzing the transference and linking the feeling to the genetic figures.

THERAPIST: As soon as your anger comes, it gets channeled into anxiety. You have all these defenses you use that keep the anxiety down: laughing it off, the generalizing, the rationalizing, the avoiding. The defenses are against the anxiety, but underneath the anxiety is anger. And this seems to be linked in some way with an expectation that you should please.

The therapist must monitor the time carefully and keep within the alloted time bounds. The first half of the session should be summarized and the session closed. Following a break of 15 minutes, the session recommences.

THERAPIST: So how did you feel and what did you think over the break?

[Investigating what occurred to the patient over the break is a good test for how accessible the unconscious of the patient is. For example, many patients report intense feelings or fresh associations or feelings toward the therapist.]

PATIENT: I kept thinking about the anger and the sexuality. Oedipal stuff, I suppose. I started to feel like I was exploding, somewhat sexually, mixed with anxiety. Everything about me just doesn't want to let go. I feel turned on, sexually aroused.

The therapist recapitulates the core issues touched on during the session: the critical, smothering mother and distant father and the patient's labeling of her mother as the "bad guy." The patient then reported that, while she was in graduate school, her mother confided to her that her father was impotent. "I was dying! To think my mother told me this!" She then reports an incident that occurred at age 14. She was sleeping in a one room cottage with her parents and heard them have sex. She reported feeling terrified. As the capacity for intimacy with the therapist deepens and the defense system is partially restructured, the patient's relevant communications multiply.

PATIENT: I was a virgin at 33. I mean that is not normal.

THERAPIST: So up until 33 you avoided sex. (*Patient looks angry.*) So what's there?

PATIENT: I'm angry with my mother about that (*quiet voice*).

THERAPIST: But do you notice how quiet your voice is?

PATIENT: It's like tragic, really. And I still don't have a normal, fulfilled sexual life. I feel like I'm cheated. I feel like my mother really screwed me up there. I'm aware of the sadness. Because other people were brought up with the same sexual code, and they're not screwed up.

THERAPIST: Did you masturbate?

PATIENT: Only inadvertently.

The patient discusses how she made a conscious decision to be nice [reaction formation] to her parents because they would die and she didn't want to feel guilty when they did, so she avoided anger. She then mentions a "promiscuous" friend who had sex with her boyfriend. The therapist challenges this perception of promiscuity, and the patient agrees that this alone is not indicative of promiscuity. The therapist refocuses on the anger toward the mother that has never been resolved. The patient discusses how impatient she was with her mother's illness before she died. Her mother was complaining about not feeling well, and the patient became irritated. "She saw herself as a martyr. Instead of feeling sympathetic, I would feel angry."

The next vignette focuses on the mother's death. It is quite common for personality disordered patients from all clusters to have impacted grief when a genetic figure dies. *The therapist should help mobilize the grief process so that buried feeling can be metabolized.* This often allows deeper work to occur. The therapist may return to the pathological grief later in therapy after the core issues have been addressed, which will allow a fuller experience of the grief process.

THERAPIST: So what was the last interaction with her like?

PATIENT: She looked awful. She was just so bloated and everything.

THERAPIST: What did she say to you?

PATIENT: I had stenciled this little hoop thing. That's how oblivious I was to what was going on. I was being reassuring. I was trying at that point to not fall apart, to cry. That intimacy, to say that I loved her. I was trying to not fall apart.

THERAPIST: So for you, becoming emotional would mean falling apart?

PATIENT: That intimacy. I couldn't imagine talking to her, not with a real connection. Not with an acknowledged emotion. It was like you had to protect people from that.

THERAPIST: What was her funeral like?

PATIENT: I remember, consciously saying to myself that you've got to talk with him about this, to my father. I know that I deny things, and I just wanted to talk to him about it. I couldn't. Just what he felt about dying. I managed a little bit [*painful wave of grief-laden affect*]. But he's so goddamn remote (*anger evident*). It was some opportunity for me to connect with him. I remember not wanting to bury it like everything else. Some of the sadness is for her but some is for the relationship with my father; it is just so pathetic (*intense grief, patient crying*).

THERAPIST: So it is very painful that there is no closeness between you and your father. And that even in your mother's death there is no accessibility. Showing feelings is something you just didn't do. What was your good-bye to her?

PATIENT: I've been thinking, my poor little mother. She just had such a lousy life. She never got what she wanted from him, and then she had all that pain and suffering. I was relieved, too. I was always afraid of what we would ever do if something happened to my father, and she had to live with us, and how we would ever survive. It's a sadness that the relationship was not better. If she had her dream, I would have lived in her home town, Sunday dinners. I fought that.

She then returns to a current incident with her father where she felt criticized, but the details are vague. This is indicative of the need for further defense restructuring. Her avoidant style is firmly entrenched in her personality, as she avoids almost everything conflictual.

THERAPIST: So you see with emotional things the details sort of evaporate. And that's another way that you keep away from your emotions. Whether it's a fight with your husband that happened last month, or this incident with your father where he was judgmental and critical, or your son when he is being oppositional and difficult, or whether it's me in here where you feel like I'm pushing you.

PATIENT: That does happen.

THERAPIST: What are you feeling right now?

PATIENT: Like, here we are at an impasse, again.

THERAPIST: You see your defense system goes into operation around strong feelings. Not just anger, but also sexual feelings, grief. All your feelings are in a way constricted by this defensive system that you built up over the years, which is paralyzing you and kills the intimacy in your relationships. But we have a little bit of a glimpse at what is at the bottom of this. One, you had a very distant father–daughter relationship where he was emotionally unavailable to you, and you have strong feeling about that. And the other is that you have this relationship with your mother where she was very critical and controlling, holding onto you in a way, and dismissing and putting down your sexuality.

PATIENT: And my father always thought she was kind of a jerk. He always kind of put down femininity. He would make fun of femininity. I can remember thinking she was not too bright and not wanting to be like her for that reason.

THERAPIST: So are you saying that you rejected her to gain his approval? You rejected aspects of your femininity?

PATIENT: I think I felt he always wanted a boy.

The patient explores her relationship with her father and then reports she feels tired. This illustrates the depressive mechanism at work, a common defense for many personality disordered patients. Usually this is anger turned inward, but other feelings may be closer to the conscious experience, especially grief. The patient's feelings are being channeled into fatigue and tiredness. More defense work is undertaken to mobilize her affect, and she becomes sad.

PATIENT: I did remember sitting in his lap and stuff when I was a kid, when I was little, maybe 6 or 8. I think it was when I got to adolescence or puberty that it all went to shit.

THERAPIST: Let's look at sitting in his lap; how did it feel?

PATIENT: I have this image of sitting in his lap fiddling with his hair, happy. I think he was more comfortable then.

THERAPIST: What did you feel toward him?

PATIENT: Love.

It emerges that when the patient was entering puberty, her father withdrew his affection. The focus then becomes this link between paternal withdrawal and sexuality.

PATIENT: That made me a woman that he didn't approve of. If I saw him as disapproving of femininity and I wanted to attract boys, he would disapprove of me. I gave up on goddamn femininity because of him! (*wave of grief and anger*) But I never thought of it in terms of trying to please him.

THERAPIST: He couldn't tolerate women because of his own mother. Or, to be more specific, he couldn't tolerate his own daughter's sexual development, and at that point, you lost him. And you denied your sexuality for 30-some years in hopes that—

PATIENT: Under the guise of, nice girls don't do that sort of thing.

THERAPIST: Nice girls might be loved by their father if they're asexual because they are not threatening. So you see that there is something very important that happened between you and me. Do you remember when you started to get in touch with your anger toward me. What did you experience?

PATIENT: (*soft voice*) Some sexuality.

THERAPIST: And what did you do as soon as you started to experience the sexual excitement.

PATIENT: I got anxious. I shut down.

THERAPIST: And what's the first relationship where a girl experiences her sexual excitement? Was it that your sexual feelings caused your father to abandon you?

The focus is then on oedipal attachment toward the father, her fear of incest, and her total denial of her sexuality. It includes the loss of the already distant father at puberty and denouncing her sexuality in an attempt to maintain her link with him.

PATIENT: I never saw how remote he was. I thought *she* drove him (*flings arms out*).

THERAPIST: What was she looking for?

PATIENT: Something—love.

THERAPIST: So how did she feel?

PATIENT: Isolated and denigrated. So when I would come home she would glom onto me, and I would feel suffocated by her.

THERAPIST: So she tried to get the attachment from you. And what did she get from you? Nothing. Even when she's dying, you're showing her stencils when she's on her death bed. But you had built a massive wall with her and had identified with your father.

PATIENT: I really felt sorry for that. I can see how we both shut her out.

THERAPIST: Which must have made her more frantic. And then even as an adult she tried to talk to you, and you didn't want to hear it.

PATIENT: I think she must of been so desperate to even bring it up [father's impotence] because that wasn't in her code. You don't talk like that in our family; you just don't discuss that with your daughter. Sexuality wasn't displayed; it wasn't anything ever acknowledged.

THERAPIST: By whom?

PATIENT: By anyone.

THERAPIST: Well your mother acknowledged it. At least she said, "Don't do it." But there was at least an acknowledgment.

PATIENT: That there was something *not* to do.

THERAPIST: That is an acknowledgment that you're sexual. It wasn't a total denial of your femininity and sexuality. Your father just cut you off.

PATIENT: I'm feeling what a shit I was to her, guilt. Guilt is also the number one theme in my life.

THERAPIST: At some point you must have been very angry at your mother to cut her off. And then in continuing to try to please your father, you denied your sexuality because that was your link with him. But in the interim, you lost your mother. You pushed her away, and she became more frantic.

PATIENT: What I did to try to separate was move far away.

THERAPIST: You never stood up to her.

The therapist starts to bring the session to a close and explores the patient's feelings toward the therapist and what was covered in the session. The therapist explores the patient's positive feelings, which she has difficulty describing. The patient is asked how many sessions she thinks it would take to resolve her difficulties. A treatment schedule is then drawn up.

THERAPIST: Any other reactions to the trial therapy today?

PATIENT: I'm surprised, and I'm *not* surprised at the strength of my—the pervasiveness of my defenses. I've seen it. [This is an indication that the defenses are becoming less ego-syntonic.] I feel like I've felt it more; that's a good feeling, it really is.

THERAPIST: We scratched the surface of many of feelings today, but I think your feelings are much deeper than that, and if we can get to the full intensity of them, I think the whole system can be changed. The goal of therapy is that you get a total resolution. If we get the outcome we are looking for, you would have a full intimate emotional and sexual relationship with your husband. And the issues at work would totally resolve, in terms of your self-esteem about what you do.

PATIENT: That sounds too good to be true.

Two weeks later, sessions five and six (two back-to-back sessions) are scheduled and begin as follows:

PATIENT: (*smiling, looking strikingly more feminine*) So I start, right?

THERAPIST: Usually with the first thing on your mind.

PATIENT: I guess what was on my mind is how many things were on my mind.

THERAPIST: Why don't you list the things? Then we can plan what the focus is today.

PATIENT: I think the first think I've was aware of is being more aware of my body sensations.

The patient's unconscious is clearly open, and resistances are lowered. The patient is relating in a much more straightforward manner. She is not giggling or laughing in the same way she had during the trial therapy. She reports thinking about her mother's death and remembering more about that and also her grandmother, who was a significant figure: "I think her death was a really major, major event." Then she reports that her grandfather dropped dead when he was taking her mother to the hospital to give birth to her. Her father was away in the service at that time. The funeral procession passed by the hospital: "If I hadn't been born, other people would probably not blame me for his death." She associates her birth with her grandfather's death. Her mother was very close to her grandfather and was grief stricken when he died. She remembers the devastating feeling of loss when her grandmother died but not feeling she could talk about it. She also reports seeing parallels between her husband and her father that she talked to her husband about. She reports enjoying sex more with her husband: "I felt freer." The next focus is on the patient's anger as well as positive feeling toward the therapist for his persistence.

PATIENT: Feeling that in the past I got away with avoiding a lot of things. Wishing maybe that I had picked up on more things.

THERAPIST: In terms of me, there was some anger that I was being so persistent and confronting your defenses, but on the other hand, there was a feeling of gratitude.

The focus is then on the transference. The patient reports she is irritated because of the therapist's lack of emotion. The therapist has not commented on her appearance, which is stirring up strong feeling related to her father's avoidance and belittling of her sexuality and femininity. The interpretation is not made, but the therapist uses this to guide the process to her anger.

PATIENT: I want you to react to me in someway.

THERAPIST: React in what way?

PATIENT: Some smile, some acknowledgment of—I think you did that a little last week when—

THERAPIST: So how do you experience the anger that I'm not smiling or reacting in the way you want.

PATIENT: Anger, anger. I feel like I'm being tricked. I don't feel it. I can't just turn it on. I feel like giving up.

More defense identification and analysis are undertaken. The patient's resistances are in operation. The focus then shifts to a incident where she got angry toward her husband but again cannot remember the details. The connection between repressing her feelings, especially anger, avoiding conflict, and becoming depressed (depressive mechanism) is pointed out. The patient is asked to describe an incident in which she remembers being in a massive rage. She describes her infant son defying her by destroying his slippers, and she became enraged and pounded a railing.

PATIENT: Absolutely unleashed rage; I guess I could kill him.

THERAPIST: If that part came out how would you do it?

PATIENT: Just pummelling him.

THERAPIST: How would you feel immediately afterward?

PATIENT: I don't want to think about that. I feel stupid. To sit here and picture hurting my son. He would be screaming and terrified and afraid of me. Picturing this wild woman!

THERAPIST: So if that wild woman came out what would be the damage?

PATIENT: There would be emotional damage. I guess anybody's ultimate with rage is somebody ends up dead. I'm not aware of feeling that, but that would be the natural conclusion. How do you think anyone would react if they killed their kid? I'm feeling manipulated, fantasizing stuff like that.

THERAPIST: Murder. You're really afraid of the part of you that has destructive impulses, and you want to portray yourself as only having nice impulses.

The patient then recalls an incident when her father broke her favorite doll in a fit of rage, but she is not able to get in touch with her feelings toward her father. She places this incident around the time her grandmother died. The focus is on the relationship with her grandmother. When she died, her mother would not allow her to go to the funeral. "My whole world fell apart. She meant the world to me." She never had an opportunity to say good-bye.

PATIENT: I can feel it now how much I missed her. I remember feeling like she was my refuge when my parents would argue. I was special to her. I was the special grandchild. [Grief-laden affect surfaces.] When I was a little girl, I never felt like there was anyone I could talk to.

THERAPIST: You weren't able to say good-bye to her?

PATIENT: She just loved me (*crying*).

THERAPIST: So there was a great deal of grief and anger that she abandoned you.

PATIENT: She was my refuge. There was a time when my mother told me they were thinking about divorce. I could go stay overnight. In my mind she was perfect. I knew that I was special. I always felt that she loved me.

She then discusses her feelings about her grandfather's death and the impact on the family. Apparently, he was much beloved.

THERAPIST: Do you think your mother blamed you?

PATIENT: In order for me to come into the world—I was demanding to be born.

THERAPIST: Because you're talking about a very special relationship with your grandmother that you usually have with your mother. That special mirroring relationship. Because if your mother was depressed—

PATIENT: She was devastated. I think some aunt told me. Why would that have been kept secret if it weren't a terrible thing? She probably wasn't able to nurture me.

THERAPIST: So in your unconscious there is a strong association between death and birth. She was grieving while she was attaching to you. Why would you ever let yourself get close to anyone? It kills them.

PATIENT: When she died [grandmother], it was like my mother died.

Step 5: Encourage more adaptive patterns. (a) Encourage activities, challenges, and positive adaptive patterns that were previously avoided. (b) Process patient's experience and reaction.

During the middle phase of therapy, the patient is encouraged to deal with avoided situations. For example, she is encouraged to engage her husband instead of avoiding him and withdrawing. She is encouraged to try her newfound skills at work and in relationship with her children, particularly her son, who has been passive and defiant. She is also encouraged to deal directly with her husband instead of withholding sex.

Summary of Remainder of Process

As the therapeutic process unfolded, other issues came to light that had not been discussed in the initial phase of treatment. The patient expressed a concern about her alcohol consumption. The use of substances during therapy is discussed more fully in Chapter 10, but suffice it to say that using drugs or alcohol slows the therapeutic process, as the deep restructuring cannot have the required intensity.

Apparently, for a number of years, the patient would come home from work and have a few glasses of wine and retreat to her room while her husband worked on his hobbies. She eventually saw the destructiveness of this pattern and reduced her alcohol consumption dramatically. It was also noted that her father had developed a drinking problem and that she would often consume alcohol with him in an attempt to be accepted. It also became clear that the patient suffered from a rather severe case of vaginismus throughout her married life. This was resolved almost entirely during the first block of treatment. Therapy was terminated after 38 sessions with good results. A 6-month follow-up was scheduled. However, after 2 months, the patient phoned and requested to be seen. There was evidence of regression, and the therapist and patient agreed to complete another round of treatment. During this phase of treatment, severe dependency cravings were worked through that seemed related to preoedipal attachment issues. This block of therapy lasted 34 sessions. Restructuring proceeds at a slower pace when the patient narcotizes his or her anxiety. In this case, the patient's unacknowledged alcohol dependence protracted the treatment beyond the usual length expected. The fact that the therapy with the personality disordered patient has multiple foci is highlighted in this case. With such a patient, each focal issue needs to be elaborated and derepressed. The core genetic structure unfolded as follows:

Core Genetic Structure Highlighted

The patient's core genetic structure followed the following pattern:

1. The patient's grandfather died taking her mother to the hospital to give birth to the patient, who was an only child. Her father was overseas at the time. The patient's mother formed an insufficient bond with her infant because of her grief, causing a narcissistic wound.

2. The parents' marriage was troubled. The patient often overheard them fighting. Later, the patient found out that her father was impotent and that her mother was sexually unfulfilled.

3. The patient had an affectionate bond with her maternal grandmother who died when the patient was 8. She was devastated and had a pathological grief reaction.

4. The patient's father was emotionally distant and denigrating to his wife and to women. However, the patient experienced him as somewhat affectionate toward her until puberty, when he cut her off. She renounced her sexuality in a futile attempt to stay connected to him.

5. The patient's mother attempted to have a close relationship with the patient, but the more she tried, the more distant the patient behaved, stimulating more of her mother's desperate attempts to cling to her.

6. The patient's mother died and again there were signs of a pathological grief reaction.

EVIDENCE FROM CLINICAL FINDINGS

These two cases highlight a number of issues that must be taken into consideration with the Cluster C patients.

1. Repressed hostility toward the genetic figure(s) is almost always part of the core genetic structure, as well as pathological grief over unresolved losses.

2. There are often mixtures of disturbed attachment issues and oedipal conflicts.

3. The initial picture of the core genetic structure will often change as the unconscious becomes more fluid, and defenses are partially restructured. The genetic formulation unfolds and becomes clearer with each cycle of derepression and working through. However, it remains crucial to have a working formulation to begin with.

4. Other problems not mentioned at the onset of therapy will emerge as the therapeutic alliance is enhanced and trust is deepened.

5. The emphasis with this cluster is almost always going to entail heavy defense restructuring.

6. Even though the patient may appear to be functioning well to outside observers, severe disturbances of life functions are almost always existent.

7. Personality disordered patients' genetic structures have multiple foci. Resistances and defenses return with each core issue that is uncovered.

8. Maintaining as much therapeutic neutrality as possible facilitates the intensity and rapidity of the transference phenomenon. This is the stance of choice, especially with patients who have a high degree of motivation.

The next case presented of an avoidant personality highlights important differences that indicate the need for a less ambitious and comprehensive approach. This can be conceived of as a module of treatment that serves as the basis for a deeper working through at a later point in time, if the patient so decides. This case is not presented in as much detail as the previous case. The differences in approaches will be discussed to highlight some of the technical differences.

STEPWISE APPROACH WITH A HIGHLY EGO-SYNTONIC AVOIDANT PERSONALITY DISORDER—THE CASE OF THE MAN WHO FEARED HE WOULD BE VIOLENT

The patient was a married man in his late 20s who entered treatment after participating in a depression screening clinic at a local facility. It was recommended that he be seen for psychological treatment. He reported a mild level of depression since adolescence. He appeared highly ego-syntonic. In the initial interview, it became apparent that the patient suffered from an avoidant personality disorder. He was very concrete (no evidence of organicity) and did not seem to have even a rudimentary capacity for psychological mindedness. His wife recently had had a second child and was feeling overwhelmed and unsupported due to his lack of involvement. He appeared very hesitant, blushed easily, and was very defensive about his concerns. His eye contact was fleeting. He seemed to want to keep things on a surface level and discussed some general complaints about his job dissatisfaction. He frequently was pushed around by other employees even though he held a job of some responsibility. He had no close friends, although he did report some positive attachments. The patient was highly detached and yet very anxiety ridden. He spoke in a halting and soft voice, nearly a whisper. His motivation for treatment was assessed to be low. He had some difficulty formulating the goals he wished to achieve, although he did want to feel better.

Assessment

Although the patient had sufficient ego strength to tolerate a rapid uncovering approach, his motivation to sustain an in-depth restructuring was assessed to be low. He thought he could probably resolve things in a few sessions. A time-limited framework was agreed upon because of low motivation to work on characterological difficulties. With patients who show this degree of resistance, it is important to set a predetermined number of sessions, or the patient will likely terminate prematurely and never experience the termination phase. It was explained to this patient that often a great deal can be accomplished in a short period of time, but usually 12 sessions are required. He was offered a 12-session treatment to attempt to resolve the depression, which was the issue for which he wanted assistance, and he agreed to this. However, it was clear that major characterological disturbance was fueling the depression and that eventually we would have to broaden our focus.

Course of Treatment

The initial session was spent exploring the phenomenology of the patient's depression, establishing treatment goals, and educating the patient about the treatment. The patient agreed to be seen weekly for 45-minute sessions.

The main focus of the first session was to develop a positive therapeutic alliance with this patient, which was a challenge. In order to enhance the alliance, a careful phenomenological evaluation of the patient's depression, its variations and onset, were explored. This slightly increased the alliance, as the patient felt that the therapist was interested in him. Gradually, his pattern of avoidance in the transference was pointed out, such as his avoidance of eye contact, unwillingness to talk about issues, taking a passive position, and withdrawing when anything painful emerged. His avoidance was extremely ego-syntonic, and this was demonstrated by showing how the avoidant pattern manifested itself with his wife and colleagues. Early in the treatment, each session felt like starting over, but the patient eventually responded. A thorough history was taken that revealed some of the sources of this man's disturbances, which were related to unresolved feelings about abuse by his father.

Cognitive Restructuring

This patient was emotionally sealed over and could not relate on an emotional level. Cognitive restructuring was utilized as the first approach by asking him to give examples of times and incidents when his depression seemed worse. It emerged that this was related to situations of interpersonal conflict.

THERAPIST: When was the last time you noticed an increase in your depression?

PATIENT: Thursday, I felt more depressed after work.

THERAPIST: What happened in work?

PATIENT: I had an outstanding order that the client was pressuring me to come up with, but our purchasing department manager never ordered it. I always have problems with her.

THERAPIST: Can you describe the incident and how you reacted?

PATIENT: I called her and asked her what happened, and she gave me the run around.

THERAPIST: How did you react?

PATIENT: I went back to work but felt like going home.

THERAPIST: So you had certain feelings toward her but you reacted with depression and then wanted to avoid work. Is it possible there was some anger toward her?

PATIENT: Yes.

THERAPIST: Do you notice a tendency to avoid your anger in other situations?

PATIENT: Yes, with my wife sometimes.

It becomes clearer to the patient and the therapist that the pattern of avoidance and withdrawal has been long-standing, since adolescence. This patient suffered from a great deal of anxiety when he was an adolescent and essentially avoided situations that would activate his anxiety. The pattern of anxiety, avoidance, and depression was extremely entrenched. The therapist moves from incident to incident identifying the sequence of conflict, repressed feeling, anxiety, avoidance, and depression. The repressed affect is not mobilized, only identified. The patient begins to develop more insight into himself and his reactions but he is still disconnected emotionally. Finally, after a number of incidents have been reviewed and the corners of the triangle I/F, D, and A labeled, the therapist then attempts to mobilize the affect.

The therapist also focuses on the patient's cognitions: "I must control [overcontrol] my anger or I will be damaging like my father. *Anger is dangerous and is to be avoided.*" The first step in cognitive restructuring is to provide intellectual insight into the nature of the patient's psychic apparatus, the defensive structure, feelings, and anxiety. The next step, which begins to desensitize the patient to his/her impulses and makes it acceptable to talk about them, uses fantasy portraits. This serves to bring the affect closer to the surface, to demonstrate that the therapist is not afraid of strong impulses, and further restructure the defenses by showing the patient he/she can withstand the forces within him/herself without resorting to characteristic defensive patterns.

THERAPIST: Can you describe an incident where you became angry?

PATIENT: Yes, the other day my son was not doing what I told him to do, and I was angry.

THERAPIST: Can you describe the incident?

PATIENT: Yes, my son was playing with his food, and I told him to stop. He spilled his milk, and I yelled at him.

THERAPIST: How did you feel?

PATIENT: Angry.

[No indication that the patient is in touch with his feelings.]

THERAPIST: In fantasy, what would have happened if you had totally lost control?

PATIENT: I felt I could have hit him, but I would never do that.

THERAPIST: But if you went over the edge?

PATIENT: I would have grabbed him by the neck and hit him in the face.

THERAPIST: If you did hit him like that what would happen to him as a result?

PATIENT: Like that! I would have injured him severely or worse.

THERAPIST: You mean murdered him? What would he look like if you had lost control and in a fit of rage killed him?

This cognitive restructuring activates the patient's emotional schema. He begins to show signs of sadness related to the yelling and mistreatment of his son. He feels guilty and insists that he never wanted to treat his son like that. The thought of losing him intensifies the grief, and his eyes begin to tear. He then recalls an incident when he was 8 years old.

PATIENT: My father was violent. One time my mother wanted to do something he didn't want her to, and he lost control and punched her in the face.

THERAPIST: What did you do?

PATIENT: I froze.

We then begin to get a clearer picture of the roots of his passivity and avoidance: "If I avoid my father, I can reduce the chance of him blowing up and becoming violent." He then discusses the fact that his father, who was an alcoholic and alienated everyone, was also quite explosive and violent. The patient developed an avoidant defense system so that he would not be the target of his father's violent outbursts. The grief and anger over the disturbed father–son relationship became the main focus of the treatment. The patient then began to deeply mourn this relationship and the impact on his development. He vowed never to hurt his family the way his father did and spent his energy avoiding conflict. However, this approach was creating havoc in his life. A T–C–P interpretation was made linking the avoidance of closeness with his wife to that of his therapist due to the association between violence and intimacy. His secret fear was that if he did get close to anyone he might become destructive.

During the midphase of therapy, a tragic event occurred in the patient's life. A male employee with whom he had a positive relationship was murdered. Because of the work that was done prior to this, the patient for the first time in his life experienced deeply felt grief over this loss. This led to his deeper mourning of the father–son relationship that was always troubled and lacked affection or closeness.

During the last phase of therapy, the patient was showing less avoidance with his wife who encouraged him to enter marital therapy to improve their relationship, to which he agreed. The last phase of the treatment was devoted to termination, the loss of the therapist, who was one of his only close male attachments in his life, and his plan to overcome his longstanding avoidant personality. He was given the option of returning at a future time for an in-depth restructuring that was explained to him. He declared that he was not yet ready for this but would consider it in the future.

This case highlights the fact that in a circumscribed treatment of 12 sessions, avoidant personality traits can be modified, and the patient can be made less ego-syntonic and more psychologically minded.

COMPARISON OF LAST TWO CASES

Although any short-term dynamic approach emphasizes personality change, the increments of change expected depend on many factors that have already been reviewed. The therapist cannot expect the same results with everyone. Although there are many similarities in some of the technical aspects of the way the last two treatments were conducted, there are important differences.

• If the patient has little awareness of his/her difficulties, is not psychologically minded, and has low motivation for change, it is often best to offer a time-limited approach, defining the number of sessions before commencing.

• If the patient does not clearly opt for personality change, then the emphasis on defense analysis and restructuring has to be used judiciously, or negative outcome will result.

• The experience of a positive bond with the therapist that deals with the process of termination so quickly mobilizes strong affect, so often, affective restructuring can be used. Completing a comprehensive restructuring, however, involves multiple derepressions and extensive working through. For some patients, this can be achieved in very brief periods of time.

• More time has to be spent on history and phenomenology with resistant patients who are poorly motivated, so that the core issue can be formulated without having the benefit of material that emerges from derepressions of the unconscious.

• With highly resistant and poorly motivated patients, the therapy is going to entail more grief emphasis than anger, which is more threatening. The therapist can do cognitive restructuring to prepare for more work with anger at a later date.

CONCLUSION

The cases presented in this chapter are fairly representative of the spectrum of characterological disturbances represented by those patients who fall within Cluster C. It is often difficult to determine what makes one patient respond to a very brief intervention and another require more systematic effort and time. This issue will be discussed in greater depth in Chapter 11.

CHAPTER 9

Cluster B Disorders: The Mixed-Results Group

I was, at first, ready to sink down with surprise, for I saw my
deliverance indeed visibly put into my hands, all things easy, and a
large ship just ready to carry me away, whither I pleased to go.
—DANIEL DEFOE, *Robinson Crusoe*

The Cluster B personality disorders include the antisocial, borderline, histrionic, and narcissistic personality disorders. "Individuals with these disorders often appear dramatic, emotional, or erratic" (American Psychiatric Association, 1994, p. 630). These disorders generally present a challenge to the short-term therapist, and yet the application of short-term methods can have profound effects with certain patients from this group. Unlike the Cluster C patients presented in Chapter 8, there is significant diversity in the Cluster B categories, and especially significant are their differential responses to treatment. This chapter is subtitled "The Mixed-Results Group" because, although patients do improve, it is not at the same pace or with equivalent depth of change often witnessed in the Cluster C disorders.

Treatment with this cluster is more difficult than with Cluster C because of the greater diversity of characterological and developmental issues. Of the four personality disorders in this group, both clinical practice and the scant research indicate that the histrionic is the most amenable to STDP. I present this group first, with a detailed case example. The narcissistic group also usually responds well, except for the extremely malignant

199

ones who often have sociopathic traits. Cognitive restructuring is indicated for most borderlines. Managing the self-destructive behavior that is commonplace with this group is initially best done by a team of therapists, with the use of support groups and behavioral contracting (Linehan, 1993). The defense and affect restructuring methods can be used in the treatment of borderlines once the acting out is contained, but until this occurs, derepressive work should not be attempted. I have found that flexible scheduling can be an excellent format for borderlines. I establish a relationship and let them decide when and how frequently to return for booster sessions.

The antisocial group has many degrees of severity with varying levels of sociopathy (Stone, 1993). I have used STDP with patients who have sociopathic features with good results, but full-blown antisocial personalities are unresponsive. I will focus on the subgroups that are most responsive.

COMPREHENSIVE TREATMENT OF A PATIENT WITH A HISTRIONIC PERSONALITY—THE CASE OF THE WOMAN WHO WAS ALWAYS A VICTIM

The patient entered treatment at the recommendation of a friend who had been successfully treated with STDP. The patient, in her early 30s at the time of treatment, had a history of depression and chronic suicidality, for which she had been treated with individual psychotherapy and medication.

Stepwise Approach

Following an initial evaluation, the patient was judged to be an unsuitable candidate for an in-depth, rapid restructuring. Because of the chronic nature of her suicidality and reports of previous treatments, during which she had been told by one clinician that she would need medication and psychotherapy all her life, an empathic phase of treatment was initiated to test her capacity to form a collaborative relationship and to insure a sound alliance before proceeding with more anxiety-arousing methods. She was seen twice a week for seven sessions. The following assessment was completed during the first consultation with the patient.

Assessment

Presenting Complaint

The patient presented saying, "I've been in therapy for 3 years unsuccessfully[1] with a number of different psychologists and psychiatrists."

History of Past Illness

The patient reports experiencing a combination of anxiety and depression for 5 years. During this time she was seen by numerous social workers, psychologists, and psychiatrists for "problems with anxiety." She had a number of somatic symptoms, the most notable of which were stomach pains, which were evaluated by a gastroenterologist. She was treated with various psychopharmacological agents. She became depressed and suicidal, began to hear voices, and cried all the time. The patient had been hospitalized for 2 weeks on an inpatient psychiatric unit.

Mental Status Examination

The patient is oriented and ego functions appear intact. There is no evidence of hallucinations, delusions, or thought disorder. On the Sunday prior to the evaluation, the patient said that she had thought about slashing her wrists and threatened to kill herself but made no overt gestures. She is currently on antidepressant medication (Prozac) and has a history of depression that ranges from mild to severe. She also has a history of panic attacks, particularly when she goes into a crowded room or elevator. She is fearful in interpersonal relationships, particularly with men. She has low self-esteem and feels unworthy. She has a fear of getting fat. She also has a history of irritable bowel syndrome. Her affect was sad, and she seemed fearful and anxious. She described feeling discouraged with therapy and felt that her previous therapist encouraged her dependency on him and "hadn't addressed the issues." A friend who had been treated with STDP had recommended the therapist.

First Phase of Treatment

During the first phase of treatment, the patient was seen twice weekly to establish a therapeutic relationship and to make further assessment because of her complex admixture of characterological disturbance, psychophysiological disorders, history of clinical depression, and suicidal preoccupation. At first sight, this patient appeared to be a very poor candidate for STDP. However, this case underscores the necessity of viewing every patient with a fresh perspective and not being deterred by the severity of previous evaluations and/or diagnostic labels. Evaluations and previous history are important to consider, but clinicians should suspend judgment until clinical contact with the patient. Although this patient was initially discouraged from pursuing a short-term approach, it soon became apparent that she was motivated to make changes, and she requested that the approach be attempted. Her evaluation from the hospital noted that she was organized at a neurotic level and that her unconscious was accessible. She also appeared to be intelligent and had a desire to understand herself and to recover. She was likable and genuinely sought to make contact.

The first phase of the treatment was not audiovisually recorded, so that transcripts of the sessions cannot be presented. However, this treatment phase of the stepwise approach was characterized primarily by empathic attunement, that is, mirroring, exploring phenomenology of her depression and anxiety, and cognitive restructuring. The cognitive restructuring focused on making connections between the patient's depressive reactions and withheld anger. No major exploration of the past was undertaken, as this could overload the patient if the defenses are not first restructured.

During this primarily cognitive phase of treatment, the therapist provides information to the patient about how feelings are avoided and channeled into symptoms and defenses. Beliefs about "unworthiness" and being "unlovable" are explored and related to low self-esteem. After the initial phase, there was no evidence that the patient was borderline or that her ego was compromised. She responded to the approach by becoming less depressed. She requested STDP, and an extended session was arranged with the understanding that she might not be able to tolerate the approach and might have to resume a more supportive approach.

Extended Session

The extended session was 3 hours in length with a 15-minute break halfway through. This session and subsequent sessions were audiovisually recorded. The remainder of the treatment consisted of eight 1½-hour sessions every 2 weeks. Follow-up was conducted a little past the 6-month (from termination) point and was also audiovisually recorded. A 2-year follow-up was conducted by telephone. Excerpts of these outcome interviews are presented in Chapter 12. The following is a summary of treatment time frame:

> Initial consultation—45 minutes
> Supportive dynamic phase—six 45-minute sessions, twice a week
> Extended session—four 45-minute sessions
> Course of treatment—eight 90-minute sessions, bimonthly
> Follow-up—6 months after termination, 90-minute session
> Total number of sessions—28 45-minute sessions including follow-up
> Two-year phone follow-up

We now go to the opening of the extended session. The patient has brought a book on anger with her.

THERAPIST: What were your thoughts and feelings about the extended session today?

PATIENT: I still am nervous abut it.

THERAPIST: You have some anxiety?

PATIENT: A little.

THERAPIST: And what is the anxiety related to?

PATIENT: Being in a situation where I don't feel like I'm in control.

THERAPIST: What about this situation makes you feel like you're not in control?

PATIENT: I guess I always feel that way with doctors. I know nobody forced me to do this, but I feel like I don't have complete control.

The initial phase of this session immediately focuses on the patient's transference feeling—anxiety related to her feelings toward the male therapist. This should be thoroughly explored and brought out into the open. The therapist's interest in understanding the meaning of this should be conveyed with gentle questioning.

THERAPIST: It's important that we examine it because you come here with a certain anxiety, and the thought in your head is there is something about control or not having full control when you're with doctors. What are your thoughts about that?

PATIENT: Past experiences.

THERAPIST: Which past experiences come to mind?

The therapist actively encourages the patient's associations by asking, "What are you thinking?" "What comes to mind?" or "What are your associations to that?" When the patient responds to these inquiries, it is one indication that the resistances are at a low level, and there is a good therapeutic alliance. Resistances and defenses will emerge as the process deepens and feeling is activated over the core issues.

PATIENT: I guess from the time I had the ectopic pregnancy. Actually before that, the fact that I was so wrongly diagnosed, for such a period of time and treated like I was an ignorant little girl, in many cases, by many doctors.

THERAPIST: You had a lot of negative experiences with doctors? Was there one in particular that comes to mind?

As rapidly as possible, the therapist wants to anchor his/her discussion to a specific incident so that the restructuring phase of the therapy can proceed and defense constellations can be observed and brought to the attention of the patient.

PATIENT: I don't know his name. At Planned Parenthood, I guess a month before I got pregnant, I was having severe cramps all the time. And he was laughing at me saying, "Why don't you get on the pill and get rid of all these problems?" That was his solution, I mean after examining me and not being able to find anything. And that's the kind of male attitude I experienced as a kid from my father. You know, that you're just stupid, and you don't know what you're doing.

THERAPIST: So some of the anxiety that you have has to do with being humiliated by people in authority and that you have some loss of control. What other things caused your anxiety today?

PATIENT: That's the main one.

The therapist discusses having received the patient's records from her hospitalization and the fact that there were no contraindications for short-term psychotherapy. The patient then questions her diagnosis. The therapist asks the patient to review the issues and symptoms that she wants to address.

The following issues are identified and explored in a collaborative atmosphere: *anxiety*; *depression* (her depression seems to have lifted "for the most part"); *lack of self-worth/low self-esteem* ("I think there is something definitely wrong with me. . . . Just liking myself is a big issue; I never have"); *anger* (the patient says she does not know how to deal with anger); *anorexia* ("Starving myself, I just don't deserve to eat. I don't want to get fat so I don't deserve to eat"). The patient declares, "I want to just get better and go on with my life, and that's why I really want to focus on what's bothering me."

THERAPIST: What's happened since we got together?

PATIENT: I've been having very strange dreams. I'm so sick of them. One dream that I had, my sister was in it; she must have been picking on me or teasing me. I got so angry I finally went to punch her (*demonstrates with hand*), and I actually did punch.

THERAPIST: You never have had a dream where you're violent?

PATIENT: I'm always a victim.

THERAPIST: Have there been any times over the past few weeks when you were angry?

This is a common characterological trait in patients who are severely disconnected from their anger. They often are victimized and gain some gratification in the power they hold over the victimizing figure.

The patient describes an incident where her cat jumped on her and scratched her back. The patient was clearly not in touch with her anger, but she describes feeling tension. The therapist addresses the difference between tension and anger, but it is not clear to the patient. She describes other incidents where she thought she was angry, and she begins to see the pattern of unexperienced, repressed feeling and the channel to anxiety and character defenses—passivity, submissiveness, pleasing, and helplessness. Usually, with each incident reviewed in this manner, there is a slight increase in true anger; it begins to build. This is like stoking a smoldering fire by using bellows to add oxygen. The patient will respond by becoming more engaged if this is done methodically and the defenses are not prematurely stressed.

The patient next describes an incident in which she was pushed down by a boyfriend and her reaction of shock. Other incidents are explored and cognitive restructuring techniques are utilized, clarifying for her the difference among defense, anxiety, and anger but with only mild defense analysis. The focus then becomes the transference feeling.

PATIENT: Maybe I'm afraid to get angry—I just feel like if I get angry I'm going to take it out on you. I mean you're the perfect person to do it to; you're a male.

THERAPIST: Is there some anger toward me right now?

PATIENT: Not really towards you.

THERAPIST: So one thing you say is that there is an issue with anger towards men, and that I'm a perfect target because I'm a male. But whatever it is, we should get to your feelings *today*. Besides your fear of letting me get into your innermost self, you're also terrified to get in touch with this angry part.

The patient is again asked to describe an incident in which she was angry. Each time a new incident is described, more defense restructuring is undertaken, in a gradual fashion. Each time an incident is reviewed, the patient's reaction and defenses are elaborated. More and more irritation is built up, and greater evidence of this is manifested by greater responsiveness, increased tonicity in body posture, and greater congruence among facial appearance and hand movements, and emotional state. She is beginning to look angry. The patient's defense constellation is pointed out [defense restructuring] as she begins to build up greater irritation toward the therapist and concomitant defensive responses.

THERAPIST: Right now what are you feeling?

PATIENT: Irritation.

THERAPIST: So let's see how you experience this irritation?

PATIENT: It confuses me; you want me to describe something, I have no idea.

THERAPIST: So this is the way you want to go through your life.

PATIENT: NO! I guess I'm going to have to get over it. I feel like throwing something at you right now. Is that a feeling?

THERAPIST: It's a thought, so there is some anger inside of you that you want to hurt me, but how do you experience the rage inside you right now?

Patients are often confused between their feelings and fantasies. For this patient, the thought of throwing something at me is equivalent to experiencing anger. For many personality disordered patients, anger and violence are seen as one and the same.

PATIENT: Just the tension; my body is tensing up. . . . I don't allow it.

THERAPIST: (*points out fists*) You become so terrified of your anger, you push it down, you become tense, you withdraw, and you distance yourself.

The patient recognizes her habit of pushing her anger down and reports experiencing nausea. She talks about how she is fighting not to block the therapist out and disassociate.

THERAPIST: I now that you are saying you are angry, but my experience with you is that intellectually you're angry, but emotionally the systems are not connected for you. So when you say you're angry, you're not feeling anything; your face looks flat. It's very important that we get to your feelings. There is a part of you that seems very detached, like your emotions are somewhere else.

PATIENT: Well, how do I get in touch with them?

The above intervention highlights two important points. One is that the patient must have a clear understanding of the importance of being emotionally connected and seek this condition so that patient and therapist can undergo the disruptive aspects of the defense analysis. Otherwise, the therapist can do damage if he/she proceeds. The second point, highlighted in previous vignettes, is the depth of emotional disassociation in the personality disordered patient. The therapist is generally one of the few people in the patient's experience who values the patient's emotions, and this by itself can be highly anxiety arousing. The genetic figures probably showed limited interest in the patient's emotional life, so that an interested figure reactivates longings and other mixed feelings.

The focus shifts to a psychiatrist who was "cruel" while the patient was undergoing treatment for infertility. She is able to portray how she would have choked him if she had "let the beast inside her out." For the first time, this patient is able to discuss her violent fantasies, but affect remains at a low level (cognitive restructuring). This technique eases the patient's fear and anxiety concerning her aggressive instincts, which for most people are natural reactions to being attacked or humiliated. The patient has never talked with anyone like this. She acknowledges feeling some guilt, since actually attacking the psychiatrist would be an overreaction. The importance of helping this patient get in touch with her anger is crucial to a positive outcome. Patients who are subject to victimization have not learned how to stand up for themselves and, thus, tend to be repeatedly victimized by others.

THERAPIST: What else are you feeling right now?

PATIENT: I just think this is funny. Me planning to hurt someone.

THERAPIST: Is it funny, or is it that you have a lot of trouble talking about your aggression?

PATIENT: I guess I have a lot of trouble talking about it.

THERAPIST: There is a lot of anxiety for you, to talk about your aggression. But if you're honest, wasn't there really a part that wanted to hurt him after he treated you like that?

PATIENT: Yeah, but I took it out on myself instead.

THERAPIST: So this is one pattern that you have: You swallow your rage and take it out on yourself. If you had done that to him, how would you have felt?

PATIENT: I wouldn't have felt like hurting myself.

THERAPIST: You wanted to hurt yourself after that?

PATIENT: I was going to slit my wrists over the course of that week.

She then describes how her psychiatrist told her she would be on Prozac for the rest of her life and how upset she was about this. As she discusses this, she is getting more in contact with her anger. She then discusses how she would attack him, but this time it is with a true display of affect. However, her defenses return, and she backs away. Next, she talks about how she would stab him in the heart. She then declares, "I don't like men" and links this to her father and "not being wanted." When asked for an incident she says, "I blocked everything out." She next says the only time her mother paid any attention to her was when she did something wrong. She then talks about her brother who was abusive toward her.

The patient recalls an incident at age 3 where she said she was going to leave, and her mother packed her suitcase for her and told her to go. She describes feeling very empty, and there is the first sign of sadness. "What did I do that was so wrong that made people not want me?" She then talks about her feelings toward her psychiatrist and her feeling that he was standing in her way of getting better. She reports that he never remembered what she told him and was "patronizing" toward her. "He was working against me." She then displays some sadness over "trusting someone" and not having it work out. The focus then becomes intimacy with the therapist and the patient's tendency to associate any intimacy with sexual intimacy.

THERAPIST: Are there any thoughts that this relationship could become sexual?

PATIENT: Not really, I guess it is—

THERAPIST: So let's see what your thoughts are: How would this become sexual?

PATIENT: That is the only way men like me or ever wanted to talk to me.

THERAPIST: So the only reason a man would ever get to know you or to have an intimate involvement with you is to use you? What are you feeling right now?

PATIENT: Sad (*affect sad*).

THERAPIST: You must have had a tremendous craving for intimacy and closeness to put yourself in that position.

She then discusses a relationship with a psychologist who treated her, "And I did open up, and I found him attractive because here is someone showing genuine interest and caring. I told him I was physically attracted to him and that was the biggest mistake in my life." She described how the therapist tried to explain it as transference feeling, but he became more distant, "like a doctor." "I'm afraid I'm going to be let down again. I don't want to have sex with you," she says, referring to the current therapist. The importance of this issue is discussed, and the first 1½ hours of this session is closed.

This segment of the extended session highlights the importance of immediately creating an open atmosphere where all aspects of the patient's transference phenomenon can be discussed. If the therapist is uncomfortable discussing or tolerating the development of sexualized transference, then deeper-level work will be very difficult. The sexualized feelings must be derepressed in a safe environment. The histrionic patient, as is highlighted in this case, has an overly fused tangle of affectionate and sexualized feeling, which is usually related to unresolved feelings about an important genetic figure. At this point, it is not yet clear who this figure is, but as already noted, this tangle of sexualized feeling has been replayed with significant male figures and has developed as a transference phenomenon with other therapists. Often, such patients request a hug, which might frighten the therapist, but the situation is easily addressed without injuring the patient. The therapist should identify the feeling of affection or the longing for closeness, which, when brought to the surface and identified, is acknowledged without saying "no." If the patient insists on being hugged, the therapist can explain that it is important to understand these natural longings and cravings but not to gratify them in this context. Following a break of 15 minutes, the session recommences.

THERAPIST: So what were your thoughts over the break?

PATIENT: I thought about leaving, but I didn't. . . . We really did touch upon something that has bothered me. I can't accept a man being nice to me.

She then describes how her previous psychologist invited the patient's significant other for a session. In the session, the patient was instructed to: "Explain what was going on . . . that I was attracted to Dr. X. I didn't know why he was ever brought in." Again the issue becomes how she buried her anger toward this therapist. Instead of getting angry because "He wasn't really there for me," she became tearful.

PATIENT: I just wanted somebody to treat me like I was okay. I wasn't asking him to have sex with me. I wasn't asking him to do anything (*sad affect*). I guess he humiliated me. He wanted me to open up. It was like game playing.

THERAPIST: You started to talk about some positive feeling toward me, and then you were reminded about your relationship with Dr. X. Have you experienced some physical feeling toward me?

PATIENT: Yeah. I guess that I just felt comfortable talking to you and that the only way I was going to get any attention back was to have a physical relationship.

THERAPIST: What was the feeling that you experienced physically? Something sexual? In what part of your body did you experience it?

Derepressions and decathecting unresolved feeling are enhanced if the experience can be linked to the actual physical sensation in the body such as genital arousal. Feelings are often first experienced physically, in the body.

PATIENT: (*sighs*) [Patient avoids describing feeling or image of sexual attraction but acknowledges the importance of topic and then describes another incident in which she was sexually attracted to someone who showed her attention. She then describes the fantasy.] There is something wrong with me. I associate attention and love with sex. I guess I was looking for the attention I never got from my father.

THERAPIST: Do you think I'm interested in you?

PATIENT: No, I hope not.

THERAPIST: I don't mean sexually. I mean in terms of your development, in terms of you getting better, in terms of you resolving what you—

PATIENT: Yeah, I think you are because you don't strike me as the kind of doctor who just wants someone to keep coming in for the rest of their life. You seem genuinely concerned about people getting better and going on. It makes me feel more comfortable, but still in the back of my head I remember nobody's ever done that.

It is almost always the case for patients in Cluster B that they were used narcissistically or physically by ineffective or disturbed genetic figures. The child is usually forced to take care of parental needs. A normal developmental experience of a nurturing, giving caretaker is limited or absent.

THERAPIST: Okay, so there is something in the back of your head, and what is that in the back of your head?

PATIENT: My father could have never sexually abused me? I start wondering about that too. Maybe I also did it to get back at him. He never would have condoned this kind of behavior. He would think I'm a disgusting tramp.

This is always a delicate juncture. Histrionic character development always involves some degree of sexualization of the father–daughter relationship, sometimes at the level of overt incest. The therapist should let the facts emerge from the patient. If the patient has been sexually abused, it will emerge within a derepression.

The patient then discusses her anger toward her father, and she is asked to describe an incident in which she was angry toward him. She is now more emotionally in touch and describes how she would kill him. She is encouraged to fantasize about how she would do this in as vivid terms as possible, to amplify the feeling. She describes how she would stab him repeatedly. She states that she would then do the same to her mother. She is able to tolerate this with no signs of regression or distancing. This indicates that sufficient restructuring has taken place, and the treatment may proceed with further anxiety-arousing techniques.

PATIENT: I've never given myself a chance at anything because of him. I've been self-destructive. I did anything to get attention. I did drugs—they didn't notice that. I tried to kill myself—they didn't notice that. I drank—they didn't notice that. They never noticed anything.

She then describes an incident at age 16 in which her mother became violent and discusses how destructive her relationship with both parents has been. She imagines her father's death: "I think I'd feel bad because I never had a father, that's about it. Sadness for myself, sorrow for him that he was such a miserable human being. How can I grieve something I've never had? I've never had a father." The patient cries softly as she discusses this profound loss. She then discusses how her father read two things, the newspaper and *Playboy*, "which was like a bible to him." She mentions that he treated women as objects.

THERAPIST: And both times [you killed him in your fantasy] there was stabbing in the heart.

PATIENT: Because that's where the pain is felt by me in the heart (*holds heart*). For not wanting me and pushing me away for all those years, and criticizing me.

THERAPIST: So do you think this is the root of some of the rage you have toward men?

PATIENT: Yes.

THERAPIST: Do you think that you have been replaying that pattern over and over?

PATIENT: Yes. And I'm worried I'm doing that with Al [significant other]. Things are going all right, and I can't deal with that.

THERAPIST: What do you think would happen if you could resolve all these feelings that we touched on today?

PATIENT: Probably go on with my life in a healthy way. Get off of Prozac. Stop taking things out on myself. Deal with anger more effectively. Feel good about killing my father (*looks sad*).

THERAPIST: So if we could stick with this focus you would be able to resolve these things and live a free life?

PATIENT: I would hope so.

The rest of the session focuses on the patient's relationship with her mother and how her mother dated another man when the patient was 16. She had yelled at her mother then, and "she denied it. My mother always insinuated *I* was screwing around." Apparently, her mother would project onto the patient her own feelings in an abusive manner. "She accused me of being a lesbian when I said I hated men." She then returns to the incident in which her mother banged her against the wall. She then fantasizes how she would smash her mother's head and "keep beating her until I felt better." She then states, "All my life I did nothing but try to please the two of them. She was an emotional cripple. She'd spend weeks in bed. She would fight with my father and then go to bed, and I'd always make sure she ate and take care of her. Then she would accuse me of trying to take care of him."

PATIENT: I've never had a normal relationship with—I can't be friends with a woman because then I'm a lesbian, and I can't be friends with men because then I'm a tramp.

THERAPIST: All intimacy was tied to sex. All closeness was tied to sex. Your father with his *Playboys*, your mother with her innuendos and accusations—

PATIENT: And always coming off as perfect, Miss Wonderful. She did exactly to me what she said her mother did to her. Except she never told me to go kill myself, she didn't have to.

THERAPIST: Have you thought about her death?

This technique, focusing on the genetic figure's death and funeral, accelerates the emergence of the impacted grief over the disturbed mother–daughter relationship. The patient reports that she contacted 5% of her rage during the session. She now understands how her defense system works. The comparison between her defenses at the beginning and end of the session are contrasted. The focus is then on her experience of anger toward the therapist. She is now much more animated: Her hands are active, as manifested by a strangling gesture. She is able to stay with this and discuss how she would "bash the therapist into the wall." "I probably would have killed you!" She then contacts a sick feeling—guilt—that she "had done something like that." The therapist then discusses her positive feelings, and she declares, "I cannot trust there are no ulterior motives, that you're not going to have sex with me. I guess that part of me wonders why you don't want to, what's wrong with me?" This is linked to her desire to get back at men and her self-destructiveness. The therapeutic contract is discussed and the task recapitulated.

PATIENT: I would feel grateful if you were able to help me.

THERAPIST: Is there anything else that you want to say before we stop today?

The extended session ended at this point. A contract was made to meet every 2 weeks for 1½ hours. The transcript has highlighted a number of important issues that are reviewed in the following section before we continue with the case.

Sexualized Feeling

Although sexualized feeling can emerge in the treatment of many personality disordered patients, it is more prominent in the Cluster B disordered, especially the histrionic and borderline patients. This transference feeling will develop early and must be derepressed by encouraging the patient to acknowledge and experience this feeling if it becomes obvious in the transference. The sexualized feeling often serves multiple psychic functions. First, it has often been a substitute for intimacy and is fused with longings for closeness, both physical and emotional. Second, it is often a means of expressing anger toward the opposite sex and retaliation toward the genetic figure—in this case the father, who was distant and tended to objectify women. Third, it also becomes a vehicle for self-destructive impulses, which are a manifestation of internalized rage and guilt over its expression.

Sequence of Derepression

Often the sexualized feeling, which has a defensive function, must be derepressed before deeper layers of rage, guilt, and grief can be reached. If the sexualized component of the transference is not brought to the surface early on, the therapist often becomes immobilized by the erotic aspects of the therapy, which become a reenactment of the original trauma (too much sexualized feeling and insufficient nurturing or abuse with genetic figure).

Importance of Boundaries

The therapist must be very cautious about engaging in any form of physical contact, as this often is loaded with sexualized transference feeling. The therapist should make it clear in all aspects of communication that the boundaries are firm and that the therapist can tolerate the patient's most intense feelings and longings without becoming distant or seduced. Strong countertransference feelings should alert the therapist to the extreme pull that exists, whereby the patient believes gratified love will heal the injury.

Opposite-Sex Patient–Therapist Match

The transference feeling will develop quicker in opposite sex therapeutic dyads. Same-sex matches will create more competitive issues in the transference, but the same issues can be addressed by focusing on relationships with the opposite sex in the patient's life.

Disturbances with Both Parents

Patients in Cluster B will manifest a higher rate of disturbances in relationships with both genetic figures and siblings. Each figure must be derepressed and worked through until the feeling is at a high level of felt experience. In the above case, the patient went from a very low tolerance for affect to a higher one in the course of the trial therapy.

Increasing Intensity and Tolerance of Affect

With each derepression and metabolizing of associated affect, the patient's tolerance for affect should increase. As can be seen in the case above, the patient was increasingly more comfortable talking about her "dark side," her aggressive fantasies, and impulses to destroy. She also became less anxious, more animated, and more emotionally tolerant of her deeper self.

Achieving Deeper Understanding

When the therapy and therapist are on task, the patient achieves increasingly deeper levels of understanding and insight—the patient "gets it." There is a resonance between the patient and therapist that keeps the treatment on track. If the alliance is not sufficiently strong, the therapist must improve it before continuing, or the therapy will bog down, and recovery will be difficult.

Loss of Focus

In an extended session, there are so many issues to attend to that it is not uncommon to lose focus temporarily. If this occurs, the therapist should summarize the session and restate what has been *mutually* understood or restate the patient's issues or goals. In the above case, there was one point where the therapist thought the focus was lost and proceeded to recapitulate the issues. The patient asked the therapist why he was doing so and said she was on the issue of her anger toward her father. The therapist accepted this correction and returned in a more focused fashion to the chosen issue.

Past Therapies

Many patients in this cluster have had a history of previous therapy. The therapist must explore the nature of these relationships so that what has been learned or reenacted can be understood. The repetitive transference phenomenon will almost always emerge and the feelings, positive and negative, should be brought to the surface, otherwise the bond with the current therapist will be more difficult to establish.

Shifting Therapeutic Stance

In this case, the clinician was able to shift from a type 1 therapeutic alliance to a type 2, from an empathic, supportive style to an abstinent one. This kind of flexibility helps maximize the therapeutic results. However, shifts in the type of alliance should be discussed with the patient so that he/she is aware of what is occurring and understands that a change in approach is called for. In this case, the patient requested a more rapid in-depth approach.

The first session after an extended session is usually a good test of the potency of the initial intervention. Usually dramatic change is reflected in both the patient's physical appearance and in his/her manifestations of unconscious activation. It is always an exciting interview because the results of the previous work will be strikingly apparent if quantum change movements have been activated, and few patients do not experience something powerful after the extended session.

Two Weeks Following the Extended Session

THERAPIST: So what's been happening since the last time we met?

PATIENT: My sister and I went out to dinner, and we were talking about how my mother never contacts me. And I'm the only one who can get along with her. Since our last meeting, I really noticed how mad I am at her, and I don't feel so mad at my father anymore. Could that be possibly because we got a lot of it out?

In the opening phase of this session, we can see the results of the therapeutic effort. The patient appears energized and ready to begin by focusing on her relationship with her mother. She has a greater awareness of her own dynamics and seems to want a deeper understanding of herself. However, as the session proceeds, it is clear that her defenses are in operation, serving to keep the therapist, as well as her feelings, at bay. This is not unusual, even after a successful extended interview. The restructuring process must continue, and the therapist has to reaffirm the therapeutic task.

THERAPIST: What else has happened since we met last time?

The patient discusses her upcoming wedding and the fact that she is not going to invite her family. She also said she cut back on her medication, and "I don't feel depressed."

THERAPIST: What do you think we should focus on today?

PATIENT: My mother.

The patient is quite capable of selecting the focus because her unconscious has been activated and the alliance is strong. The focus, however, quickly shifts to her relationship with her fiance and anger toward him. It is usually better early in the treatment to activate the patient's affective schema by focusing on a current conflict. If the therapist moves too quickly to the genetic figure(s), in this case her mother, it will be much harder to activate feelings and achieve a derepression. The genetic figures (P corner of the triangle of persons) are the hardest to tackle. In this case, the patient's defenses were up, and she became argumentative when feelings were elicited. It is often helpful to recall and summarize an incident from the previous session in which the patient's affective schema was successfully activated.

The patient describes in a vague way how her family never showed her respect, how she has always tried to please them, and how this has been self-destructive. The therapist then summarizes the *core issues,* as extracted from the extended session.

THERAPIST: Last session, we talked about some of the factors that have gone into this. One is that your relationship with your father was a crippled one: He used women as objects, wasn't able to allow you to get close to him, and was interested in controlling you. Your mother, on the other hand, had this dishonest relationship with you where she would get panicky about anything sexual, and then, when you were 17, you found she was out with another man all night. You have a lot of feeling built up toward them.

PATIENT: I'm fighting distancing myself right now.

The patient reports a dream that she had last night. It is a complex dream with no obvious manifest content. She is asked what she makes of the dream.

PATIENT: . . . my family doing something to embarrass me, and me getting back at them but not hurting them by hurting myself, by getting drunk possibly staying with someone.

THERAPIST: So you get back at them by acting out.

The focus then returns to the incident with her fiance where she felt humiliated, and more systematic defense restructuring is undertaken. She is resistant to attempts at eliciting her emotion, but it is clear via her body posture and animated expression that her feeling is close to the surface.

PATIENT: There are times when I get mad at Al, and I think about grabbing a knife to get even with him.

THERAPIST: Before you started seeing me?

PATIENT: Yes.

THERAPIST: You're very sensitive to humiliation. You turn off [anger], turn cold, and withdraw, but that is crippling you.

She then says she would choke her fiance but would like to borrow someone else's hands. She then portrays what would happen if she unleashed her fury and murdered her fiance for humiliating her. She says that she feels guilty for standing up for herself. "Part of me keeps telling myself that I'm not worthy and I don't deserve to be happy." She accesses grief over thoughts about murdering and losing her fiance.

Course of Treatment

The course of treatment following the extended session was fairly straightforward. The core issues that were established during the extended session remained the focus of treatment. During the early phase, the patient discontinued her medication. Her progress was remarkable and underscores the importance of what can be accomplished with complex character disturbances and mixed symptom constellations when the patient is motivated and displays a readiness for change.

In Chapter 12, I present portions of the termination session, the 6-month follow-up session, and 2-year phone follow-up from this case.

TREATMENT OF THE NARCISSISTIC DISORDERS

Patients with narcissistic sectors to their personality and full-blown narcissistic disorders present a challenge to the short-term dynamic therapist. Patients who have a narcissistic sector to their personality can usually be handled with the standard restructuring approaches, but a premature use of defense restructuring can be severely disruptive. The clinician must possess an understanding of a "developmental model" (the importance of an adequate caretaker, who is capable of mirroring the emergent self) in order to understand the function and the structure of narcissistic defenses.

Millon (1992) has described two variants in the pathogenesis of narcissism. One is primary, where the child is elevated by parental figures to a position of being special, so that the grandiose narcissistic phase of development is unrealistically reinforced, resulting in a classic narcissistic presentation. The other results from a deprivation of the child's emotional needs, so that the child prematurely looks to the self for the sustenance and feels valued by *reflecting the caretaker(s)' needs.* This is a faulty or reversed mirroring in which the child becomes too much of a narcissistic object for the parent. In my clinical experience, the latter type is more common and often less easy to spot. These patients are not the "brash, exhibitionistic, self-assured, single minded," individuals who exude "an aura of success in career and relationships" that Masterson (1988, p. 90) describes. When they enter treatment, they are usually deflated, a result of a change in their external situation and a lack of mirroring of the grandiose narcissistic "false self."

There are important clinical differences between two groups of patients that one encounters in clinical practice, patients with narcissistic personalities and patients with a personality disorder with a narcissistic sector or features. If the patient has the experience of a positive relationship with one significant figure, then the patient will usually not develop a full-blown narcissistic personality. However, if there is a lack of available figures, then the personality is usually severely compromised. This is not a categorical situation; the variants are infinite, but the treatment decisions by the short-term therapist will effect the outcome. The therapist must know when mirroring is required and when defense restructuring is called for. What makes this approach different from standard psychotherapy is the judicious use of defense analysis and anxiety-arousing techniques to derepress the system more rapidly. The following case serves as illustration of this technique.

Treatment of a Man with a Narcissistic Personality—The Case of the Stunted Man

The patient is a highly intelligent engineer in his late 20s, who had graduated from a prestigious university. He was referred by a psychologist who had treated the patient and his wife for severe marital disturbance. The patient is separated from his wife and young children. The marital therapist and the patient's wife were concerned about his high-risk behavior, including substance abuse (alcohol and marijuana used while driving) and unprotected sex with prostitutes. The marital therapy seemed stuck, and much of this was related to the patient's characterological difficulties. The patient was referred for a consultation in hopes that he would benefit from STDP. He was seen for a 45-minute consultation during which his presenting problems and history were reviewed. He agreed to an extended session, 3 hours in length, which was audiovisually recorded.

Extended Session

The patient begins the session discussing the fact that he is feeling optimistic about the therapy. (*Patient is slouched and has head supported by left hand. He appears surprisingly comfortable.*)

THERAPIST: Can you review what you see as the difficulties in your life?

PATIENT: Well, there are certain behaviors. The thing that comes most to mind is the dangerous behaviors that I'm unable to control. Seeing prostitutes I guess is the most dangerous thing, substance abuse, pot and alcohol.

THERAPIST: So number one is the self-destructive behaviors. Number two, what would you say?

PATIENT: Is the confusion, or what I think of as emotional retardation or not being able to process emotions very well. In other ways, I'm like a small child. A low-grade chronic depression that I think is under the surface all the time.

THERAPIST: What do you think the most important one is?

PATIENT: The self-destructive things because they could kill me. That's the critical one because if I don't do something about that, then the others are moot (*laughs*). Potentially soon.

THERAPIST: Did you notice that when you said that you laughed? I don't know what the laugh meant. You find it humorous?

PATIENT: Why I was laughing was that I find that turn of logic amusing. I don't know why, I just—

THERAPIST: That you find your own self-destruction—

PATIENT: But I'm not relating this to me.

The patient's comment, "I'm not relating this to me," is definitely the case. He is dangerously on the edge of destroying his life, and he is totally removed from what he is saying and doing. Prognostically, this is a poor sign because he is not suffering over what he is doing. This is a good example of ego-syntonic defenses in full operation. For the most part, he is protected from dysphoric feeling and anxiety. When these do threaten to emerge, he turns to substances or sex as a mechanism to stay away from his feelings.

THERAPIST: Do you notice that right now you appear detached? We listed a number of serious problems, but it appears as if you are watching TV right now (*referring to the patient's body posture and manner*). Do you have a tendency to be detached? It's almost like it creates a barrier or wall. You could be talking about someone else's life rather than your own. For a man with your intelligence, your potential, to be doing this to himself seems like a big tragedy. Because this part of you, that self-destructive part, means there is a need to defeat and sabotage yourself.

PATIENT: You mentioned that last time. The way you put it was, you said there was some powerful need to destroy myself, and that's obvious, that has to be true.

THERAPIST: That need to defeat yourself could come out with me today, to actually sabotage your own will to get to the bottom of the difficulties and resolve them.

PATIENT: I feel like right now and over the last few minutes the barrier or wall is beginning to come down, and I just want to tell you that the very direct way that you are addressing me is frightening to me, and I take it very personally. I'm frightened of the way you are saying things. I feel very disoriented right now. I feel humiliated to say this, but it reminds me of the very direct way my parents used to deal with me. [The patient shows no sign of fragmentation or loss of orientation.]

At this point it is not clear if the patient is organized at a borderline level. However, some borderlines would show severe fragmentation with this level of defense analysis. It is only later, as treatment unfolds, that the therapist becomes aware of the intractable nature of the patient's self-destructive behavior throughout his life. One can already see the process begin to take hold as the patient is getting in touch with his fright. We are at a crucial diagnostic point in our ego assessment: If the patient leans more toward the neurotic structure, he will be able to handle this level of anxiety arousal; on the other hand, if we are dealing with a primitive borderline phenomenon, we may see fragmentation of the ego and will have to switch approaches. We can note the high level of ego-syntonicity present at the beginning of the session and how the patient became frightened when this was observed. We return to the first half of the extended session.

PATIENT: I can't imagine why an organism would want to destroy itself (*crying*).

THERAPIST: There is a lot of feeling there. Do you know what it is connected to? We are not talking about an organism, we are talking about a man destroying his life and putting his family in jeopardy.

As with borderlines (Akhtar, 1992), one of the important aspects of treating the narcissistic patient in short-term therapy is to address the self-destructive behavioral repertoires that the patient uses to keep him/herself away from the emotional pain. The core issues cannot be systematically derived, derepressed, and worked through as long as the patient is acting out in self-destructive patterns. For many patients, this is not possible in short-term psychotherapy. For others, such as this patient, it is. Since the patient's ego system tolerated the anxiety without regression or fragmentation, the anxiety-arousing defense analysis methods are used. At this point, the process emphasizes cognitive restructuring, asking the patient to discuss incidents of importance in the C area of the triangle and then clarifying the I/F and D areas. This process offers a cognitive understanding of the psychic system, and each time the therapist presses for more feeling. In this session, only low levels of affect are contacted, and anxiety remains at a low level. Low levels of negative feeling toward the therapist are mobilized, and the therapist tries to elicit these, as well. At this point, a 15-minute break is taken.

The patient is now asked the standard question about what he experienced over the break. He reports that he put most of what was discussed out of his mind (this is a sign that his defense system has an extremely strong hold on his emotional self). until he was returning from a coffee break. He also asks for reassurance that he can freely talk about what he desires. He is encouraged to be "open and honest and say whatever is on his mind." The defense work and restructuring has mobilized significant affective material, as is seen in the following vignettes.

PATIENT: It occurred to me that, I feel in a lot of ways, that the way I was raised destroyed me in a lot of ways, and so maybe that's the pattern I'm living out as an adult (*sad and tearful*).

THERAPIST: And I can see that you have a lot of feeling about that.

PATIENT: I do.

THERAPIST: It's very painful to look at that.

PATIENT: I don't know if it is true. Well, that's the way it feels, that's all I know. And I think that when I was telling you about not being able to catch up [developmentally], is one part of it.

THERAPIST: How would you feel if you were able to catch up? Not only catch up but emotionally thrive?

This is the beginning of elaborating the patient's narcissistic core. He has a vague sense that something has been lost in his development. The injection of hope from the therapist is very important.

PATIENT: (*sadness and tearfulness continues*) I don't think that I was helped by my parents in some of the things that I needed. And some of the things that I needed were maybe not things everyone needs. I have images of not being cultivated. I feel like a house plant that has had all its leaves and branches pruned. Kind of left like a bonsai; even worse though, a bonsai is still whole. It's possible that this pattern has manifested in the self-destructive behavior.

THERAPIST: What are you feeling right now?

PATIENT: I'm afraid.

THERAPIST: But you also seem to be in a lot of pain. I get the sense that you are trying to clip your own branches right now, emotionally.

PATIENT: I don't know if what I'm saying is right or I'm just being a jerk. Maybe this is something I've dreamed up to blame my parents for the way I am (*controlled sobbing*).

THERAPIST: We are not here to blame; we are here to get to the truth of your life and get to the bottom of this, so we can get to the engine of it.

PATIENT: And I feel like that's the engine (*intense sobbing and waves of grief*). I'm really mad about it. I know that my mother was smoking when I was in the womb, and I know that my mother is emotionally crippled. I just believe from the time I was in the womb, and then from the time I was born, and then all throughout my infancy and childhood, that my mother was not there for me in the capacity that I needed.

THERAPIST: So this was a very deep injury to you.

PATIENT: That is where what I call my weird attitudes about women come from. It only stands to reason that a person who has been denied that basic sustenance would be compulsive about getting it. That's why I have this compulsion for approval and compulsion for physical contact. So between that and never being able to catch up intellectually with my parents.

[Even when the patient was a young child, his mother competed with him intellectually and crushed his emerging self-esteem.]

I can talk for hours about what it was like not being cared for when I was real little. When my son was 2 months old, my mom was babysitting for a little while. When my wife came back to get him, he was in hysterics—screaming, yelling out of the playpen. So my wife went to pick him up. My mother said, "Don't pick him up, he has to learn how to deal with this himself." He was only 2 months old! I know that's what she did to me. That (*screaming and yelling*) was to me, in my mind, I was 1 or 2 years old in the crib, and I was hungry, and my mother wouldn't come to get me, and I was mad and angry about it. So all of those things to me are as close as I can get.

This patient spontaneously reported how he observed his mother interacting, or rather not interacting, with his 2-month-old son. The sight of this reinflamed his deeply entrenched narcissistic wound and gives the therapist increased insight into the nature of this injury. I occasionally ask patients to observe how their parents interact with their grandchildren. Much can be learned about parenting styles, comfort with affection and capacity for nurturing. Narcissistic cores are more intractable than those in patients with defined trauma, which often require more metabolizing by the therapist to adequately reconstruct the core trauma. Having the patient review pictures from early childhood and baby scrapbooks are methods for helping the patient understand the emotional tenor of his/her early life and contacting early aspects of the last or damaged self (Trujillo, personal communication, September 11, 1996).

THERAPIST: All of those things are very important. You mentioned quite a few issues, and I think it's going to be important for us to get a focus. You said your father died, and this was quite a powerful experience for you. Another is the issue of the child–mother relationship, and you sense that this has been a crippled one, that you have a lot of unresolved feeling toward her that we really need to focus on. You said anger before, but you brushed over that very quickly, and certainly there is a lot of grief there because you missed something very important to your development. And there is a lot of feeling right now as I'm saying this. What are you feeling right now?

The therapist has to constantly reestablish the focus so that the therapeutic process does not turn into a long-term model. This is difficult when there are so many core wounds. Frequent summarizing is helpful, and asking the patient to select a topic of focus is a way to keep on track. The therapist should try to stay with an issue until it seems that all the feeling has been fully experienced, expressed, and dissipated.

PATIENT: (*crying*) I'm imagining that if I'm going to get better I'm going to have to say good-bye, put down, kill, whatever the expression, a lot of

224 PROCESS AND TECHNIQUE IN TREATMENT

what has fed me, these self-destructive behaviors and whatever they entangle with. And that's going to be like a death of me.

THERAPIST: So you're saying that as we continue to move on here, you are aware that you are going to have to say good-bye to the crippled you, to leave that behind.

PATIENT: But it's me (*sobbing*). Maybe it's crippled, but it is the only me I know.

THERAPIST: You have a tremendous amount of grief with that.

PATIENT: (*another wave of sobbing*) Yes.

The patient starts to rationalize hurting himself and how the human brain processes such events. The therapist moves back to the task at hand.

THERAPIST: You are at an important juncture here. You can continue to pursue this path of hurting yourself. I hate to put labels on this, but in some ways, there is a very masochistic element to what you're doing. A need to punish and hurt yourself. A need to be used over and over again. There is a lot at stake here. To maintain that crippled part you need crutches, drugs, alcohol, and prostitutes.

The patient declares his will to continue the process.

THERAPIST: What issue should we should focus on for this half of the session?

PATIENT: I feel like if I had some help (*holding back tears*).

THERAPIST: Where were your parents?

PATIENT: I don't know. They were around, but they weren't with me. The way we're together now, they weren't with me at all.

THERAPIST: You mean you didn't have this kind of intimacy with them?

PATIENT: Not at all, I never have. Even just before my father died. We knew that he only had a few years to live, a year before he died. And before that we knew he was sick, his heart, caused by smoking and just his general lifestyle. And I'm on the same path that he was.

THERAPIST: So in other words he was a self-destructive man.

PATIENT: Oh yes, absolutely! I'm on exactly the same path. And we knew he was going to die in a matter of days in the last weeks.

THERAPIST: Can you tell me about the last time you saw him before he died?

We then focus on the loss of his father and visiting him in the hospital. He did not want his father to die alone, and he spent a night in the hospital with him. "We talked about a lot of things" (*sobbing*). "I asked him about his father, and his father abandoned him when he was a baby. He was very much at peace except when I brought his father up. He had a grimace on his face." (This is reactivating tremendous grief in the patient, and he is tolerating this with no defenses.)

We discuss the patient's anger toward his wife whom he felt tried to "blackmail" him. Apparently, she told him there was some news (his father had died), but she was not going to tell him unless he made a particular confession about his behavior. The patient's rage proves inaccessible, and his grief surfaces. He then talks about the funeral and how he wanted to view his father's body before he was buried. "He looked young. He was only 60. I said good-bye, but I didn't really say good-bye." (*The patient sobs with genuine grief-laden affect.*)

THERAPIST: What we know is that your father had been abandoned by his father and, in a sense, your father wasn't there for you—there was a kind of emotional abandonment in your relationship with him. And you must have a lot of feeling about that in addition to the grief. And there is a strong identification with his self-destructiveness.

PATIENT: When my marriage was really blowing up earlier this year, what I thought about was that 60 years ago my grandfather had a marriage that was blowing up and walked away, and I saw what it did to my father. And I have made a very clear decision not to do this to my children. It's very important to me.

THERAPIST: We have spent some time talking about the tremendous grief that you have. That your father went to the grave without having a close father and son relationship that would have been beneficial to your psychological and emotional development. At this point, what do you think that we should focus on to get the most out of today's session?

At this point, the therapist summarizes what has transpired and makes links between the patient's current patterns and previous ones. The patient is very involved with the therapist and emotionally present. The remainder of the session focuses on his relationship with his wife. He focuses on an incident and is able to contact his anger in contrast to what was observed in the first half of the session. He is energized and animated. He describes how he would murder her with an ax. "If we were back in the stone ages, she'd be dead." He discusses what would happen if the more savage part of him emerged, and he reveals mutilation fantasies. "What I did was monstrous. The reality is that I could be executed for this or put away for life." The session closes with a recapitulation of the patient's areas of disturbance and how the core issues generate and relate to these patterns.

Two Weeks Following the Extended Session

THERAPIST: Usually, the way we start the session is with the first thing on your mind.

PATIENT: Two things are on my mind. One is that, I happen to be in a lot of pain today [congruent with appearance], but I noticed that, since our last session, that I'm enraged all the time. About a week ago I acted out by getting some pot and saw a prostitute, but before then I know I've been feeling rage all the time. But since then I have been feeling a certain confidence that I'm not going to do this anymore. It occurred to me that I don't want to destroy myself.

THERAPIST: But it is important that we look at this because a part of you *does* want to destroy yourself. What we talked about last time is that there are two parts. One part has a tremendous self-destructive impulse to ruin, destroy, to kill yourself.

PATIENT: But I feel like this self-destruction is a method to anesthetize this rage and this pain. But then I had an interesting experience last night. In fact, where I have had a lot of contact with my wife very much of it has been very positive, although there's been some of the same old negative stuff. My reaction in the past would have been, "OK, go out and have some drinks," which would have led down that road [prostitutes] but it was, like, "No." In fact, she [wife] told me she didn't want to see me, but I went and saw her, and I confronted the situation, and I didn't act out in screaming or anything like that. It would have been less painful to go out and have drinks or whatever.

The patient discusses some difficulties he is having at work, where he bombards associates with too much new material, and his realization that this is driven by rage and wanting "to get them up to speed." He asked for feedback and found that his associates did not find helpful his behavior of acting like a "madman," sending them memos, and calling excessively.

PATIENT: I am processing this feedback in the light of my personal life and am getting a view of my character. I thought the day would come or the process would come where I would have to say good-bye to the me that I've known all my life. I feel like I am on the threshold of at least one aspect of that.

THERAPIST: So, in other words, what you are saying is the grief that you're experiencing is related to saying good-bye to a part of you that you have known for many years.

PATIENT: (*sad affect*) That I relied on and thought was me and thought was good. I'm realizing there is something there that is not good.

This is an important phase of the recovery process and an indication that the extended session was successful in making his defense system and self-destructive patterns less ego-syntonic.

The Working-Through Phase

The working through focused on the two core issues that were exposed during the trial therapy. The first one was that the patient had a very poor attachment with his mother, what Winnicott described as the "not good enough mother." Fortunately, the patient's mother was living, and the patient was living with her, so that his current relationship with her was a way for him to observe the mother–son relationship with the benefit of his new awareness. It did bear out that his mother, raised in a well-to-do family, had limited emotional capacity and, furthermore, was very competitive with her gifted child. His intense craving for human contact, intimacy, and closeness had never been sufficiently fulfilled. He had found substitutes in a pattern of drug use and visiting prostitutes as a partial attempt to get something but also as an expression of his rage for his mother and his wife, both of whom withheld affection. The cycle of drug and alcohol use and visiting prostitutes continued with less frequency. Each time he engaged in this behavior, he felt deeply ashamed and expected to be told not to return to treatment. Each time, the build-up of feelings prior to his acting out was elicited.

The other issue was the patient's relationship with his father, which had been virtually nonexistent. However, he had idealized his father, who was a prominent professional, and identified with his self-destructive characteristics. He also disclosed that in his search for a father substitute, he had been seduced by an older male who used him sexually. This was a traumatic and devastating experience to the patient and had to be worked through, especially in light of his transference feeling that the therapist might do the same thing.

Follow-Up

Approximately 1 year after termination, the patient returned and reported that he had been drug- and alcohol-free for 6 months and was seriously committed to his sobriety. He had not seen any prostitutes during this period. He had made a job change, was still separated from his wife, but more involved with his children. The following year he filed for divorce.

Patients with Full-Blown Narcissistic Disturbances

These patients often enter treatment after a business failure or threat of divorce from their spouse. Many of these patients have a disdain for mental health professionals, and consulting one adds to their sense of inadequacy and shame. With some of these patients, I have found that a time-limited approach is the most effective. Giving clear parameters to the treatment seems to ease the patient's anxiety so that some reparative work can be accomplished. If this is successful, the patient will often return to treatment with the therapist at a future point. The treatment goals should be to establish enough of a holding relationship to keep the patient in treatment for the prescribed number of sessions. I find that between 10 and 12 are best: Any more and the patient will resist; fewer than 10 sessions does not allow for the attachment–separation issues to be mobilized. Cognitive techniques can be very useful because they are nonthreatening and provide some intellectual insight into the patient's defensive operation.

The Case of Gino

The patient came to treatment because of concerns over his marriage. Gino made a classic narcissistic presentation and had little motivation for in-depth treatment. He wanted his wife "straightened out," reporting she refused to continue ironing his clothes. He was indignant when it was suggested that maybe she was reacting to the manner in which he described treating her. He was offered a short-term treatment of 10 sessions, which he agreed to, although he was not sure what the therapist could do for him, given the fact that his wife "needed to do what she was supposed to do." The goal was simple: Have the next session and attempt, in spite of his entitlement and demands, to form a positive relationship with the patient.

The goals were limited, but what unfolded was striking. The patient revealed a deeply held and shameful secret that his father, a celebrity, had had an affair, and his mother carried this shame. Also, as is common in narcissism, his mother had elevated him to the "little prince" status. During the treatment, he was able to contact feelings of grief over the loss of his mother who held a position akin to a saint for him. The 10-session model allowed the patient to experience an intimate relationship for the first time. He appreciated the therapist's frankness about his manner of presentation. Once, he asked to use the therapist's photocopier for something personal and was told, "No." He was outraged but seemed to come to some acceptance after much discussion. Following termination, he reentered therapy with a colleague because of insurance limitations.

Two years later, in a follow-up interview conducted over the phone, Gino offered some observations about the treatment process. He said the type of psychological problem that he was dealing with was "like a cut." "You were trying to compress the time. I don't know if you can speed up a cut healing. If you have a lot of problems that are layer upon layer, they have to be peeled off." He said that after the therapy, "I was a little better" and that he wanted his wife to change but that "I'm not perfect." He seemed to feel that any further change would precipitate a major disruption in his life, and he was not prepared for this. He concluded by saying, "You should have let me use the copier."

The Case of Ray

Ray entered therapy for the first time in his 40s as a consequence of a deteriorating second marriage. An athletic, energetic executive, he was shaken by the depression and apathy he was experiencing for the first time in his life. He was having trouble performing adequately at his high-profile position. Ray had a degree of arrogance even in his suffering and bristled when his defenses were pointed out. Because of his reaction to defense analysis, the focus became his feeling about admitting his vulnerability and entering psychotherapy, which was a clear indication to himself that he could not handle everything alone. As he began to describe his situation, the severity of his marital difficulties became apparent. Ray's wife, an attractive woman, a few years younger than he, was functioning at the level of a child. She did not work, clean the house, or assume any disciplinary role with their children. She was a prolific spender who used up the resources as fast as he could earn them. It became clear to him that, if he were going to have any life of his own, he would have to leave his wife, and he was grief stricken about abandoning her.

The core issue was revealed rather quickly. Ray, too, was an only child (in my clinical experience this form of narcissism is more common with only children). Ray's father was practically an invalid. He spent almost all his time sitting and watching TV. He had virtually no relationship with his son. He did not participate in his life. Ray learned to ignore his father and to rely on his mother who seemed to get her emotional needs met through Ray.

During treatment, which lasted 20 sessions, Ray experienced a number of derepressions of grief and anger over the loss of his mother. He also remembered a "forgotten incident." Apparently, after his mother had died, his father became depressed and Ray invited his father to live with him, his first attempt at getting close to his father. During the first week of his stay, Ray's daughter was molested by his father. Ray immediately placed him on a plane, and his father died sometime after this and was buried by the state. Ray did not even know where. He had not attended his mother's funeral, either. During the course of treatment, he accessed the most painful grief over these losses. He found out where his parents were buried and went to visit their graves in an attempt to achieve closure. He also contacted his rage toward his father. Ray's demeanor changed dramatically during the course of treatment from the somewhat classic presentation to a softer, more emotional and likable person. At 2-year follow-up, Ray was very happy with his life. He had divorced his wife, was living alone, and feeling excited about a new business venture.

The Case of David

David, a very youthful man in his 40s, had recently given up an almost 20-year history of alcohol dependence with the help of Alcoholics Anonymous. He had done well in a career that was somewhat below his ability. He was referred for short-term treatment. When defense analysis began, with his detachment and rationalizations being pointed out, he responded in an outraged way. This response differs from anger: It has an angry part but is more like a howling of someone in pain. Instead of a defense analysis, a more empathic mirroring approach was used. The patient's affective tone during the sessions was communicated to him by saying, for example, "You appear sad." "Your eyes have some painful feeling in them." "I sense you're feeling angry." The patient responded positively by bristling less. Once this empathic bond had been strengthened, some mild defense analysis and cognitive restructuring were undertaken that led to some derepression of core material.

The patient was the only child of a very depleted woman who had chronic physical and emotional difficulties. The patient, although the center of her life, never felt as though there was enough of her. He constantly feared her loss as there was no extended family. He developed an inflated self to protect him from his fear of abandonment and anxiety. He found drugs and alcohol in his early years and continued this pattern until his life began to show signs of major trouble. During therapy, he mourned the death of his mother and made connections between the dyadic nature of his early relationships and his reliance on depleted women to supply all his needs, creating a maladaptive repetitive pattern. During treatment he said, "I am always managing the safe zone between abandonment and engulfment."

Patients with Narcissistic Sector to Character Disturbance

Patients with a narcissistic sector may initially appear to be syntonically defended, but when defense analysis ensues, the patient may react as if he/she is empty or at a loss. Often, the clinician will discover the narcissistic sector of the personality only after attempts at restructuring finally succeed, and undifferentiated affect is accessed. Undifferentiated affect is somewhat difficult to describe. It is like depression and is often described by the patient as feeling lost or empty. In these cases, the therapist must modify his/her approach and use more self psychology techniques, such as mirroring. Exploring the patient's developmental history becomes crucial. The therapist and patient should attempt to get as clear a picture as possible as to what occurred in the patient's early life. These preoedipal influences can often explain why the patient is feeling this emptiness. It is often an abandonment depression that is deeply felt.

For example, one patient who was primarily an obsessional character, did not react to defense analysis with an activation of his affective schema. It became clear in treatment that the patient had missed an early bond with a nurturing figure. This was discovered when it was pointed out that the patient consistently avoided eye contact. When he was asked to attempt to maintain it, a mixture of anxiety and sadness was evident on his face. From his developmental history, we had noted that he had spent the first 2 months in an incubator and probably had very little human contact. He reacted to this with increased signs of grief. As compared to treatment of the histrionic personality, as well as the Cluster C personalities, *narcissistic personalities require a major dislodging of unresolved grief that must be completed before anger can be metabolized.* This unresolved grief is a result of the major abandonment that the patient has experienced by the genetic figures.

Also, later in his development, this patient described a void of intimate contact, having received neither affection nor emotional interest from either parent. If the therapist and patient make the correct formulation, more feeling will be derepressed and is treated in the same fashion as any other derepression—by intensifying feeling and providing enough time for the patient to metabolize it. The use of affective restructuring techniques is helpful. For example, the clinician may ask, "How deep within you does that feeling go?" or "What physical sensations do you notice as you talk about this?"

Some of the issues that have emerged in my work with this group of patients are summarized below.

Lack of Paternal Figure or Substitute

Almost all patients with full-blown narcissistic disorders have an absence in their developmental history of a relationship with a father or a father figure. Most times, the father is never acknowledged, and if he is, he is passive and childlike. The therapist must help identify this crucial loss and access feelings and fantasy about what happened to the father. This is what Maine (1991) so aptly identifies as "father hunger," and the narcissist's grandiosity may be an attempt to regain the lost father. A balanced approach combining defense analysis and empathic attunement is often effective.

Search for the "Good Enough Mother"

These patients have not had sufficient nurturing and often have become the emotional caretaker of the maternal figure. Representations of this state can often be observed from the patient's transference responses to the therapist. For example, the patient described earlier in the chapter with the substance abuse/prostitution pattern always expected that he would be humiliated by the therapist when he reported his behavior. This was pointed out and linked to the humiliating fashion in which his mother often related to him. Patients may search for this early comforting bond through addictive behavior.

Educating the Patient

If there seems to have been some narcissistic injury, I often recommend two books that many patients report have powerful effects on them. One is Alice Miller's (1983) *The Drama of the Gifted Child,* and the other is James Masterson's (1988) *Search for the Real Self.* Miller's book has been especially useful for patients who have been narcissistically used by incomplete or disturbed parental figures. This often helps access the affect, and the standard restructuring attempts are made. If possible, the therapist should link this to an incident either from the past or one observed with a child. The object is to frame the injury as a lack of sufficient maternal supplies and to intensify the feeling so it can be processed.

Patients with Low Motivation

With patients who have low motivation, it is best to use the time-limited approach. The patient can learn that therapy does not have to be a humiliating event and this may set the stage for his/her return later.

Addressing and Labeling the Shame

The patient's shame must be identified as soon as it is evident and brought to the surface. The potential intimacy with the therapist will quickly reactivate the shame around the core issue of not being good enough. If this is identified early, the therapy will proceed more smoothly. Particular emphasis should be placed on exploring the patient's feelings about seeing a therapist and the shame associated with that.

Long-Term Prognosis

I agree with Kernberg (1986), who believes that the best way to evaluate the effectiveness of treatment with narcissistic disorders is long-term follow-up. I have not conducted any with my patients. The very act of aging increases narcissistic vulnerability and is likely to lead to deterioration in the untreated patient. This is a strong call for those of us in clinical practice to learn effective methods of engaging these patients and for developing increasingly effective shorter-term treatment approaches.

BORDERLINE PHENOMENON: A POTENTIALLY VIOLENT BORDERLINE MALE PATIENT

The patient, a male in his late 20s, was referred by an employee assistance program (EAP) therapist when the patient threatened to murder a family member. At the time he was seen, it was clear that he was indeed capable of carrying out his threat. The family member was informed, and the situation was very tense. Hospitalization was considered, but because of the high degree of resistance to this option from the patient, it was not chosen. This patient did well with empathic cognitive restructuring conducted intermittently, chosen because his work schedule required him to be out of town. For some borderline patients, being able to regulate the dose of therapy gives them a desperately needed sense of control. During the course of therapy, the patient's wife left him, and he was able, with difficulty, to continue working. He was almost chronically suicidal and homicidal but was able to control the impulses to act on these feelings. Any real or perceived threat, however, could trigger a massive explosion. He was able to benefit from very low-grade cognitive portraiting of what would happen if his violent or suicidal impulses broke through. Discussing them seemed to drain off some of the energy for this patient. Throughout the therapy, he was able to link his own violence to his early life that had been filled with parental violence, alcoholism, and neglect. The patient would not stick to a regular therapeutic schedule but scheduled appointments when he felt he needed to talk. Short-term therapy was not the treatment of choice in this situation, but in the absence of a commitment on his part to do more regular sessions, short-term interventions and flexible scheduling were used by default and successfully stabilized his condition.

Short-Term Techniques after Patient Is Stabilized

The use of short-term restructuring techniques can be very effective for patients after they have their self-destructive patterns, such as substance abuse, parasuicidal behavior, and sexual acting out under control. I have used these methods in the course of longer-term treatment to accelerate the process.

Danger of Regressive Episodes and Acting Out

None of the anxiety-arousing short-term techniques should be used until the therapist has developed a solid therapeutic alliance, and even then the borderline patient may react negatively to the use of these techniques. I have used these techniques in an experimental way with patients who were in serious danger and had not responded to other, more traditional approaches, such as the borderline male patient presented first. This should not be attempted with more primitively organized borderline patients until one has received the necessary training.

TREATMENT OF THE ANTISOCIAL PERSONALITY: "THE SEVEN RINGS OF HELL"

Patients with antisocial personality disorders are considered untreatable by mainstream psychotherapy. Many clinicians consider it futile to attempt short-term psychotherapy with this group. However, I think there are various factors that therapists should consider before they write these patients off as untreatable, except in a contained environment.

Patients with Sociopathic Traits

Many personality disordered patients have antisocial personality traits that coexist with other disorders. These patients need to be evaluated carefully before treatment begins. Stone (1993) reports 22 categories of antisocial personality with increasingly higher levels of malevolence. The clinician needs to be able to differentiate among the more virulent forms of antisocial or psychopathic personality and those patients more amenable to treatment.

Substance Abuse

There is a high level of substance abuse in those diagnosed with antisocial personality disorder. It is crucial for the therapist to determine the nature of the patient's substance abuse and the contribution this makes to the personality disorder. Many patients with severe and milder personality disorders enter treatment after or during a period of sobriety. Long-term substance abuse has severe negative effects on characterological formation. Many patients may have antisocial features and mimic full-blown antisocial personality disorder.

The Case of the Sober Male Patient

The patient, a male in his early 30s, entered treatment at the urging of his AA sponsor. He had 5 years of sobriety at the time he was first seen. Many of his defenses were brought to the surface, and affect over the lack of positive parental figures was accessed and derepressed. He entered an extended phase of mourning. His identification with antisocial lifestyle was interpreted as an attempt to find his manhood related to massive rejection by a cruel and abusive father. He also faced his guilt concerning many antisocial acts. The patient seemed to make good progress and made a touching termination. However, he refused to pay for his last session, and the bill had to be sent to a collection agency before he finally paid. Unfortunately, he did not fully experience the depth of his sadistic feelings toward his genetic figures because of their neglect and abuse. Such mixed results characterize my work with this group of patients.

CONCLUSION

This chapter presents a diverse group of patients falling under the rubric of Cluster B personality disorders. Some of these patients make substantial gains in personality integrity with the use of short-term restructuring methods, whereas others, such as the antisocial and borderline personalities, achieve fewer gains. Many who consult short-term dynamic therapists have been treated before, and this has improved the patient's object relatedness, preparing the patient for a more intensive derepressive course of treatment. This is a factor that many short-term therapists do not discuss; instead, they attribute the lack of cure to the fact that traditional longer-term treatments are ineffective. I think that this misses the point. What we are doing is building upon the work of previous therapists. I think there needs to be more dialogue between the long-term and short-term therapists. I am pleased that Gustafson (1995) discusses the differences and the common ground in his book *Brief versus Long Psychotherapy: When, Why, and How.* Although there has traditionally been animosity between the classic analysts and the short-term analysts, I think a rapprochement would be useful for the future of all psychoanalysis.

CHAPTER 10

Cluster A Disorders: The Treatment-Refractory Group

A man must see and study his vice to correct it; they who conceal it from others, commonly conceal it from themselves; and do not think it close enough, if they themselves see it: They withdraw and disguise it from their own consciences. Why does no man confess his vices? Because he is yet in them; 'tis for a waking man to tell his dream.
—MICHEL DE MONTAIGNE

The Cluster A disorders, which include the schizoid, paranoid, and schizotypal personality disorders, have generally been thought of as unresponsive to STDP. Probably the least likely to benefit from STDP is the schizotypal personality, which also seems to have the strongest biological substrate. I have not had the opportunity to treat many of these patients and will not include any cases from this category.

This chapter begins with a synopsis of an extended interview with a patient with a schizoid presentation who demonstrates a borderline organization. This is followed by another case of a patient with a schizoid personality who is more ego-syntonic and solid structurally. In the first instance, the therapeutic approach was shifted from defense analysis to a more empathic one, because it seemed that the patient had substantial regressive defenses. He was then treated with a longer-term approach. In the following chapter, I present a 2-year follow-up research interview with this man. Another patient was referred by a marital therapist who felt the treatment was stuck because of the patient's personality disorder. The final case presented is of a man with a paranoid personality.

THE CASE OF THE MAN WITH THE SKELETAL VIEW

Initial Consultation

The patient was a married accountant, referred by his EAP because he was having difficulty functioning at work. He was seen for a 45-minute consultation. He reported that at work he felt immobilized and sat at his desk for hours writing the words "help" and "die," and then crossing them out. On one occasion, he curled up under his desk in a fetal position. He appeared depressed but was not in a major clinical depression. He agreed to be seen for an extended session.

Extended Session

THERAPIST: So how did you feel after you processed our first session?

PATIENT: (*very stiff posture, head hangs down, and voice in monotone and tremulous*) In some ways it was unsettling, and we discussed that a little last week. I'm looking forward to proceeding. I guess the one thing that surprised me was how quickly you perceived it as an emotional problem. It wasn't a complete surprise, but I have memories back from the past, but not from the recent past.

THERAPIST: What were those memories?

PATIENT: One was roughly 10 years ago. A woman who I was dating, whom I liked very much and she wasn't as fond of me, said as we broke up, said in effect that I needed treatment, that I held too much in, that if I didn't make those changes, that I would have severe problems in the future and in particular would never love someone and marry someone. In fact, I have a wife and I do love her and in some ways felt like sort of beating her [previous girlfriend's] prediction.

The patient then focuses on his severe social avoidance and feelings of awkwardness. He says "I feel like there is a shell, and inside the shell I'm very limp."

The defense analysis is undertaken by pointing out his helplessness and barriers. The patient reacts slightly but is largely unresponsive. He reports he has no close friends and dreads going to parties.

PATIENT: It used to be a constant source [of hurt] that there was something wrong with me that I couldn't enjoy [life]. The beer commercials on TV with all these people having a good time, are pure hell to me, and I avoid that completely. That kind of person who is portrayed in those commercials is who I'm not and what I don't think I can be. One side doesn't want that any more, but it still nags me.

THERAPIST: It's a very important choice if you want to change that kind of pattern, because you can live like this for the rest of your life. It's not a matter of life or death.

PATIENT: I hope not; I used to be in a suicidal depression. I don't now, but I would hate for that to start again. It's not inconceivable that it would change. In a sense, that is life or death.

He expressed concern that if he did not change, it would cripple his relationship with his daughter. He is worried his daughter may not like him.

PATIENT: It brings up my parents. I don't have a very emotional relationship with them at all. I think it hurts them, at least my mother.

THERAPIST: It seems like you're still on the fence here.

The focus becomes the relationship with the therapist and how they will have to establish a close, open relationship. The patient says that he does not know whether he wants to make big changes but that now that he is out of the crisis (he had a better week), he does not have the motivation to change. He admits that he suffers greatly. He talks about how he wants to discuss his sex life but feels as if it would be a betrayal of his wife and so does not want to talk about it.

He talks about how much he hurts his wife with his quietness and then begins to sob. He then begins to discuss his relationship with his wife and an ex-girlfriend more openly.

He discusses how his mother talked to him about her emotions and once said that she should not have married his father. He said that he is very much like his father in appearance and personality.

Developmental History

During the course of the extended sessions and subsequent sessions, the following issues emerged. While the patient was in his first year of college, he had experienced a major depression and suicidality. He left school on a medical leave and saw a private psychiatrist for outpatient treatment. His therapist, an older man, died during his treatment. For the first 6 months, after leaving school, he isolated himself in the bedroom and compulsively masturbated. His parents did little to intervene. He finally emerged, got a factory job, and then returned to college to finish his degree at an Ivy League school. He had no close relationships during his childhood, and entering college seemed to increase his sense of alienation and aloneness.

He recalled an incident from his childhood in which his father told him the story of his own life. His father, who had come from an impoverished background, had to clean up the men's room after fraternity parties. His father shared his impression that there are two kinds of men—the kind who get drunk, throw up, and urinate everywhere and the kind that clean it up, to which group he belonged. His father, who had a prominent position in the community, had virtually no relationship with the patient. He remembered no affection or closeness from either parent, and he was not close to his sibling.

Treatment Summary

During the course of treatment, his depression increased, and he was placed on a variety of medications that seemed to have limited benefit. He became increasingly suicidal and during one phase became extremely regressed. At one point, he described the therapist as a skeleton with eyes. The deep disturbance in his level of object relatedness was clear, and the approach was modified to twice-a-week supportive dynamic therapy. Often, it is difficult to determine which patients will respond to a short-term approach, and response to treatment is often the best indicator. However, *if the patient becomes massively regressed and severely suicidal, the clinician should rapidly shift to a more empathic approach.* Also, emergency measures should be taken such as involving support systems, considering hospitalization, and contracting with the patient. This does not mean that restructuring methods cannot be utilized, but intensive defense analysis should not be used until and if the ego is strengthened. The first phase of treatment consisting of defense restructuring lasted 20 sessions.

The patient's condition worsened when he and his wife decided to buy a more expensive house in an affluent community. He was at times frozen with anxiety over this decision. The patient became very suicidal and regressed, not wanting to leave his bed in the morning. He made a pact that he was going to kill himself at the end of the year and shared this with the therapist. He seemed to be reenacting in a dramatic way the period of time when he was on the verge of suicide and his parents were helpless. This deepened his sense of abandonment. He was afraid that the therapist would not react. Contracting and emergency sessions were used to communicate concern. The patient was asked to make a commitment between sessions not to act on his suicidal impulses, which were quite strong. At times, conjoint marital sessions were held to stabilize the marriage, which was suffering as a result of the stress of his deterioration. The patient was also given material to read that described schizoid disorders, which he found valuable, as it helped him to know his limitations. Seeing the patient more frequently seemed to provide the patient with the required ego support during this very difficult period.

Analysis of Case

This case required a multimodal approach. Psychopharmacological agents were used to mend biological defects, and conjoint therapy was also used. This underscores another important point with patients in this cluster: *A flexible approach should be used incorporating various treatment modalities to stablize the patient.* At the time, it was difficult to tell whether the use of STDP had worsened the patient's condition or helped to engage him more deeply in the process. It now seems that both effects occurred: STDP facilitated a therapeutic alliance but also overly stressed the patient's poorly functioning defenses. His suicidal phase was reenacted in a powerful recapitulation of his rage and abandonment and his expectation that he would again be abandoned. For research purposes, a 2-year follow-up was conducted and is presented in the next chapter.

THE CASE OF THE MAN WHO JUST HEARD THE WORDS

The next case is similar diagnostically to the one just presented, but in contrast, the patient seemed to have less of a biological loading for schizoid personality and depression and had better ego adaptive capacity, as well. He was an athletic man who used his prowess to his advantage to gain some positive sense of worth. In fact, he was very successful in his athletic pursuits. He was self-confident and had a commanding presence.

　　In the initial extended session, the patient appears apathetic and detached. There is little facial expression. He is slouched and has his head on his hand.

Extended Session

THERAPIST: So what seems to be the problem?

PATIENT: We've been going to Betty [marital therapist] for about a year, Lisa [wife] and I. Lisa is basically very upset about my interaction with her, in a sense of responding. I mean I know I'm more introverted than I should be. I've always been that way. Betty thought that this therapy would open things up more quickly. We're kind of in a log jam. She's [wife] unhappy with our relationship, and I am too. She's the one that always initiates it. I have a tendency when I'm confronted with something to withdraw rather than confront it. It's the biggest problem I have. I kind of avoid conflict. If there is a minor thing that bothers me, I just don't tell her about it. I just don't think it's worth telling her. I just live with it. I think eventually what happens is those things build up until I resent what she's doing. In our relationship, I just don't think it's an equal thing. It's a point where she keeps bugging me, and I just shut it off.

THERAPIST: So you shut down. What happens after that?

PATIENT: She gets upset with me. I mean, the reason why I love her is she's so emotional; that's what I liked about her the most. I think it gets to a point where it doesn't feel comfortable. That's the only way I can describe it. I just don't respond to her sometimes.

THERAPIST: So you say the main issue that you've come with today is that you're introverted?

PATIENT: Well, I don't think I'm introverted as a person. I'm outgoing, and I can communicate pretty well. I think in the relationship, because I really haven't had—I got married 4 years ago when I was 40. The relationships I had before that, I mean I wasn't really running around or anything like that, but there wasn't any long-term relationship that I had. There was never a serious relationship, I don't think, before Lisa. In that sense, I haven't had a long term relationship, in a sense that Lisa was married before, and she was with that person for a long time, and she's that kind of person, that has that type of relationship. This type of thing just seems to be something I can't deal with.

THERAPIST: You're introverted more in the relationship with your wife and less outside of that relationship?

PATIENT: I don't know if introverted is the right word.

The patient at this point is very hard to follow. (In fact, this tape was very difficult to transcribe because of the patient's idiosyncratic way of expressing himself.) He is vague, contradicts himself, and does not finish his sentences. He mumbles so that it is hard to capture what he is saying. From what he has said so far, it appears that there is major ego-syntonic character pathology, but the exact nature of it is unclear.

PATIENT: What I meant is that I just kind of internalize a lot of my—Instead of telling her what I think, whether it is positive or negative, I keep it inside and just expect she knows it.

THERAPIST: Can you give me an example of how this problem manifests itself?

The patient continues to discuss the marital therapy in a vague way, but does not provide any detail. They were in marital therapy because of his wife's frustration with his lack of communication.

THERAPIST: How are you feeling right now?

PATIENT: About the relationship? I feel fine.

THERAPIST: What were your thoughts about coming here today?

PATIENT: Um, I was curious about what's going on. I'm kind of leery about the whole thing, but at the same time—

THERAPIST: When you say leery, what do you mean?

PATIENT: Well, I just don't see psychoanalysis as a science. I think it's something . . . I think people are well educated and well meaning, but I just don't think there is a basis, it's not like the physical sciences.

THERAPIST: So in a way you say, you're leery about this. We should look into that.

PATIENT: I think there are different ways of achieving certain goals, but in a way I'm not well versed in your profession. Most sciences, there is a right and wrong, and people prove things.

THERAPIST: In terms of being here, today?

PATIENT: I think that therapy could work. I'm positive about it.

THERAPIST: It seems like you're mixed about it. Part of you is skeptical, and part of you thinks it could work.

PATIENT: I think I've always been someone who's handled things himself. I never had anyone I've spoken to about how I feel.

The patient then discusses a previous therapy with a social worker, which he felt had been a positive experience. However, he lost interest and stopped going, which was typical of his attachment difficulties. As can be seen by the transcript so far, *patients in Cluster A exhibit so many malignant defenses that it is very difficult for the therapist to establish a clear focus.* In these cases, the therapist wants to immediately address both the character defenses and treatment resistances. This is demonstrated in the following segment.

THERAPIST: So, the first issue that you and I are going to have to face is your ambivalence about being here.

PATIENT: I'm not going to hold anything back, and my therapist thought that this was a good—

THERAPIST: I notice that you have a tendency to ramble a lot. Go around in circles. Because, up until this time, you still haven't identified to me what it is that you would like to resolve.

PATIENT: I guess what I would like to see me do, as a person, is grow into a relationship, in a sense of interrelating with Lisa in a loving and caring way.

THERAPIST: That sounds very intellectual or canned, in a way.

PATIENT: I guess it's hard to explain because . . . I don't want to ramble again. I have always been in charge of what I do. I am an administrator; I can run things. I guess the problem is I don't have any guidelines.

THERAPIST: You have driven a long way, and are paying a lot of money, and spending a lot of time for something. But it is still not clear what brings you here to do this.

PATIENT: I think if I knew what the exact problem was and knew how to deal with it, I wouldn't have that problem because I'd take care of it.

THERAPIST: So, in a way, you don't know what the problem is?

PATIENT: I don't know what the causes are. I know what the results are.

THERAPIST: But in terms of the problem, it doesn't sound like you know what you're here to do. Which really puts us in a difficult position because up until the time we have some identifiable problems, there is no way we can have a plan to resolve them.

PATIENT: I thought I said the problem was relating to the relationship.

THERAPIST: Relating to the relationship?

PATIENT: Relating in the relationship.

With this degree of character pathology it is difficult to even establish a current incident, so the therapist must continue on the D corner of the triangle of conflict. One can get a glimpse of the pervasiveness of the "communication difficulties" this patient has with his wife. It is not uncommon, in cases such as this, that the patient has not really entered therapy of his/her own free will. This usually results in the patient going through the motions but remaining highly resistant. If this issue is overlooked, early unplanned termination or poor outcomes will result. Again, the sooner we can establish an actual incident, the easier the therapeutic task will be.

THERAPIST: Can you give me an example of that because that's vague, "relating in the relationship."

PATIENT: You mean the things that Lisa doesn't like.

THERAPIST: The issue is, are you here because Lisa wants you to be here or because you see some problem?

PATIENT: I see problems. I think what she is saying about me is correct.

THERAPIST: Is there a part of you that tends to take a very passive, compliant position?

PATIENT: No. Maybe I should go back a little way. I've been a very independent person in a sense of being by myself—

THERAPIST: But again, you're ruminating right now. Are you aware that you do this in relationships? Up until the time that you can identify something we can work on, I don't see how this is going to be a success for you. The other thing I noticed is that you appear to be emotionally detached. There is a barrier in our way. I'm going to have to pursue you to get more focused.

PATIENT: I think I'm open. I don't think I'm rambling because I'm trying to hide something. Maybe I am. Maybe that's one of my defenses, but I don't think I am. I mean if you ask me something, I think I feel comfortable talking to you.

Patients with this degree of character pathology have great difficulty distinguishing between thoughts and feelings. They use the words as if they are interchangeable and often become confused if this is pointed out.

THERAPIST: But again, that's a passive position, to come and wait for me to ask you the right questions. You know yourself better than I do; I just met you 15 minutes ago. You have been living like this for 44 years.

PATIENT: But I have also built up these defenses to protect myself from interacting. I have never really had a close friend. I don't talk about anything.

Now we get a genuine communication about the nature of his core pathology. He has gone through life without being close to anyone. It is advisable to stay with the character analysis until feelings are intensified and closer to the preconscious zone.

THERAPIST: So one problem is intimacy and closeness. In this case, to let me into the intimate center of your life.

PATIENT: Yeah, I think that is true more so with Lisa. I think that's what she wants and needs. I think that is what a relationship is for. I don't think

I've ever done that. What you said was interesting because a number of people say that about me, people who don't know me. But once the people know me they say, "Oh, he's a nice guy." I protect myself a certain way that people pick up pretty quickly. I have always thought that it was just the way I looked or acted—it wasn't me. Obviously, when people say that, you get more and more aware of what people are thinking, but I don't feel that way. I don't feel I'm detached.

His communication at this point is much more coherent and direct, but his defenses quickly regain their hold as he then undoes what he has said. This highlights the ebb and flow of the patient's defenses, as they attempt to regain control and kill the process of developing intimacy, as has happened countless times before in this man's relationships.

THERAPIST: Right now, you're rambling. Do you notice?

PATIENT: No.

THERAPIST: And then a smile comes.

PATIENT: I don't think I'm rambling (*mumbles*). If you say so.

THERAPIST: Do you notice you're smiling?

PATIENT: Yeah, why? I shouldn't be?

THERAPIST: What is the smile? And then you look out of the window. How do you feel when you look into my eyes?

It is often very helpful with patients who have major attachment disorders to encourage them to look into your eyes and notice how their body responds. Because of their defenses, they rarely receive feedback from others that would increase their self-awareness. Thus, attachments are made and lost with very little growth occurring along the way.

PATIENT: In what way, how do I feel? I think you're confronting me, and that's fine.

THERAPIST: But that's a totally intellectual response.

At this point, the therapist summarizes the patient's defense constellation as consisting of detachment, intellectualization, rumination, smiling, generalization, and passivity, and the barriers that it creates are underscored.

PATIENT: I agree. I don't think there is any question about this.

THERAPIST: The issue is that you come this far, and then it seems like you are going to sabotage your own effort.

The therapist continues to focus on this barrier and to point out how it ruins his relationship with the therapist.

THERAPIST: Are you defeating this before you even give it a try? You've already set it up so that it is going to fail?

PATIENT: I haven't consciously done it.

THERAPIST: Conscious or unconscious doesn't make a difference. We have to examine the truth of you. Is it that you've come here to defeat me? The smile comes again.

PATIENT: I'm just thinking if I say "No," then you say, "Why are you doing what you're doing?" It's a catch 22. I mean, I can't say, "I came here to get defeated." Then why am I here? If I say, "I came here to get better," then why are you protecting yourself?

THERAPIST: But it is very important that you examine it, either way. And to see whether this is something not only to do with me but is in your other relationships, one with your wife, your therapist, I don't know whom else.

Using the phrases "Let's examine this," or "Let's look into it" develops the observing ego. Many patients want to argue with the therapist about his/her perceptions, but this ploy must be avoided, or the patient's character defenses will turn into resistance, and the therapist will be nonconstructively engaged. The use of appropriate language to emphasize the dual nature of the process—"let's," "you and me together"—strengthens the alliance. This is especially important for patients in this cluster, as many of them have never experienced an intimate, caring relationship.

PATIENT: I know it's there! It's one of the things that I have to work on. I know I protect myself.

THERAPIST: Again, you use protect. But is it protecting or crippling you, denying you a full emotional life?

PATIENT: I don't know what words to use to describe what I am doing to myself. I know it's destructive. It's not positive.

THERAPIST: So then there is a self-destructive element in your character.

Patients from this cluster often have tenacious, self-destructive behav-
ior patterns that drive them toward greater levels of misery, which must be
brought to awareness. They are generally less aware of the destructive nature of these patterns than patients from the other clusters.

PATIENT: Yes. Yes.

THERAPIST: Is this something you want to get to the bottom of? Because we have some time together, an allotted period of time, to see if this type of therapy is going to be effective for you or not.

The therapist should remind the patient that time is limited. This puts greater pressure on the patient to participate more fully.

PATIENT: I think we have to get to the bottom of it. That's what I want to do.

THERAPIST: You want to do that? Because it's very important that you have the *will* to do this, because it's going to be a lot of hard work.

At this point, most patients have no real sense of the amount of pain that is being contained and managed by their defensive constellation. Part of the therapist's function is to educate the patient about what is to be expected by previewing the process (Trad, 1992, 1993).

PATIENT: I just don't see it as hard work. Yeah, but I'm willing to do whatever.

THERAPIST: So you don't think this process is going to be hard? But you have to be willing to be totally open and honest and look at your life and yourself.

PATIENT: I think I can do it. I know I can do it.

The core conditions of openness and honesty are necessary if the therapy is expended to attain depth of focus. These requirements, or values, are communicated in words and through empathic, nonjudgmental responding. No matter what is said and how horrendous it appears, we try to understand and to help process its meaning. The fantasy life of patients in this cluster is often quite horrific, and sometimes patients act out, or come close to acting out, and limits should be set, if necessary.

The patient appears withdrawn now, and this is pointed out. The therapist notes that the patient avoids his feelings and is "cut-off from his emotional self." He responds by saying he has no emotions.

THERAPIST: You're cut off from your emotional self. Your intellect is here and your emotions—

PATIENT: Not there (*smiles*). It's not there.

THERAPIST: You're saying that you're an emotionally dead man?

PATIENT: I know I have emotion, strong feelings. They're not there in a sense that they're not available.

The question is posed to the patient if he has a capacity to be defiant and stubborn. His communication again deteriorates.

PATIENT: I'm not black and white all the time, but I'm more comfortable with things being black and white, good guy/bad guy, that type of thing. I think most people—the grey areas, I don't like those areas. I like to make it good guy/bad guy.

THERAPIST: The thing I am aware of is that we haven't established a partnership yet.

The primitive nature of his object relations is apparent. The therapist again summarizes the patient's defense constellation and mentions avoidance, pushing his feelings down, and evasiveness. The focus then returns to what the patient sees as the problem, and he says, "Not knowing my emotions." He is asked for a specific incident but he "goes blank."

PATIENT: I'm blank right now.

THERAPIST: So when I ask you to be specific, you go blank.

PATIENT: I go blank . . . I think I'm aware of you telling me how I ramble, so I don't want to ramble, so I'm trying to be more precise about it (laughs).

THERAPIST: So when that doesn't work you go blank, which is another defense, which really keeps me at a distance from you. See the smile comes, almost like you're getting some gratification out of sabotaging this.

PATIENT: No, I'm not. It's more of a frustration, that I don't. . . . Obviously, I've gone blank for a reason. It's interesting that I've done that. I usually don't.

One can see how the alliance is increasing and his observing ego is developing. If this patient's defenses were not actively addressed, he would completely derail the therapeutic process, and the therapist would become frustrated. The therapist's understanding of the defense system and how to restructure it keeps the process flowing and deepening. The therapist must always place the decision to change in the patient's hands. Some patients will decide not to pursue STDP, and that must be expected.

The patient says there are plenty of incidents of problems in his marriage but that he is again blank and cannot remember any. He then starts to withdraw. This is pointed out. He then describes an incident that occurred with his wife while he was watching TV. His wife accused him of being physically present but emotionally unavailable. He was hurt but "tried to ignore it." He said he was angry, but he withdrew. The incident is used to begin the affect restructuring.

He is asked to describe an incident in which he displayed a massive rage. He describes an incident that caused him to "just snap" 18 years ago. He was watching TV, and his roommate was "bugging" him, playing around. This roommate pushed him, and the patient went blank and attacked the roommate in a state of violent rage: "I was taking his head and smashing it into a wall." Other roommates had to pull him off. The therapist attempts to access the emotion. The patient admits he is terrified of this happening again. He does not know what happened between the time his roommate was "wrestling around" and the moment he began smashing his head. He admits that if no one else had been around, he probably would have killed his roommate: He is asked to visualize the murder and his reaction. "I would have been horrified about myself."

THERAPIST: What are you feeling right now?

PATIENT: I feel chilled. Like I've got goosebumps. I feel chilled. I just visualized him. As you said, I can visualize killing him. Those type of things only happened a few times, when I was younger, getting in street fights. I would have felt massive guilt. Like, "How could I have done it?" It's inexcusable, that type of violence. I was out of control. There's no question, I was out of control. At the same time when I was doing it, I didn't think. I remember this clearly—I remember smashing his head, and I don't remember, him. It was just an object, kind of. I remember I was hitting into the wall, and the wall was giving. There wasn't any blood or anything. Bringing it back, I don't—

THERAPIST: So you actually remember the feel of his head going into the wall?

PATIENT: I also remember that I didn't think I was doing serious damage to him. I mean, obviously I was doing serious damage.

The patient is emotionally engaged at this point and more animated. The therapist asks, "What kind of funeral do you think they would have had for him?" The patient physically reacts by pulling back as if the question shocked him. He admits trying to push his feelings down.

THERAPIST: You seem to be always trying to push your feelings down.

PATIENT: I do.

THERAPIST: But that's going to really slow down our work here.

PATIENT: I guess what I'm saying is I don't know how to push it back up. I've always put them down. I always have. I've never had a way of expressing. I never had somebody to talk to, or I've always talked to myself. So you talk to yourself so much, you intellectualize . . . You do all the things I've been doing, defenses-wise. That's why when I went to Donna [past therapist], it was good she brought up stuff with my family I thought was always a bunch of—

THERAPIST: Words are a way for you, sometimes, of distancing yourself from your feelings. Because there is a lot of feeling right now. And obviously you're not a dead man.

PATIENT: I don't think I am.

THERAPIST: But why is it that whenever your feelings come you want to push them down with me? Because there is feeling in your eyes right now. What is that feeling right now?

PATIENT: Frustration, I want to tell you. But it's like you said, it's almost like it's not part of me. It's almost like a disconnection. Yeah. I've always known I've had the problem. I just have never known how to deal with it. I've dealt with everything else myself, and there's never been, a situation that's, directed. You can't read a book about it.

The therapist returns to the focus of the funeral of the patient's roommate. The patient talks about how horrible he would feel and how it would have ruined his life. He relates how he wishes to avoid the "idea of me snapping and making stupid decisions of me being out of control." The patient is visibly fighting his emotions, which can be seen in his face.

THERAPIST: What are you aware of right now inside?

PATIENT: I feel stimulated.

The therapist continues to bring him back to the possibility that he could have murdered his roommate and how he would have felt. Each time the patient relates on a deeper level emotionally, exhibiting more feeling: "It's even hard to think about how horrible it would be."

PATIENT: I know I've had that thing that clicks.

THERAPIST: You say that thing?

PATIENT: That anger. That rage.

THERAPIST: Now, have you ever wondered what was at the root of that rage?

PATIENT: (*sighs*) I just thought it was part of me.

THERAPIST: You took a sigh when I said at the root of that rage. What do you think is the—

This is a sign that anxiety is starting to be mobilized, and the psychic system is allowing more anxiety to the felt experience, underneath which are the patient's feelings. Anxiety is like smoke, and the feelings are the smoldering fire that is being stoked.

PATIENT: The cause of that rage? It's only occurred through physical contact. It hasn't occurred through verbal or anything like that. I think it's just instinct, protective instinct. You feel threatened—I just react to it, because I'm not used to it, because I'm always in control, and all of a sudden, it's out of control, and I feel threatened.

THERAPIST: But do you think we should get to the bottom of it?

The patient keeps describing a sense of emptiness, and this is related to his sadness, "which seems stuck." *Patients in this cluster, as well as those from Cluster B, with narcissistic disorders, often describe emptiness as a core state.* It is often a sign of extreme object loss that must be metabolized by activating the grief, which we will see later. When feelings start to emerge, the patient's defense system pushes it down, resulting in a deadened self and interpersonal style. The therapist now describes how the patient's avoidance of intimacy with the therapist limits his full emotional capacity. This ends the first half of the extended session.

The second half of the session resumes following a 15-minute break.

THERAPIST: What were your thoughts over the break?

PATIENT: The only thing, I think I've realized, at least a little bit, what it's going to take, a sense of commitment and stuff like that. I think I've been aware of problems getting in contact with my feelings. I really feel, almost handicapped.

THERAPIST: It's as if your emotion is buried under cement.

We can see the results of the increased therapeutic alliance and the defense restructuring. The patient's motivation is enhanced, his observing ego apparent, and his communication and contact improved. He is relating in a dramatically different manner with more interest and less cynicism about the process.

PATIENT: There was one point where I wondered whether I had any—kind of like you asked, was there anything there. At one point I was going out with someone. I questioned if I had that feeling; for a long time I didn't think I did. I just didn't feel I had what it took to get close to somebody. I almost felt like there wasn't anything inside of me to give the other person.

THERAPIST: What are you feeling right now and what were you aware of over the break, in terms of your emotion?

PATIENT: Surprising, it's much more of a physical thing. I have, like, an ache in my mouth.

THERAPIST: An ache, in what part of your mouth?

PATIENT: My jaw. I have a sense of, it wasn't light headedness, a lightness.

THERAPIST: Like you were feeling relieved?

PATIENT: Well, I think it was more aware, of some of the things about me. We were talking about . . . I think I've always been aware of some of the things you talked about.

THERAPIST: You've been aware that there's been a barrier and that you're emotionally cut off. A barrier between you and other people that has affected your relationships.

PATIENT: But I mean something worthwhile. Maybe I just didn't think there was something worthwhile there, to "substain" [pronounciation is patient's].

The patient then discusses his relationship with his wife and how she has complained about his detachment. The focus shifts to his sexual relationship. The therapist summarizes the issues and reviews the accomplishments so far.

THERAPIST: One of the issues is that you have a number of defenses, part of your character, part of your personality, that are ways that you distance other people from you, that you were faintly aware of, and you use this as an emotional barrier. Because how can anybody get close to you with that kind of wall? The detachment's there, the rumination, the rambling, intellectualization, cutting your feelings off, swallowing your feelings, avoiding conflict, emotionally withdrawing. These are defenses that you built up over the period of your life that have sabotaged intimacy and closeness. And, obviously, this is one of the issues in your relationship with your wife. It sounds like your relationship with your wife has become one of her nagging and provoking you, and you withdrawing from her more and more.

PATIENT: Exactly, exactly, right on.

The issue of the self-defeating aspects of his life are summarized. Further, the meaning and function of this process, and the need to get to the root of it, are underscored.

The patient presents an incident in which his wife criticized him. His wife told him to wash the kitchen floor because they had guests coming. "At times, I feel like she's the mom, and I'm the son." The focus then becomes his anger: "I didn't even let myself feel the anger." The Dr. Jekyll/Mr. Hyde metaphor is used to account for the patient's fear of his anger and his split, with the good guy on the surface and the monster underneath. He admits he was going to "direct it [his anger] in a socially positive way" during the Vietnam War, and "I would have gone into one of those special groups." He then recalls an incident 15 years ago in which he physically grabbed his girlfriend. He returns to the incident with his wife with the focus on his anger. He then portrays how he would grab her by the shoulders and smash her into the "sheetrock wall," and "I don't think I would have stopped." He is still far away from being connected to his anger, but is more involved and animated than previously.

He describes his need to "protect himself from being hurt," which is triggered "by somebody not appreciating me." The therapist asks who that is and he responds, "My parents." He is asked which one and says, "Both, actually."

THERAPIST: Both parents? Which one seems—

PATIENT: My mother, I guess. She was very distant, and I never got the sense . . . I knew they cared about me, but they never showed it. There was never any contact, never any kissing or hugging between the kids or the parents. I was always kind of independent. There was never any emotional . . . I mean the only emotion we had in the family was when my mother got mad at my father or when we broke something, and she got mad at us.

Apparently, his mother had a lot of knickknacks, and when he was a teenager, he had accidently broken a statue. She had responded by yelling and screaming at him. He had felt sorry for breaking it. She then started crying because he had broken something she cared about. Again, he avoids his feelings, although he acknowledges he was hurt and angry. He wanted to yell back, but he did not and then said that his father avoided her, too. She used to hit the children and "hurt her hands from hitting us so hard." The therapist observes and points out some feeling in the patient's eyes.

THERAPIST: What are you feeling right now?

PATIENT: I feel good.

THERAPIST: Good?

PATIENT: I feel good talking about it. I do. Just airy. It seems like we're getting somewhere. It seems like there's a direction of where we are going. The questions that you're asking are stimulating, in a sense of fantasizing certain things and trying to figure out what I'm going to say. I'm not making it up.

The only time this patient's mother had shown any emotion was when she was angry. His father "took what my mom gave him." He was "basically steady." The patient has identified with his father's stoic nature. He acknowledges that his relationship with his wife is starting to mirror that of his parents. He then starts to discuss his daughter, with whom he has a strong connection, and starts to get teary. He fights it back, and this is pointed out. He continues to rationalize why he buries his feeling. The therapist describes the psychic cost of burying his feeling (see Chapter 6 on the importance of affective contact). The patient declares that it might hurt very much but says that he wants to work this through. He then describes how much he loves his daughter and discusses how he wants to do better for her than he has for himself.

THERAPIST: So maybe it's time to change, so the next generation doesn't grow up—

PATIENT: Handicapped.

THERAPIST: Handicapped. You could resolve your problems so that she would grow up in a household where this troubled marriage doesn't get replayed, again.

PATIENT: That's why I'm going to do whatever I have to, either make it work or realize it's not going to work.

He talks about how he was attracted to his wife because of her emotional nature, and he was "taking and taking and not giving anything back" until she stopped giving. He discusses how he really never had intimacy. "It's mainly things I have to work on, to break this thing down and find out what it is." The adaptive nature of his defenses are explicated as a way of protecting himself and his parents.

THERAPIST: We are not going to totally modify that in one extended interview, but it seems like we've made a good start.

PATIENT: I feel like it's going in the right direction.

He then discusses how he was not holding back. He is asked if he can cry. He says, "Yes." He then discusses how one of his students was killed and how he fell on the floor crying when he heard. Yet he had only known him for a short time. He describes his internal experience of the grief "as if all my organs are gone." The link is made between the qualities he saw in this student and himself. The one difference is that this student had a loving, supportive family. The therapist reiterates that the patient missed the support and direction from his parents.

The time comes to end the session. The patient asks for the therapist's opinion about the treatment. The therapist responds that he thinks the patient had a positive response to the therapy and that it could work.

PATIENT: I think I was resisting at first. I don't know why. I think it is much more productive than [previous treatment]. You direct things and confront them much more.

In the next section, the patient's progress is examined with a vignette from the eighth session.

A Snapshot of Progress at the Midphase

Three months later, in the eighth 90-minute session, the patient continued as follows:

PATIENT: It's been a good 2 weeks (*affect brighter*). A lot better than the last one. Right now, I'm not focused.

THERAPIST: But you said that things have been going better over the last 2 weeks? How have you been feeling?

PATIENT: I just feel more awake, I guess, more aware of people. I see people reacting more. I see what they're feeling, whereas before I just heard the words.

The therapist asks for an example of an incident, which the patient provides. He says, "The person kind of came out."

THERAPIST: So in other words, what you're saying is there's less of that wall, that has separated you all your life from people and from emotional contact.

PATIENT: Yeah. It's more fun, more alive.

THERAPIST: So there is an increased feeling of being alive?

PATIENT: Yeah, there and even at home doing things.

Course of Treatment

The patient continued therapy and was experiencing a positive treatment response. His marriage started to improve. The core issue, the lack of bond with either of his parents, was uncovered and repeatedly worked through. However, his character pathology was very entrenched, and frequent incorporation of defense analysis was required to get to his feelings. It emerged that there were two events that had played a central role in the early adult consolidation of his character pathology.

The first event had occurred while he was in college. He had had sexual relations with a girlfriend, and after he had terminated his relationship with her, he learned she was pregnant. She chose to have the child, but even with pressure from her family, he refused to be coerced into marriage. His ex-girlfriend had the child, quickly married and moved to another state. He was ordered by the court to pay child support, and he did so for 18 years. He had no contact with his son after birth. This issue was revealed during the first block of therapy, but the patient dismissed any feeling about this by saying he always wondered whether the child was really his.

The second event also occurred while he was in college. After a party one night, a group of friends left together in a car. At the last minute, he decided not go join them but instead followed in his own car. There was an accident, and when he arrived at the scene and went to see if he could help, he realized that it was his friends, two of whom were dead. He did not react and never grieved their deaths, even at the funerals. During the therapy, he was able to contact this impacted grief and realized that this further strengthened his resolve to be a loner.

After 12 double sessions, the patient missed a scheduled session and discontinued treatment. He returned 10 months later and resumed treatment. His relationship with his wife had begun to deteriorate again, and she had urged him to return, threatening divorce. During this phase of treatment, which lasted for 18 double sessions, the patient contacted his anger in a profound way. He was discussing an incident with his wife in which she accused him of not taking good care of their daughter, which seemed unfair as he deeply cared for his daughter and felt very protective toward her. During the session, his defenses were analyzed, which served to increase his irritation with the therapist. The patient became seized with a violent impulse to attack the therapist: He lifted up the therapist's glass-topped coffee table and smashed it down again. It was an aborted episode of violence, as he avoided smashing the therapist with the table. After this event, which was uncharacteristic, the patient reported a feeling that was like a bolt of electricity through his nervous system, which seemed to unblock him in a significant fashion. He had never felt anything like it before. High levels of anger had always resulted in violent outbursts on the two or three occasions when he had experienced this before, but he would black out. This time, he experienced the rage in a very frightening manner but did not resort to violence. His grief and guilt began to be unblocked. He began to grieve deeply the losses in his life.

During this midphase of treatment, the patient began to come to terms with the loss of his relationship with his son and developed more empathy for his son's loss of him as a father. He wrote a letter to him, and his son responded. They scheduled a weekend to meet in a distant city where they both had events planned. This was quite a profound encounter. They talked all night, and he came away feeling positive but aware of his sadness. He enjoyed the young man whom he had fathered but had never met.

Unfortunately, his marriage seemed to be losing ground. Although he was improving, it seemed that his wife had reached her tolerance limit, and his changes had come too late. The therapy was extended to help him deal with the first real experience of loss. She could not see or was not willing to see the changes in him. He desperately needed validation and her support. He made many attempts to win his wife back, which were rebuffed. They were encouraged to return to marital treatment, but the wife seemed too angry and refused. During the second phase of treatment, his wife asked for a separation. His attempts at saving the marriage were rejected, and he suffered excruciating pain at losing his daughter and wife. This loss of his family protracted the treatment that would have otherwise ended earlier.

At one point, while living alone, the patient was again struck with a suicidal impulse and felt deep despair. He suffered from the deepest despair he had ever known and longed for his family in the most painful way. Yet he managed courageously to face his loss and to learn from it. By the end of treatment, this man was a feeling and sensitive human being who expressed deep appreciation to the therapist for working so hard with him.

CASE COMPARISONS

The two cases presented above have many similarities but also important differences. Both patients lacked any evidence of close relationships with parents, siblings, or friends. In both cases, there was a lack of a nurturing or "good enough" maternal relationship, and this effect was not mitigated by the paternal figure. In *The Case of the Man Who Just Heard the Words,* there was some nurturing from his grandfather, who took him places and spent time with him. He was also able to romanticize his lone position as a strong one so that he did not feel so different. In *The Case of the Man with the Skeletal View,* more extensive therapy was required along with medication to help mend developmental defects.

As can be seen from these cases, the treatment of the Cluster A personality disorders is often characterized by a stormier course of treatment. In the next chapter, we discuss what to do to reduce the pitfalls.

Patients with paranoid personalities, for obvious reasons, do not often come to the attention of mental health professionals, especially in private practice settings. Often, when they do, these patients terminate early. However, some patients of this type can be effectively engaged in short-term psychotherapy, as will be demonstrated in the next case.

THE CASE OF THE MAN WHO WORE SHADES

The patient was seen for a 45-minute consultation scheduled after his girlfriend had terminated their relationship.

Extended Session

The patient is wearing shorts, a T-shirt, and prescription sunglasses. He has taken his shoes off and looks quite relaxed. He mentions that his girlfriend is going to another city to spend the weekend with another man.

PATIENT: It's just hard. I'm not the kind of guy who sits back and lets things happen (*fighting back tears*).

THERAPIST: And what are you feeling right now?

PATIENT: Frustration. I want to do something.

The patient puts his feet up on the coffee table and his hands behind his head. His casual attitude is pointed out to him.

THERAPIST: What were you thinking when you took your shoes off?

PATIENT: (*mumbles*) The only thing that went through my mind was that I hope you don't mind.

THERAPIST: I wonder whether there is a part of you that has a defiant nature?

PATIENT: Sure.

THERAPIST: Do you think you're here to do something about your difficulties?

He states that his motivation is to get back with his girlfriend. Then he says, "This is probably a good thing to do regardless." His tendency to "devalue" the relationship with the therapist is pointed out.

THERAPIST: Do you tend to put up a wall of defiance and arrogance?

PATIENT: I respect that. I remember taking this exact pose in business meetings. Like I don't care.

His girlfriend has asked him to see therapists before. "The motivation came from her," he said. The issue of his will is brought into the fore by asking the patient whether he wants to do it for himself. Again, it is brought to his attention how his defiant attitude, stubbornness, and "I don't care" attitude ruin his relationships. The dual nature of the therapeutic process is stressed. The patient then goes on to explain his history of "closeness."

PATIENT: Not an emotional closeness; maybe for brief periods of time. I think sometimes if I let anybody in too far, they have privileged information which can be used against me. Even if it's someone I'm supposed to be in love or friends with. Maybe that's the reason why I can't open up. I think sometimes, too, if I'm pressured into sharing—

THERAPIST: I'm not here to drag it out of you.

The therapist confronts the patient's contradictory communications and asks whether he notices this with his girlfriend, too.

PATIENT: Sometimes I lie, outright lie.

THERAPIST: You mean you outright lie about things?

PATIENT: (laughs) Yeah.

THERAPIST: Are you aware that you laughed when you said that?

The fact that he is sarcastic is pointed out, and the patient says he recognizes this. He says that a lot of things that are being pointed out are also true in other situations.

PATIENT: One time, when she suggested that we go to a counselor, I said we don't have a problem, we have differences. That's the kind of resistance I've had before (laughs).

THERAPIST: And do you notice the laugh comes?

PATIENT: I can't do anything else.

He acknowledges that going to see a "shrink" makes him appear weak. He then discusses an incident in which he became enraged with his girlfriend and violently shook the steering wheel while going 65 miles per hour. He then discusses a homicide–suicide fantasy, with a violent crash into a gasoline truck. He then relates that once he struck his girlfriend. The patient contacts some grief; there are some tears over the loss of his girlfriend. This half of the extended session is summarized and closed.

The next part of the session resumes after a 15-minute break.

THERAPIST: What were your thoughts during the break?

PATIENT: (*very low voice*) Thoughts or feelings?

THERAPIST: Both.

PATIENT: I feel it's pretty slim. You're probably not going to help me out. Probably too late for me to do anything about it. Too set in my ways. And my thoughts were—

THERAPIST: What are your feelings? You have a lot of difficulty with your feelings; you're a man who distances himself with this stubborn, defiant, arrogant self.

The patient mentions his mother who is a nurse but smokes three cartons of cigarettes a week. He recognizes self-destructive features in her, and it angers him. His mood seems more somber at this point. He appears distant and detached and is avoiding direct eye contact, which is pointed out. He says his boss pointed this out, as well. The therapist continues to point out the patient's defenses and how they deaden the process. The first sign of a therapeutic alliance is noted. The patient sits forward attentively.

THERAPIST: When people put demands on you, you get really furious with them. Not give and take. Then when you want it, you get it, and when you don't: "Leave me alone."

PATIENT: Can't this be changed? What can help the process? How do I help the process?

THERAPIST: The issue is whether you're willing to be totally honest, willing to look at things even if they're very painful.

PATIENT: (*laughs*) Oh, I can't wait.

THERAPIST: But is that sarcastic?

Discussion ensues on the subject of the patient's wanting to avoid his pain, and how this increases his anxiety. The laugh, he says, is his way of reducing his anxiety. He seems increasingly more engaged. He is not sitting cross-legged in his chair, as he was during the first half of the session. He begins to discuss some problems he had in a previous relationship: "We used to argue about a lot of things. It was stimulating to a point." He talks about a fantasy of blowing the world up in a massive conflagration. He says it's not hard to imagine these things and discusses killing elementary school kids: "You can go to the nursery and get the newborns, they are a little more tender and cook properly." He becomes very sarcastic toward the therapist and the process. He finally declares he is "pissed" toward the therapist. The therapist points out how his defenses serve to repel people. The patient says that he wants to modify his style.

THERAPIST: Are you following me when I say this wall is like concrete? You shouldn't agree with what I say if it doesn't fit because everything is not going to fit. Your job is to evaluate what I say and decide whether it fits. What I've noticed in my interaction with you today is that you have a tendency to be stubborn. The defenses create your interpersonal wall: stubbornness, defiance, arrogance, sarcasm; you have a tendency to rationalize, minimize your feelings, and to avoid. When you put all those together, it puts a massive barrier between you and me.

PATIENT: Sometimes, I even call them up intentionally. I catch myself when I do it. Knowing that [wall] was there; that this has filtered down to my basic structure.

THERAPIST: But that's what we are here to look at, the basic structure of your self.

PATIENT: (leans forward, emphasizes with hand) Thank you for pointing it out, and that's not sarcastic.

THERAPIST: What are you feeling right now? When I say "feeling," you physically recoil.

PATIENT: I'm not aware of that.

The patient then focuses on his relationship with his girlfriend and why she left him. He used her and mistreated her and her children. He begins to cry for the first time in the session. He is asked what is the cause of his tears. He responds, saying that his father had been "perfectionistic," and his high school girlfriend had rejected him. He then describes how his girlfriend rejected him, and he shows sadness.

THERAPIST: You distance people from you because you don't want them to get too close. You are stuck in this paradox. If you let someone close to you and hurt you, you blast them. The wall cracked some from your relationship with [girlfriend].

PATIENT: Maybe the part about having some distance isn't necessary any more, but maybe that was true in earlier years. Kind of shy and intimidated by people. Maybe a flying buttress for the anger.

The patient is relating in a much more genuine way, although the distancing quality of his basic syntax and semantic usage is apparent in the vignette above. *When defense analysis is effective, the patient will begin to relate more positively, and there will be enhanced access to the unconscious in the form of relevant communications and affect.*

The next topic is the death of his father, who died 10 years earlier of cancer. The patient's last encounter with him while he was alive was discussed. He had no grief reaction to his father's death, which is often symptomatic of a disturbed relationship with that figure. If there are deeper layers of unresolved feeling, then the grief has difficulty emerging and, in actuality, the defenses become more fixed. The patient starts to cry.

THERAPIST: You have a lot of feeling right now, but you notice how you want to dampen it.

PATIENT: *(leans forward, puts his head in his hands, and intensely sobs for about 10 seconds in an outburst of grief, but immediately closes it off with a violent jerk of his hands)* So, she went to get my brother who was in the room—

THERAPIST: Now a minute ago, when I said, "let yourself experience the intensity," you had this tremendous display of feeling and then shut down. What were you experiencing there?

PATIENT: *(laughs)* What did it look like?

THERAPIST: I see a mixture of tremendous frustration and sadness.

PATIENT: Well yeah, the guy's dead, and you couldn't do anything about it.

He begins to talk about his concern for his mother at the time of his father's death. He had put his own feelings "on hold for a while," presumably to be more available for her. He talks about his mixed feelings and says that he was relieved when his father died. He was angry his father had not gone to the doctor when he coughed up blood. "Maybe he was scared as if he didn't want to admit it. There was no resolving-type final good-bye or anything." His mother said she was glad he was gone: "He was a pain in the ass anyway."

THERAPIST: What was their marriage like?

PATIENT: Nothing spectacular one way or the other. Yeah, I can remember the fights. Nothing really stands out, just arguments. It wasn't an overly loving relationship.

THERAPIST: Your father could be explosive at times?

PATIENT: He'd keep things bottled up. Would he explode? It seemed like it.

My mother says I'm just like him; I keep things bottled up. He was pretty bitter.

THERAPIST: You have a chance to change things if you don't destroy yourself first.

PATIENT: I hope so! I've thought about these things—they aren't resolved yet. Maybe I have to look at them a different way. I have no experience dealing with these things. I'm a little bit too involved to really see it objectively, in all cases. I've got to say that, I just can't. So I ask for somebody's help and assistance. (*soft voice*) Yeah, I want to change it; I want to change it.

One can see after a period of defense analysis that the therapeutic relationship has dramatically changed. The patient's most malignant defenses are receding as the alliance deepens.

THERAPIST: Do you feel hopeful that if you and I work together we could change it?

PATIENT: Like I said, this is new to me. So far I've expressed more to you in a couple of hours than some people do all their lives. Is that a breakthrough right there? I suppose it's significant, to a degree. Do I feel, I mean do I believe it's hopeful? Yes, I wouldn't waste my time on this.

He discusses that he still has the safeguard that the therapist is a professional, and otherwise he would not be as trusting in revealing himself. The issues and goals are summarized and agreed upon.

PATIENT: You just held up a mirror in some respects. Thank you, thank you honestly, I like it. The way it came across is very nicely done.

Two Weeks after Extended Session

The patient's presentation is strikingly different. He is dressed professionally, his posture is erect, and he appears serious. He is not wearing sunglasses.

PATIENT: I've been thinking about two things on the way up here. One concern, and one thing I forgot to mention. The thing I forgot to mention last time, that could have probably got me in this situation, was, I kind of think of it as the lawn mower incident. I was probably about 14 or 15 years old, and I was mowing the lawn. And I remember at that time debating whether it is best to make decisions based on logic or emotion. To think things out, to work them out, to act that way, or to go with what you feel about doing things. I remember thinking about this and starting to cry (*clears throat—fighting back emotion*). My father comes over from across the yard and says, "What are you crying about?" I go, "Oh, I don't know, something." "Finish the lawn!" And I just kind of mulled it over in my mind after that. I think at that time, I don't remember making a conscious decision one way or the other but probably coming up with I'll think things out and choose a logical path rather than feeling things out. I've been pretty much an extremist all my life.

THERAPIST: This sounds like an important memory. Obviously, you have a lot of feeling right now. What are you feeling?

PATIENT: I feel sad (*affect sad*). My concern is. . . . It's just a concern, from a nonprofessional, thinking in this arena. I'm tying to do this with you, for myself, for myself, for me. At the same time, I'm trying to extricate myself from this relationship with [girlfriend].

His level of respect for the therapist and the process has increased and is evident in the genuineness of his communication.

THERAPIST: There is a lot of sadness there. If you just let it come, how do you experience that sadness?

PATIENT: (*crying*) I want to cry. I want to curl up in a ball and fall asleep.

THERAPIST: How do you experience that depth of sadness? What do you notice inside?

PATIENT: Kind of sick to my stomach. Finding out something, as if your best friend died.

THERAPIST: How deep does that go?

PATIENT: I guess pretty far. It doesn't go away; it's pretty persistent (*another wave of grief*).

He returns to the memory of mowing the lawn and wonders why a 14-year-old boy would make that kind of decision. He then talks about how he cried driving over to the office. He is very sad about the loss of his girlfriend.

PATIENT: The sadness has been here all day. 'Cause I feel safe here. It stopped, and I came to let it out (*crying*).

THERAPIST: (*silence*)

The patient is experiencing a high level of grief that is allowed to pass. He never felt this level of safety with his father. He always had to guard his emotional self from any appearance of vulnerability, or his father would pounce on him, mercilessly. The remainder of the session focuses on his relationship with his father and the fact that it was not a close one but, rather, characterized by mutual defiance and provocation. Their relationship was a competitive one in which the father would provoke the patient, and the patient would respond with defiance. A link was then made between the loss of his current relationship and the lawnmower incident. He recalled that he was emotionally distraught over the loss of his first significant relationship and had been rejected by his girlfriend, who chose a rival over him. He had wanted at that time to talk to his father about how he felt and what had occurred. His father was an unemotional man who had viewed his son's display of emotion as a weakness.

Course of Treatment

During the course of treatment, which took 39 double sessions, the patient confessed to some disturbing behavior patterns. He would, on occasion, don dark clothes, arm himself with various weapons, and dress like a commando. On a number of occasions, he sat all night outside of the house of his girlfriend's ex-husband, contemplating provoking an incident that would justify murdering him. He also conducted various clandestine operations gathering information that could be used against the ex-husband. He enjoyed occasions that afforded him the opportunity to subtly intimidate this man, who had been abusive to his girlfriend. He did not become violent but for months seemed on the verge of violence.

A link was made to an early pattern with his mother and father. His father was often abusive toward his mother. When his father had left the house to go to work, his mother would invite him into her bed to comb her hair and stroke her body. He cherished these moments with his mother because he loved being able to give her pleasure, and he hated his father for what he did to her. He felt totally inadequate for being unable to protect his mother.

When he was about 6 years of age, his mother had some friends visiting, and he stroked his mother's breast in front of them. His mother laughed at him and humiliated him in a very rejecting fashion. He was confused and enraged by her reaction and, afterward, felt her loss profoundly.

In his early teens, he witnessed a purse snatching of an old woman, and, instead of reacting as he would have liked, he became frozen. He could never forgive himself for his reaction and replayed the scene again and again, vowing he would not let a woman get hurt again by a violent man.

During the middle phase of therapy, the sessions were often charac-terized by intense mourning that would start almost immediately upon his entering the consultation room. He thought this phase would never end, and it seemed like a lifetime of deep grief had been activated. He continued to have an "off-and-on" relationship with his girlfriend but established another relationship with an old girlfriend, the one whose ex-husband he stalked.

He was able to come to some resolution with his mother, who was still living. When she required surgery, he took a month off from work and spent the time taking care of her during her recuperation. He was able to come to terms with his mother's limitations and improve his relationship with her. He was also able to find some positive aspects of his relationship with his father and to better mourn his loss.

Two-Year Follow-Up

The patient was contacted by phone for follow-up. This was not an in-depth follow-up interview, but the patient was willing to share his feelings and insight. He said as a result of therapy, "I get along with people so much better, and I can talk to people." He said that his emotional pain has been "elevated to a new level of complexity, as a result of the empathy I have." Further, he described himself as being much more tolerant of his emotions and not so invested in avoiding them. He described an increased capacity to understand where his feelings "come from, to examine them, and talk to people about them."

He described the effect of his treatment: "It's like getting a raise but like getting put in a higher tax bracket." He also said that he understood why this type of therapy was chosen for him, "If I was going to talk to anyone, you had to break down the defenses." He continues to have a relationship with his girlfriend and is very involved with her children.

Comment on Case

This case presents the treatment of a patient who would be considered by many to be outside the parameters of STDP. In fact, the treatment was twice as long as the 40-session upper limit suggested by most. However, I think without the strong emphasis on defense analysis early on, the patient would have left treatment early. As is sometimes the case when doing intensive reconstructive psychotherapy, opening up the patient can reveal a depth of psychopathology that is not evident during the early phase of treatment. I agree with Gustafson (1995) that we are not useless, just as an oncologist facing cancer is not helpless. It is only evident when the patient trusts the process and is willing to reveal his/her darker side. These patients are very courageous, and I have learned much from them. Often, a phase of empathic therapy is required to heal some of the deepest layers of self-injury.

CONCLUSION

This chapter presents cases of refractory patients for whom I pushed the envelope of selection criteria of what would be considered acceptable in a STDP modality. The treatment time frame may have to be extended, but I think that the integrative approach has much to offer these patients. Even if a clinician is primarily using a long-term treatment model, the understanding and incorporation of techniques of STDP can accelerate the treatment process. If STRP is used at the beginning of the process, it can make the patient more amenable to psychotherapy before he/she is lost.

CHAPTER 11

Treatment Pitfalls

It is only fair, after showing the effectiveness of brief psychotherapy,
to make the opposite case, that is, for situations that take thirty years
to change. Nothing is understood, in psychotherapy, without
understanding its negative. This is how we grasp the forces involved.
—GUSTAFSON (1995, p. 163)

When I first began applying STDP to personality disorders, I often blamed what I felt was my own inadequate technical proficiency and insufficient knowledge of psychopathology, differential diagnostics, and psychodynamics for the setbacks that occurred. With time and experience, however, I began to appreciate that therapeutic fractures, early terminations, treatment disruptions, and unplanned dropouts are realities in any therapeutic process, and especially so in the brief treatment of the personality disordered patient. This is not to say that some therapeutic mishaps are not iatrogenically caused. It does mean that a high proportion of incomplete treatments and unsatisfactory outcomes will occur when one is working with personality disordered patients in a brief treatment model. Some patients will have gotten what they wanted from therapy and leave treatment at this point, though the therapist may consider the termination premature. Others, however, who are making excellent progress, simply choose not to continue further for no apparent reason. Particularly frustrating are those individuals who appear to be excellent candidates for brief treatment but who decline after the extended session.

I believe that every case that ends prematurely or with poor outcome warrants careful scrutiny, so that any therapeutic mistakes made will less likely be repeated with other patients. It is important that in so scrutinizing the therapist maintain a realistic yet optimistic perspective; otherwise, there is the risk of therapist burnout. As I have said many times before, personality disorders are highly challenging and complex cases to treat. In many instances, we never know the reasons for poor outcome. When one works hard and provides high-quality treatment, poor outcomes are inevitably demoralizing. The therapist, being human, may naturally fall prey to self-doubt, that is, "If I were conducting this treatment properly, the patient wouldn't miss appointments or avoid paying," and so on. These insecurities, however, only add to the difficulties inherent in treating personality disordered patients by exacerbating frustration and souring the therapeutic alliance.

Recognizing some of the more common problems that occur in STRP and with personality disordered patients gives the therapist the opportunity to anticipate and deal with the potential problems *before* they sabotage treatment. The strength of the therapeutic alliance and the predefining of collaborative goals are two factors that have been identified as crucial to positive treatment outcome (Safran & Muran, 1995). However, there are additional difficulties with personality disordered patients. Many have been incapable of developing satisfactory collaborative relationships or have avoided them altogether, presenting the therapist with his/her first challenge. Often, treatment disruptions are the continuing reenactment of early maladaptive patterns or self-defeating character patterns and, therefore, are not within the therapist's control. If handled effectively, they can become the grist for therapy; handled poorly, they often disrupt treatment. The clinician needs to be alert to serious signs that long-term treatment is indicated.

WHEN TO SHIFT TO LONG-TERM TREATMENT

Sometimes, patients who appear to be good candidates for STDP turn out not to be. When this happens, the therapist must shift to a long-term approach. Although this does not occur frequently, some patients just will not benefit from short-term treatment modalities. The clinician should be alert for patients who manifest the following characteristics.

Severe Disturbance in the Ability to Make an Attachment

A long-standing criterion for the selection for STDP has been a history of meaningful attachment. I think that the criterion is broader in that for some patients, such as the patient in *The Case of the Man Who Just Heard the Words*, there is little evidence of any meaningful early attachment. There are some patients who have no meaningful attachment and who have probably suffered some form of early and extreme abuse and deprivation. These patients often require years of continual psychotherapy to learn how to establish trust. Some of these patients do not show signs of borderline personality but have extremely impoverished lives not apparent to the outside world.

Chronic Suicidality

Some patients suffer from chronic feelings of suicidality and have even decided on a certain milestone or age to kill themselves. Usually, this does not emerge early in treatment. This is a sign that the patient is not a suitable candidate for short-term treatment. Often, this is a life-long struggle, and therapy helps the patient to develop a resistance to act on these impulses.

Repeated Psychotic Episodes

This is another indication that the patient is not going to respond to a short-term approach. Short-term treatment is too stressful for and should not be undertaken with these patients.

Active Unremitting Substance Abuse

Patients who are in the active stages of a chronic addictive disorder are not going to derive much benefit from short-term therapy. If they can attain a sufficient level of sobriety, usually 6 months to 1 year, then they can be treated. The restructuring approaches can still be useful, but potency is severely curtailed.

Treatment-Refractory Depression

Patients with intractable depressive disorders are not suitable candidates for short-term treatment and require long-term psychotherapy to provide support and hope.

If short-term treatment is initiated and the clinician subsequently decides to shift the approach, it is important to inform the patient of the reasons for this and give him/her the opportunity to discuss his/her feelings. Most patients are relieved to learn that they will not be given a task they cannot accomplish. The clinician may want to transfer the patient to someone who specializes in long-term psychotherapy and psychopharmacological treatment.

NEGATIVE REACTIONS

Personality disordered patients display a variety of negative reactions while in treatment. Some of these are attributable to patient resistance, which is not an uncommon phenomenon in any therapeutic relationship. The negative reactions and significant resistance may indicate treatment failure or therapeutic fracture, but oftentimes, these are best viewed as forms of therapeutic communication that call attention to unresolved character patterns or the fact that the patient is not quite ready to take advantage of treatment. Before we review some common patient reactions, an understanding of resistance in its many forms is important.

Manifestations of Resistance

In Chapter 6, we discussed defense mechanisms in some depth. The concepts of defense and resistance, although similar in some ways, merit clarification. Davison et al. (1990) define resistance as "The ways in which thoughts and feelings are inhibited, restricted, and delayed." I tend to agree with them that in many cases "Resistance is evoked by a quantum of aggressive energy emanating from the superego" (p. 602). Viewed in this way, patient resistances are manifestations of defenses, expressed as a reluctance in the transference. Manifestations of resistance include: silence, inappropriate affect, closed patient posture, inhibition in recall of time, avoidance of topics, lack of imaginative thought and dreams, rituals, tardiness, absenteeism, refusal to pay, repetitive affect, acting out, and inhibition of an autonomous ego function.

Resistances demand to be and must be addressed as soon as they manifest themselves, or there will be an insurmountable build-up of negative transference feeling, causing therapy to come to a halt. *The best method of avoiding major resistance is to bring the patient's anger and other negative feelings to the surface, where the patient can work to metabolize them.*

Common Patient Reactions

Premature Termination

As we have discussed, the motivation for treatment varies greatly from patient to patient. If a particular patient is highly ambivalent about treatment and has trouble establishing a therapeutic alliance, the potential for premature termination is high. Most clinicians intuitively sense this resistance and try to work with it by exposing self-defeating character patterns and exploring what the resistance means. In *The Case of the Man Who Just Heard the Words* and

The Case of the Man Who Wore Shades in Chapter 10, I illustrated that patients who appear unmotivated and highly resistant can still be worked with, provided that defenses are dealt with immediately and directly. If this is not done, the patient may choose not to return. In some cases where defense analysis ensues, the patient may refuse to hear it.

To *reduce the possibility* of this occurring, the therapist might consider recommending a time-limited model. The time-limited model offers a framework that many poorly motivated and highly resistant patients will find acceptable. Also, the therapist can encourage the patient to commit to come in for one last session before terminating. For some patients, this commitment is useful. When a premature termination does occur, I often phone the patient to see if he/she will agree to schedule one more session or to discuss the termination. After this, I do nothing further to pursue the patient.

Unplanned Dropout

As we have discussed above, unplanned terminations are the most difficult ones to understand. The treatment seems to be progressing, and then the patient disappears without explanation. These terminations are typically the most difficult to predict and guard against. I have found that, in my own practice, many of these dropout patients have done the same with previous therapists. They seem to be searching for a panacea and present with unrealistic expectations of their role in therapy. Sometimes, these patients have a history of active substance abuse about which they are not forthcoming, so that the treatment lacks the honesty it requires to succeed.

When I notice a history of previous incomplete treatment, I quickly identify this as an issue needing examination and try to determine what led to the abrupt terminations. Although there are sometimes perfectly acceptable reasons for ending therapy, patients who jump from therapist to therapist are generally searching for the "perfect therapist" who will cure them with minimal effort on their own part.

Suicide Attempt or Parasuicidal Behavior

Suicide attempts rarely occur while the patient is in treatment. If it does happen, the therapist must carefully assess the reason why. When these instances do occur, it is generally early in the treatment process before a therapeutic alliance has been formed or a thorough assessment has taken place. Often, these patients are poor candidates for short-term treatment and require longer-term treatment. This is also the case with parasuicidality, wherein the patient habitually engages in nonlethal but potentially self-destructive activities. Many patients in treatment have suicidal feelings or self-destructive impulses. Few will act upon them. The patients who do have suicidal impulses, however, can be dealt with effectively by using the restructuring techniques.

Missed or "Forgotten" Sessions

Unfortunately, this happens all too frequently during the course of treatment (Langs, 1989). When it does, it tends to have a demoralizing effect on the therapist and engenders irritation in him/her toward the patient, especially so for therapists in private practice. Even when the patient signs a policy clearly stating his/her responsibility to pay for missed appointments, difficulties often arise.

In one case, a college-educated patient was making productive use of his sessions and seemed to be progressing well. When he did not arrive for his scheduled double session, he was phoned. His reply was, "I totally forgot." He was reminded that he still had to pay for the time. Even though he had signed a policy statement to this effect, he was outraged. He could not decide whether to come for the remainder of the double session, as he lived some distance away, and could not be convinced to come in and discuss this. As a compromise, he was asked only to pay for half of the session, which he agreed to do. The patient did not return to treatment. I phoned him some months later and invited him to return to treatment. Though he was amiable on the phone, he never called back. This patient seemed to need a showdown in order to discontinue treatment, which indicates elements of strong transference. It turned out that he had behaved in a similar fashion with a previous short-term dynamic therapist.

Most cases of missed sessions can be dealt with more easily and are less disruptive to treatment. Missing more than one session without good reason, however, raises the issue of the patient's commitment to treatment. When this issue presents itself, I discuss the patient's ambivalence, if he/she is aware of it or can admit to it. I find it is usually better to close the treatment if this is unsuccessful. A pattern of missed appointments builds up too much negative feeling in the therapist, which is ultimately damaging to the positive aspect of the therapeutic alliance. I feel it is better to close the treatment on a positive note rather than to allow the patient to wander out of therapy.

Failure to Pay for Treatment

In a private practice or clinical setting, failing to pay for treatment also results in a build-up of negative feeling from therapist to patient. Dealing directly with matters of money is, for many therapists, more anxiety-provoking than discussing sex. Patients fail to pay for their treatment for a variety of reasons that have to be examined with respect to the core issues and transference feeling. One patient, a mental health professional, entered therapy and then declared that he would not be able to afford paying for the sessions and that his previous therapist let him pay late and on a sliding scale. He became irritated with me when he was told that he was expected to pay at the time the service was rendered. He was sure this was a sign that I was not a caring person. It later became apparent that financial difficulties were related to his core pathology. He paid faithfully and when therapy was over, he expressed his gratitude for the therapist's refusal to be manipulated by him.

With this patient, it was explained that not paying for the therapy would build up negative feeling on my part, which would taint the therapeutic task, and that it was in his best interest not to create resentment in me by not paying in a timely fashion. After all, I would be working hard for his fee. The ability to feel comfortable with one's fee and openly discuss this with the patient is central to establishing a collaborative ego-adaptive alliance. The worst thing a therapist can do in this area is to allow a large balance to accrue, as the patient often flees treatment to avoid increasing guilt over unpaid debt. A collection agency may be required to recoup some of the loss, which usually marks the end of any future collaboration.

To *reduce problems* in this area, financial responsibility should clearly be placed with the patient, and this should be done at the onset of treatment. Although it is difficult to discuss these issues with a patient who is suffering emotionally, it makes a clear statement about the importance of dealing with money openly.

Increased Symptomatology

It is a common occurrence to have patients develop new symptoms during treatment. Often, the restructuring of the defense system reconfigures the patient's psychopathological dynamic forces and shifts these in a new way. For example, a patient with a severely syntonic character may develop panic attacks or experience depression or a disruption in sleep patterns. This does not mean that the patient is deteriorating, but it can mean that the patient's unconscious forces have been released and are being experienced closer to the surface.

Also common are increases in the frequency and intensity of symptomatology and destructive behavior patterns. This phenomenon, first observed by learning theorists, predicts an increase in behaviors before they are extinguished. To *reduce the possibility* of this, which works to lessen the patient's motivation for treatment, the therapist should provide the patient with an explanation of this as a common treatment phenomenon for those undergoing rapid transformation.

Increased Drug and Alcohol Abuse

Patients in turmoil often turn to drugs and alcohol for comfort during difficult periods. This can slow the therapeutic process, especially if the therapist is attempting an in-depth restructuring. The use of drugs and alcohol can retard the patient's reactivity and prevent the intensity of affect from reaching the surface, which results in a less satisfactory outcome.

Failure to Acknowledge Benefits of Treatment

In some patients who respond favorably to treatment, there is a subsequent disavowal of the impact of the treatment on their growth. This usually represents a denial of the positive feelings of gratitude and affection that have been activated during the therapeutic process (Klien, 1957). This becomes obvious when the patient acknowledges positive results but does not cite the therapy as a factor. This leads to continued repression of feeling and an incomplete affective experience. To *prevent against this occurring,* the therapist can ask directly, "To what do you attribute these changes?" This question should bring the issue into focus, and if the patient fails to give therapy any credit, this can be pointed out to him/her. Often, the feelings beneath this defensive posture are gratitude and affection toward the therapist, which, if experienced, create a sense of betrayal of the patient's biological figure, that is, "If I acknowledge that our work together has helped me make substantial changes, then how would my parents feel?"

Slowing the Pace of Treatment

We in the psychological community must acknowledge that rapid change can be very threatening to the patient and those in his/her life orbit. Some patients react to this threat by attempting to slow the process and thereby contain a measure of anxiety. If the patient experiences waves of intensely painful feeling, he/she may want to put the brakes on treatment. The patient's resistances might return for no apparent reason. Sometimes, these are caused by realistic fears of reprisal from others to the patient's change that can be potentially dangerous, as was the case of a woman in an abusive relationship with a prominent and powerful member of her community. In other cases, the patient has catastrophic expectations that have their roots in childhood conflicts. For example, many patients begin to assert themselves as a result of therapy and then become fearful of retribution from people important to them, such as the loss of love or the risk of a divorce.

To *reduce the possibility* of this occurring, the therapist can reframe using *supportive–empathic interventions*. Even though there is a high level of pain (which often continues in a powerful way between sessions), the patient can be encouraged to endure negative reaction to his/her change as part of the "healing process" that signifies he/she is metabolizing his/her feelings more effectively.

Stormy Reactions Following Productive Sessions

Sometimes, a particularly positive session will be followed by a very stormy one. One patient who did major work on his core issues and accessed deep feeling came into the following session very argumentative, sarcastic, and noncommunicative. Often, bringing this observation to the patient's attention will allow the deeper feeling to emerge, whereupon they then can be processed.

Plateauing

This is a phenomenon that I have observed in patients who have made rapid progress and then report that they do not feel like doing much in a particular session. This, too, is a form of resistance. Again, I often use reframing by describing this as a normal reaction and a time to survey how much more is left and how far we've progressed.

Decompensations

These are, along with suicide attempts, probably the most disconcerting for a therapist to face. Decompensation occurs both in long- and short-term treatment. When it happens in short-term treatment, the therapist should logically consider whether or not this is an iatrogenically induced decompensation; sometimes it is. Fortunately, careful assessment prevents this from happening frequently. When the patient does show signs of decompensation, however, swift intervention is essential. Medication, brief hospitalization, or more frequent outpatient contact may be necessary.

Common Therapist Pitfalls

The following is a list of some common pitfalls for therapists practicing STDP:

Working Harder Than the Patient

At the onset of treatment, the activity level of the therapist is quite high, higher in fact than that of the patient, but as treatment progresses, less activity on the therapist's part is usually warranted. If the therapist continues to work too hard and take an overly active approach, the therapy will quickly lose its effectiveness. A significant imbalance in the therapeutic effort usually indicates some unrecognized countertransference reaction. At this point, the therapist needs to examine his/her reaction, identify any feeling, and modify his/her approach accordingly. An extreme imbalance of this sort may also be related to unaddressed passive character traits, which would need to be identified.

Expecting Unrealistic Results

Expecting more from the patient than the patient is realistically capable of achieving can create too much pressure and add to the burden with which the patient entered therapy. Recognizing exactly what is attainable is not easy. Often, observing the patient's capacity and functioning as they react to challenges in their lives is the only available indicator. Very often, this can be discussed with the patient. The patient is in the best position to determine the veracity of treatment expectations.

Losing Sight of the Treatment Goals

Conducting therapy with an eye toward the goals of treatment is obviously easiest at the beginning of treatment. As treatment progresses, it is easy to forget the focus of therapy, thereby prolonging treatment. It helps to occasionally remind both the patient and oneself of the treatment goals in order to keep the process focused.

Not Ending When the Patient Is Communicating a Desire to Terminate

Sometimes, the patient states in an ambivalent way that he/she thought they would make the present session the last. The therapist should be careful not to ignore this, despite the perception that the patient appears uncertain, as the patient may act on this and not return. Sometimes, the patient will agree to another session, but if the termination is extended too long, such a patient may cancel and not return. Many patients have difficulty dealing with their feelings about termination. I strongly believe that it is better to end treatment with some form of closure, even an incomplete one, as opposed to losing the patient without having addressed termination.

Allowing Other Family Members to Sabotage Treatment

The family systems of personality disordered patients are often highly dysfunctional, and other family members may be very threatened by the therapeutic process. It is not unusual to receive calls from related people wanting to discuss various aspects of the patient's progress. This can be a very slippery slope for the therapist. *Confidentiality must be strictly main-*

tained. If the patient does give permission for the therapist to talk with a family member, the reasons for doing so need to be clarified. All calls should be communicated to the patient in a timely fashion. Often, the personality disordered patient has long existed with diffuse boundaries and is used to having these boundaries violated. However, even when the intention is good, boundaries must be scrupulously maintained. Communications can be easily distorted, and, therefore, it is prudent to have the patient present for any discussion with family members.

Underestimating the Patient's Capacity for Change

There is no way to predict accurately a person's capacity for change, and underestimating the patient's recuperative powers will undermine that patient's treatment. It is hoped that treatment will provide the patient with a potent source of healing power. Patients have been known to endure all sorts of abusive relationships and still survive, amazingly enough, relatively intact.

Allowing a Build-Up of Negative Countertransference Feeling

If the therapist is not aware of the patient's limitations, or if the patient violates the therapeutic contract, negative feeling will necessarily build in the therapist and have a destructive impact on the therapeutic process. Also, if the patient's character defenses are not restructured, especially the more malignant types— defiance, passive aggression, and acting out—the therapist will find that his or her irritation makes it difficult to be empathic. I often explain how a patient's negative behavior affects me and how this can interfere without work.

Incomplete Assessment Process

The assessment of the patient is an ongoing process, as more is revealed about various aspects of the patient's life and development. To be successful in treatment, the therapist must refine the structural diagnosis and his/her approach, as necessary. One patient, who seemingly presented with a masochistic personality, displayed over the course of treatment signs of a schizoaffective disorder. The treatment implications for the latter are very different than those for the former.

Not Listening to What the Patient Wants from Treatment

At times, the therapist finds him/herself in the position of offering the patient more than that patient says he/she wants from treatment. Although the therapeutic focus is malleable to some extent and can be enlarged, it can only be done so at the pace dictated by the patient. A patient in an optimal gestation period and with good ego-adaptive capacities may choose not to deal with problems that appear obvious to the therapist. The therapist is practically, professionally, and ethically bound to consider what it is that the patient wants.

Assuming Too Much Responsibility for the Patient

When therapy is "stuck" even though the therapist continues to work hard, the patient may not be assuming his/her share of the therapeutic responsibility. In one case, the therapist attempted to derepress feelings resulting from traumatic abuse. The patient, however, remained involved in an abusive relationship wherein she continually reenacted the early abuse. The abuse served to numb her and helped keep her feelings in check. The patient was clearly told that she would never be able to deal with the effects from the early trauma as long as she continued in the present abusive relationship. The patient decided to enter a support group for women who had been abused to help her keep her commitment to terminate the relationship.

Not Assuming Enough Responsibility for Lack of Progress

We therapists are notorious for blaming our patients for not getting better. When treatment fails to progress, it is easy to dismiss that failure as resulting from the patient's resistance, lack of motivation, or untreatability in order to avoid our own feelings of inadequacy, frustration, and powerlessness. This is countertherapeutic. When what we are doing is not working, we need to systematically review our treatment plan and consider other options. These options will be discussed later in this chapter.

The Illusion of Omnipotence

This is often an incipient process wherein the patient believes the therapist has magical healing powers. At times, the therapist's authoritative demeanor encourages this. This is unrealistic and dangerous for the patient to believe. The therapist can guard against this by acknowledging to the patient his/her own limitations and by fostering a collaborative, nonauthoritarian relationship.

Tolerance for Deviancy

Therapists who undertake the difficult cases of patients with personality disorders must have or develop a high tolerance for deviancy. This, too, may seem obvious but is worth examining. Personality disordered patients typically enter therapy with highly chaotic personal lives, especially with respect to interpersonal relationships. Also, as we have seen, they often have tremendous sadism and masochism that can be uncomfortable for the novice to listen to. Inexperienced therapists or those who have not worked with patients with more complex mental illnesses sometimes react in ways that stultify the therapeutic process. I view deviancy simply as an expression of the particular patient's life struggles. Reacting with shock or condemnation serves only to fracture the fragile therapeutic alliance and inhibit patient honesty. Therapists who undertake treating personality disordered patients must first be comfortable with the primitive forces in their own unconscious.

BREAKING UP STALEMATES

Sometimes, therapy just gets stuck. The patient seems unable to move forward, even though the therapist continues to work hard. If this is ignored for too long, the therapy will shift gradually to long-term treatment, and the intensity of the short-term model will dissipate. Some of these cases are very challenging or refractory ones. In other cases, the reason for nonprogression is harder to explain. However, there are a variety of ways in which the therapist can overcome these obstacles.

Consultation with Another Therapist

Not all therapists have access to other therapists (e.g., those who practice in isolated areas), but most do, and consulting another professional is often a very good way to overcome treatment obstacles. When the patient and therapist agree that therapy is not progressing rapidly enough, the therapist can suggest consulting another therapist as a way of obtaining a second opinion. I generally let the patient know I feel that progress has halted due to something I am missing. I feel it is important not to blame the patient but, rather, to express a general sense of puzzlement. This will go a long way in undoing any feelings that the patient has that the therapist is omnipotent, which often plays some sort of role in treatment of the personality disordered patient.

The therapist may have overlooked something in the patient's history or assessment that should be addressed. At other times, the therapist believes he/she is on the right track but finds the results are unsatisfactory. He/she may simply have doubts about continuing a certain approach. The following case illustrates how this can work.

The Case of the "Nice Guy"

The patient was being treated with STDP for long-standing characterological disturbance, as well as a variety of psychological and physiological symptom constellations. He believed he was unable to return to work
because of a memory problem. He presented as a very likable man to those
who had met him. Psychological testing confirmed the therapist's diagnosis
of a well-entrenched obsessional character with significant isolation of
affect. A combination of defensive, affective, and cognitive restructuring
interventions were made. The patient was not able to contact his emotions.
He began to express concern that his memory was faulty and this might be
the real problem. Previous testing did not confirm this.

The possibility of a consultation with another therapist was broached,
and the patient was curious as to why. It was explained that although he
appeared to have the necessary attributes for STDP, there might be a problem
in the therapist's approach that was making it difficult for him to progress.
The patient agreed and was seen by another therapist, who was able to
corroborate most of what was already described but added some important
insights. The patient's attachment capacity was another possible contributing
factor, which may have been affected by his spending the first 2 months of his
life in an incubator. Although this information was previously known, the
contribution of this factor to the patient's current distress was perhaps
considered more lightly than it should have been. Consequently, the consultant
recommended a phase of more empathic alliance building and grief-oriented
work, which, when effected, succeeded in advancing therapy.

Audiovisual Consultation with Patient as Consultant

When the therapist incorporates audiovisual recording into the treatment
process, the tape can later be used as a consultative mechanism. The
following illustrates this point.

The Case of the Highly Resistant Man

This patient was being treated with STDP for long-standing characterological disturbances, manifested by severely self-defeating episodes of
substance abuse. He had been through numerous rounds of substance-abuse
rehabilitation, both inpatient and outpatient, in the form of a 12-step
program. His therapy quickly bogged down because of extremely "off-putting" character defenses. His defenses included stubbornness, sarcasm, and
extreme defiance. Any tack that was taken to get through his wall was
rebuffed with the most insidious combination of these defenses. After

repeated sessions of defense analysis, the therapist told the patient point blank that if they could not progress past this point, therapy was doomed.

He was offered the option of collaborating with the therapist in a joint consultation by reviewing the videotape of the last session and seeing if the wall could be penetrated or bypassed. The patient agreed to this, albeit with hesitation. When shown a videotape of the session, he was shocked by his own dripping sarcasm and the venomous nature of his defiance. He clearly did not like what he saw. This was the first step in making these defenses ego-dystonic, and it strengthened the therapeutic alliance. Progress had been made. The root of the patient's defiance turned out to be a severely abusive relationship with his father, wherein the patient used defiance against his father's dominance. On a number of occasions, the patient had awakened to find his drunken father severely beating him on the head. The way he survived was to develop this malignant defense system, which worked to repel his father and protect him from further physically and emotionally abusive episodes. He clearly saw that it was no longer adaptive.

TREATMENT-REFRACTORY CASES

Some patients fail to improve and require more than a consultation with another therapist to address impediments to treatment. The following section reviews some of the possible strategies.

Multimodal Treatment Interventions

With extremely challenging cases, more than one therapist may be necessary to facilitate change. Remember *The Case of the Man with the Skeletal View* in Chapter 10. The benefits of working closely with a multispecialty team of mental health professionals are tremendous. Sometimes, the therapist can successfully carry out multiple functions him/herself, but better results usually occur when treatment can be carried out by a team. For example, many personality disordered patients enter treatment to resolve marital issues. Once the evaluation is made and it becomes clear that long-standing characterological issues have played a role in the troubles of the marriage, a course of individual treatment can be recommended. However, the short-term individual therapist reduces his/her effectiveness when attempting too much, that is, *both* individual and marital therapy. *Referral to another clinician for marital, group, or alcohol treatment can help keep the boundaries from blurring.*

Various combinations of treatments can also improve the overall effectiveness of therapy (Beutler & Clarkin, 1990). This is limited only by the resources and training of those available in one's community. When a couple requests treatment for marital (relationship) disturbance and they both have character pathology, ideally they often need to be seen individually by different therapists in addition to working with a marital therapist. In many locales, this is not possible; in that case, the therapist can treat one patient with time-limited treatment or a more comprehensive in-depth approach, if that is warranted, and then treat the other partner. Even utilizing this approach, it is best if another therapist does the marital work. If this is not possible, the therapist can meet with the couple after the course of individual treatment.

Another approach that has shown some promise is treating the patient individually with his/her spouse present. This has been effective in overcoming blocks created by one or both partners' defensive structures. This is usually a very circumscribed intervention, using a brief treatment model, as was described in *The Case of the Man Who Feared He Would Be Violent* in Chapter 8.

Expanding or Reducing the Locus of Treatment

When an individual, couple, or family presents for treatment, it is the therapist who is in the position to recommend a combination of treatment modalities that will maximize effectiveness and conserve financial resources. It may be clear that a certain patient would most benefit from long-term psychotherapy but, because of limited resources, cannot do so. Sometimes, the therapist will need to reduce the locus of treatment. For example, many patients are first seen for a couple evaluation. During the course of the evaluation, it may become evident that there is limited hope of improving or even saving the marriage unless one or both partners address some of their characterological difficulties. The focus of treatment during the course of a few marital sessions can be shifted to one member of the couple. The following case example illustrates this.

The Case of the Unhappy Wife

The wife of this young couple made an appointment through her EAP. They came to the first of three allotted sessions, and she presented herself as anxious and depressed. She was feeling dissatisfied with the marriage and did not want it to end in divorce. She did most of the talking, and the husband appeared withdrawn. It became clear that the wife's dissatisfaction was precipitated by his avoidant personality and social anxiety. Although he was very capable, he avoided almost everything that created social anxiety. She felt he was a good man, though she was beginning to lose respect for him and feel increasingly burdened by his behavior. The first few sessions were spent encouraging her to express her feelings and pointing out his characteristic style of avoidance and withdrawal. This type of personality was described to the husband, and he acknowledged that it had existed in him since childhood. He also recognized that it had interfered more and more in his life since he left the armed forces. The couple's resources were very limited. He agreed to be seen for three more sessions, for which his insurance provided benefits.

The focus of treatment became his avoidance. This was linked via the transference to his relationship with his father, who was also avoidant and whom he did not want to be like. During the second session, he contacted strong grief that he lacked a close father–son relationship because of his father's personality. He was encouraged to confront his boss who took advantage of his avoidance by putting him off. He approached his boss about a need for medical benefits and was surprised that he conceded. Although a full working through was not possible, he derived great benefit from the three-session intervention and reported that he and his wife were doing much better. This was a compacted treatment where the avoidant traits were isolated, feeling derepressed, interpretation made, and extratherapeutic behaviors were encouraged.

THE QUESTION OF PSYCHOPHARMACOLOGICAL TREATMENT

The use of psychopharmacological agents in the treatment of personality disorders is controversial. Much of the information on their efficacy is based on noncontrolled studies, and they are primarily case reports. A variety of medications have been cited as having some usefulness, including antidepressants, anxiolitics, major tranquilizers, and lithium. How medication is viewed by the therapist and incorporated in STDP are the subjects of even more dispute. The controversy over the use of psychoactive drugs rages between the extreme positions of those who view them as a panacea and those who consider them a crutch. Although the issue surrounding medication cannot be given the attention it deserves in this book, I will attempt to highlight some of the major dilemmas for both the medical and nonmedical therapist who treat the personality disordered patient in STDP.

A Crutch or Panacea?

There are those who view medication as a crutch on which the patient relies, preventing the full development of that person's capabilities. The thinking is that the patient will never learn to function independently with the chemical crutch. The opposing viewpoint is that drugs are necessary for the psychiatric patient, whose behavior is biologically based, much as insulin is necessary for the diabetic. Managed care supports this position as more conducive to rapid results. However, inflexibly espousing either position is, in my experience, not useful and can be counterproductive to effective treatment. Using medication to mend a developmental defect or treat comorbid Axis I conditions is warranted under certain conditions. There are drawbacks, however, in rushing to a pharmacological agent to alleviate distress. There are no hard and fast rules, and each case must be viewed separately. Each patient presents with a different threshold for psychic pain. Too little distress for some patients reduces their motivation to change, while too much distress leaves the patient without the energy to undergo psychotherapy. I will highlight some of the factors that I consider when making recommendations for psychopharmacological consultation.

How the Patient Feels about Medication

An important criterion that I use when considering medication is how the patient feels about being on medication. Some patients have strong feelings against using drugs and, in most cases, this should be respected. Obviously, if a patient is suffering from a disorder that has a strong biological basis, it is the therapist's responsibility to properly educate the patient and arrange a consultation with an appropriate expert. On the other hand, there are those patients, many with addictive issues, who view medication as a cure. If a patient insists on medication, I feel a referral to a psychopharmacologist is appropriate.

Anxiety and Depression

Comorbid anxiety and depressive disorders are often concomitant in the personality disordered patient's presentation. When possible, my experience has been that patients derive greater benefit from treatment when they are not on psychoactive agents. Patients on antianxiety medication react more slowly and less intensively to restructuring. Also, when the patient is medicated, the therapist is hindered in assessing the manifestations of the anxiety, which is so important in STDP. Therefore, I generally encourage patients on antianxiety medication to come off of it before the therapy starts. Although many will not agree, most patients do discontinue this medication sometime in the early phases of treatment.

The use of antidepressants has similar drawbacks, in that they tend to dull the patient, and emotional reactivity is lower. Also, side effects are discouraging and reduce compliance. Although most clinically depressed patients need antidepressant treatment, some respond very well to STDP and overcome the depression without medication. Some patients who show signs of clinical depression quickly see positive results when they are encouraged to contact their anger and other repressed feelings. It is helpful to get a clear picture of whether or not there is a familial history of affective disorder. In one case of an obsessional male, the patient had a depressive reaction that was clearly a response to the surfacing of a massive rage toward his wife, a rage that he had buried. When he was able to contact the feelings, his depression rapidly lifted. He had no previous history of depression but had always feared his anger.

DRUG AND ALCOHOL ABUSE

An important issue is how to deal with the patient who is actively using substances or has a history of episodic use. Substance use is quite common in the personality disordered population. Some of these patients enter treatment while in an active stage of an addictive disorder, whereas others enter treatment after 1 to 5 years of sobriety. The latter group can be treated with the standard restructuring procedures.

The group in the active stages of an addictive disorder are more difficult to treat. Some of these patients state at the very onset that they do not want to be involved with a 12-step program. Some report they have already tried it. This presents a dilemma for the therapist. Therapy will not be effective if the patient is actively in an addictive cycle. The use of substances becomes the main defense that undermines any attempt at restructuring the defenses. There are those I know in the field of addiction who would refuse to see a patient who is actively using substances. I do not agree with this approach. I think that it is crucial not to become condemning of the addictive behavior but rather to put this responsibility into the patient's hands. I emphasize my position that therapy will be meaningless unless the patient can attain sobriety. Most patients understand this and desire to change. I discuss the available options if the addictive cycle continues, commitment to a 12-step program or inpatient substance abuse rehabilitation. After repeated slips, the patient will either drop out of treatment or will make a commitment for extra help. My experience shows that the characterological style of the patient does not emerge clearly until after a year of sobriety has passed. Characterological treatment is most effective after this time.

THE QUESTION OF TIME

It may seem a bit late in the book to address the issue of time, since this book is about short-term treatment. I believe that the material that precedes this point is a necessary foundation to any discussion about time. There is currently a trend afoot in the general field of psychotherapy toward reducing the overall length of treatment. I have propounded herein many reasons why this, under the right circumstances, is a good thing. Unfortunately, this trend has resulted in a proliferation of briefer treatment approaches created by those without the requisite training and education. Certainly, competition exists in the field of psychotherapy, just as in any other profession. This competition can work to encourage research and the trial of new ideas and theories. Unfortunately, this competition can also result in damage to the advancement of clinical science and practice when it is not approached methodically and scientifically. My fear is that a whole generation of therapists will be trained in ungrounded programs and do much harm by undertreating severe disorders. Advances in the field of dynamic or any other style of brief treatment require more than a name with "brief" or "short" in it, or a plan to limit the number of sessions. Woody (1991) suggests that we counter this "quick fix" mentality, especially when the primary concern is cost containment.

In clinical practice, patients do not always follow our time frame. If the upper limit of STDP is 40 sessions, do we discontinue if the patient is continuing to benefit? We generally do not; the arbitrary setting and following of limits are not always in the best interests of our patients. At other times, sticking to a predetermined number of sessions is highly effective. What of the patient who asks to continue? The patient's reasons for wanting to continue must be carefully considered and discussed before a decision can be made.

As I mentioned earlier, there are ways to present data that do not do justice to the clinical phenomena. The most obvious is when previous treatments are not acknowledged as building blocks of current successful outcomes. So, if we say a patient had an 80% improvement after a course of 30 sessions, do we also acknowledge that he/she previously underwent an analysis? I think we need to have a more honest way of understanding and communicating these issues.

We have a long way to go in understanding what accelerates and what protracts the therapeutic process. A question I am often asked is whether the use of empathic approaches works to lengthen treatment. I think the answer is yes. But, the clinician must use an empathic approach during various phases of treatment when it is warranted. For example, in *The Case of the Man Who Just Heard the Words* in Chapter 10, the patient experienced the devastating loss of his family just at the point at which he was getting better. This could have driven him back to his position of isolation. A phase of empathic work, however, strengthened his resolve, and he continued to grow. Often, the most difficult part of treatment is knowing when to shift phases and avoid being stuck too long in an empathic phase.

Many therapists become fearful that returning to defense analysis will somehow be damaging. This is generally not the case if the patient understands and concurs regarding the treatment goals.

CONCLUSION

There are many factors that account for treatment difficulties and various standard and creative methods to deal with these difficulties when they occur. Probably the most important point is that honestly attempting to understand the problem and not place blame with the patient are the most crucial aspects. Blaming the patient because he/she is too sick serves no productive purpose. Certainly, we all experience frustration and anger, but being in touch with this prevents us from slipping into less adaptive patterns. Rather than blaming the patient, we should systematically review the possible contributing factors that account for treatment disruptions. Often, involving the patient in this process reduces resistance and increases collaboration. The main factor that accounts for positive outcome invariably is the quality of the therapeutic alliance. As we have discussed throughout this book, an inherent paradox exists in that personality disordered patients, especially those with the more severe forms, often have difficulty establishing an alliance. Actively addressing treatment disruptions in a nonpunitive, collaborative fashion is often the first step in creating an effective therapeutic alliance.

CHAPTER 12

Termination and Follow-Up: Measuring Therapeutic Effectiveness

It is only the most arrogant of therapists who would assume that as clinicians we can definitively and prophylactically "cure" our patients. . . . Patients can and do return for more therapy at different points in their lives and returning in this way is unrelated to the quality of the original therapy.

—BUDMAN (1990 p. 217)

"Treatment success basically means that intended goals are achieved" before treatment is terminated (Schulte, 1995, p. 284). In STRP, the ultimate treatment goal is almost always comprehensive personality change. What exactly is comprehensive personality change? Comprehensive personality change encompasses enhanced well-being, improved social functioning, and shifts in personality organization, which is also referred to as modification of structure (Strupp, 1978). This is, admittedly, a formidable challenge. However, it is my firmly and deeply held belief that significant personality change *can* be achieved—and in periods ranging from hours to under a year. This entire book is predicated upon this belief. I have seen it repeatedly in my own work and in that of others, whose work I have been privileged to learn from by way of videotape or follow-up interviews. Fortunately, the psychological community has a renewed interest to investigate quantum personality change events, both those naturally occurring and those thera-peutically induced. Certainly, even more research in this area is warranted.

We as clinicians, too, should be working individually to continually examine and improve our effectiveness. We learn from our results, both positive and negative. This process is the main topic of consideration in this chapter.

Because we set clear goals and establish a specific treatment focus at the inception of therapy, the progress can be measured first upon termination and then also at the time of follow-up (Lambert, 1992; Lambert, Shapiro, & Bergin, 1986). This is an important function of the termination interview. Follow-up interviews provide another opportunity to consolidate gains and explore problems. To give an idea of how the termination session can work, I offer excerpts of a termination interview from *The Case of the Woman Who Was Always a Victim* (see Chapter 9).

TERMINATION SESSION

THERAPIST: How are things going?

PATIENT: All right.

THERAPIST: It doesn't sound so good?

PATIENT: No. Some good things—I talked to my mother yesterday, unexpectedly. Which is good, I finally got it out in the open how I was feeling about things . . . We just started talking about things [about her sister] . . . I started talking about my father and the fact that I actually forgive him, and I can deal with him now. And then I looked at her and said, "I'm still mad at you," and she was like, "Oh, okay." She didn't get hostile or anything; we just talked it out. . . . Just the things that happened when I was a kid. How they used to fight and the fact that she still tries to put me in the middle of things. And I explained what she [mother] was doing, complaining and putting father down. [Triangulating patient; she then confronted her mother.] "I don't need to hear this." So she realized, "You may not mean to put me in the middle of it, but you're still doing it." She was really good, she listened! She said that she knows, in the beginning when we were little and she saw my father wasn't paying any attention to her, it really hurt her, and she tried to deal with it. She said after a while she just got so bitter and that's why it may have come across that she was trying to pull us one way or the other or get mad if we talked to him. So a lot came out, and I found out a lot more of what she went through as a kid.

THERAPIST: What did you find out?

PATIENT: Just how horrible her mother really was. She was constantly told she was no good and to go die. It was really tough on her. I said she made mistakes and hopefully I won't make the same ones you did. It was really a good talk, and when I left there I felt a lot better. When I went over there the last few times, I don't want to go near her. I don't want her touching me. I'm shutting her off a great deal, and it's uncomfortable.

THERAPIST: This sounds like an important milestone.

PATIENT: Well, I've been trying to do it for 2 months now.

THERAPIST: And it went very well. She listened, she didn't cut you off.

PATIENT: She didn't! I would have drowned her [they were at the pool] (*laughs*). No she did, she listened, we talked. The worst thing was that, I know we had some good times as kids, but I cannot remember anything . . . anything good.

THERAPIST: How do you feel?

PATIENT: Sad.

She then goes on to say that she still has concerns about her weight but knows that she is not fat. This has been a major issue in therapy. This is explored and does not seem to be symptomatic.

THERAPIST: What are your thoughts about this being our final good-bye?

PATIENT: It's kind of scary.

THERAPIST: Do you have some anxiety about it?

PATIENT: (*starts to cry*) Sad. (*pause*) It's difficult because I'm afraid of screwing up and having to come back.

THERAPIST: What makes you think that will happen?

The patient then discusses her difficulty getting pregnant and her fear that she will not be able to deal with it if it does not occur.

THERAPIST: I think you are going to be able to handle it one way or the other. . . . I think you're at a very different place than you were when you went through it the first time.

PATIENT: I know I am, in a lot of ways. Well, there is more to it. I'm afraid I'm going to get all the anxiety when I go to the doctors. They were really tough on me. I couldn't even go to the hospital without having an anxiety attack. I spent more time in the bathroom than I did getting the ultrasound or whatever. I know it's not going to happen, but it's there.

THERAPIST: How do you feel about you and I saying good-bye?

PATIENT: I'm glad because it seems like it's time. It's just scary to me; I haven't been on my own for a long time.

THERAPIST: So some of that anxiety is really a normal part of letting go and living your own life. And how do you feel about saying good-bye to me today?

PATIENT: Sad, and happy.

THERAPIST: Mixed, and what are you sad about?

PATIENT: Well, I've enjoyed coming here, for the most part. You helped me a lot and I'm going to miss that: having you to talk to.

THERAPIST: So you are going to miss me?

PATIENT: Yes. (*says her husband is busy working and begins to cry*)

THERAPIST: So you feel like you are going to lose something, and you're not sure your marriage contains it, because your husband is so busy.

PATIENT: (*quiet and sad*)

THERAPIST: So how do you feel about what you accomplished in here?

PATIENT: Good.

THERAPIST: We should review where you've been and where you've come.

The therapist and patient review her presenting symptoms and areas of disturbances. She discusses her progress but still reports mild anxiety.

THERAPIST: And obviously some anxiety is part of life.

The patient then talks more about the history of her eating disorder and her memory of her father yelling that her mother was "a fat slob." The connection between her own thinness and her longing for her father's approval was made and discussed. The structure of her defense system is reiterated. When she hears arguing, she pushes down her anger and gets more abuse. She becomes resistant and pushes down her feelings. She says she feels as if the therapist is looking through her.

PATIENT: It's more fun being healthy.

THERAPIST: But you might have to grieve some of what you're leaving behind. Don't forget this has been part of you for a long time. And usually what happens after you've been through this kind of therapy, over the next 6 months to a year, a lot of things continue to develop and expand.

PATIENT: In what way?

THERAPIST: What we started in here will continue. The development you have missed, you will begin to catch up on, in a more natural way. I think we really addressed the main issues, and time and life are going to allow your self-esteem to develop in a more positive way. . . . When you stop therapy it doesn't just stop there.

PATIENT: I know that, I know when I'm at home things will come to me. I can work them out. . . . I feel apprehensive but above all I feel really good. . . . I'll miss you and being able to talk to you.

THERAPIST: I'll miss you too. I enjoyed working with you. You have a lot of courage.

PATIENT: I wanted to get better.

THERAPIST: You did, and you have.

PATIENT: I know that.

As you can see from this excerpt, the termination session gave both the patient and me an opportunity to assess her progress. In this particular case, great gains were made.

THERAPIST'S REACTION

Despite the unplanned terminations and dropouts, there are many rewards for therapists conducting in-depth short-term treatment, especially a deep sense of accomplishment and satisfaction. I agree with Leston Havens (1989) who wrote, "Perhaps the greatest privilege and joy of doing psychotherapy is bringing the psychologically moribund back to life" (p. 32). The therapist in STRP is intensely, actively involved in the process, and so the emotional bond that has been created during the course of successful treatment is very strong. The rapid changes that occur can be astonishing and are exciting to witness. Saying good-bye is a mixed experience for the therapist, as well as the patient. Of course, it is sad to say good-bye, but deeply gratifying to know you have been part of a major, positive transformation. Many times, you have come to like and admire patients for their fortitude, not only in surviving the obstacles in the path of healthy development, but also in their spirit and courage in facing their difficulties and resolving them. With each patient you treat, you learn more about the workings of the human psyche and improve your depth of understanding of unconscious mental processes.

THE CHALLENGE OF CONTINUAL IMPROVEMENT

The concept of "continual improvement" was developed by Deming (1986); it was the fifth of 14 ways to increase the quality level of a particular system. It means an ongoing effort to modify, refine, and expand quality and effectiveness. Although the concept was originally applied to the sphere of economics, it also has application to the field of psychotherapy. In fact, the concept of continual improvement can be used to guide the development and research efforts of all therapists. In discussing the importance of quality, Dobyns and Crawford-Mason (1991) stated that, "The pursuit of quality can never stop even though it is as indefinable as love and as unattainable as justice. Quality is, therefore, rather like one of the precepts of Zen: 'There is no answer; search for it lovingly.' " I agree wholeheartedly.

The key to continual improvement is a feedback loop. The four-step Deming–Shewart loop consists of: (1) planning a change for that which you are trying to improve, (2) carrying out the change on a small scale, (3) observing the results, and (4) studying the results and deciding what new learning has resulted (Aguayo, 1991). Becoming an effective therapist, as with most everything else, is a continual process that utilizes feedback and information derived from training, reading, supervision, and accumulated life experiences. We continue to improve ourselves and advance the field in incremental steps, and this process never stops. A positive outlook and attitude are necessary. "As you improve your process, you improve your knowledge of the process at the same time. Improvement of the product and process goes hand in hand with greater understanding and better theory" (Aguayo, 1991, p. 115). The field of psychiatry/psychology is advancing so rapidly that practitioners who want to stay current must continually absorb new material. Each patient we treat is also an opportunity to learn and improve. One of the most common complaints about psychotherapy research is that it alters the context in which clinical work is conducted (Talley, Strupp, & Butler, 1994). Bridging this gap can be enhanced by the use of audiovisual techniques and follow-up interviews.

Audiovisual recordings and *follow-up interviews* are two very important clinical and research tools integral to the evolution and continued development of STDP. Audiovisual recording is a major advancement in the study of the techniques and process of psychotherapy. Follow-up interviews are imperative in assessing psychotherapy outcome (Dornelas, Correll, Lothstein, Wilber, & Goethe, 1996). Both methods allow us to continually improve. One does not have to be at a major research center to conduct research. In fact, it is something that can be incorporated into private practices and mental health clinics. The second generation pioneers of STDP, Davanloo, Mann, Malan, and Sifneos used both methods extensively in creating and refining their systems. I feel that studying their clinical case and research reports is an excellent way to get a feel for STDP and how it is most effectively used. The protocols for follow-up interviews are fairly standard, with the exception of a feature added by Davanloo, in which the patient reviews his/her videotapes and comments on the vignettes from treatment.

Audiovisual Recording

The use of audiovisual recording technology in psychotherapy has been described by Sifneos as the equivalent of the "discovery of the microscope in biology" (1990). He believes that videotapes are a major asset to psychotherapy researchers. This has indeed been a major development that has, unfortunately, been underutilized by psychotherapists, trainees, and seasoned practitioners, as well. The more traditional analytic community claims that audiovisual taping violates the sanctity of the treatment. While it must be agreed that preserving the sanctity of therapy is a primary concern, I have not found that audiovisual recording in any way violates the therapeutic relationship. Rather, it is an indispensable tool in continual improvement. There are various ways in which audiovisual recording can be used to improve and advance STDP and STRP.

Review of the Videotape by the Therapist to Enhance Treatment

Personally reviewing the videotapes of specific psychotherapy sessions is an excellent way to enhance one's understanding of the therapeutic process and to keep continually improving. The vantage point this sort of review provides is especially useful for improving the technical aspects of conducting STRP with the particular patient whose videotape you are reviewing, as well as for streamlining the process. The therapist can critically observe his/her interventions and how the patient received them. Interventions that were poorly conceived and implemented can be refined or discarded. I sympathize with Judith Jordan (1995), who said, "To chart new territory in psychotherapy is difficult at best, hazardous at worst. . . . Each generalization is fraught with complexities and pitfalls; yet trainees and young clinicians are hungry for guidelines, which so often must take the form of generalizations" (p. 269). Audiovisual review of therapy sessions can make charting this new territory far more efficient.

Review of Videotape with a Group of Short-Term Therapists

Even better than the solitary review of one's treatment sessions is to review them with a group of clinicians who are also committed to continual improvement and short-term treatment. Feedback from other therapists, when given in the spirit of collaboration, can be an effective way to improve one's skills. Further, this type of collaboration works to increase therapist motivation and keep alive the optimism and belief in the patient's capacity for substantial, rapid change. Without a support group, it is very easy to lose one's momentum and to become complacent. Treating personality disorders can be perplexing and taxing. For the therapist, STRP is extremely difficult work, not only because of the energy the therapist must put into the process, but because of the rapid assessment required, the maintenance of the focus of the therapy, and, of course, because of the accelerated pace of treatment. Demoralization is especially likely to occur when one has a number of concurrent or consecutive cases in which the short-term treatment model does not seem to be effective, and there is no one with whom the therapist can review cases.

Use of Videotaped Sessions as Consultative Aids

For those therapists in rural practices or otherwise without convenient access to other therapists, exchanging videotapes for consultation by mail can work much like meeting with a support group. The therapist, with the patient's permission, can send the tape of a session about which he/she has concerns to another, more experienced therapist for suggestions and help. Phone consultations can then be used to discuss the case in detail.

Use of Videotaped Sessions to Facilitate the Supervisory Process

This format has been used extensively and successfully in the training of short-term dynamic psychotherapists. Showing the videotapes to an experienced practitioner eliminates the subjective bias that is often part of traditional psychotherapy supervision. Instead of relying solely on the supervisee's version of the session, both supervisor and supervisee can watch the process themselves and then review aspects that are unclear.

Microanalysis of Psychotherapy Sessions

Another excellent advantage of videotaping sessions is that the clinician can focus in detail, or even in slow motion, on the nonverbal aspects of the patient's communications. This provides excellent research and training opportunities. As we have discussed earlier in the book, facial and other nonverbal communication is a critical dimension of STDP. The use of videotape in studying nonverbal communication was reported in *The American Psychologist* in the following way:

> A depressed woman participating in a research study was filmed telling a doctor how much better she was feeling in therapy. Days later she attempted suicide. Slow-motion study of her facial expressions while

talking to the doctor revealed—hidden among her smiles—fleeting, almost invisible signs of intense distress. If warning expressions such as these could be detected on a routine basis in patients with severe mental disorders, suicide might claim far fewer lives each year. This example merely hints at the potential of research exploring the emotional and motivational wellsprings of our behavior. (National Advisory Mental Health Council, 1995, p. 838)

Audiovisual Recording for Research Purposes

Even the sole practitioner can use audiovisual tapes to conduct research and patient follow-up studies. Videotapes are a rich source of data that can be later utilized for a multitude of research purposes and also for clinical papers.

Audiovisual Recording as a Third Eye

Even if one does not regularly review one's videotapes, the fact that the session is being taped can help the therapist when difficulties occur. It provides the therapist with the opportunity to review the session when treatment seems stuck. It is neither practical nor necessary to review every videotape, but it is easy to fast forward to a particular section that does merit review.

Audiovisual Recording to Establish Minimum and Advanced Levels of Competence

Certain advanced credentialing entities encourage their professionals to submit videotapes as work samples. Unfortunately, this is not a requirement in the professional credentialing of psychotherapists. I find it difficult to understand why "psychotherapists" are not required to produce work samples for peer scrutiny before they are licensed to enter practice. I believe that if this were required, the quality of available psychotherapy would be much greater. I, for one, would not want to go under the knife with a surgeon who had never been observed but who merely reported what he/she had done to a supervisor. Why should psychotherapy hold itself to a lesser standard?

Videotape Format

Many therapists express a reluctance to videotape their patients. Their first reaction is to say that they could not possibly tolerate the anxiety of working "under the lights," so to speak. This is almost always followed by the rationalization (or projection) that "my patients wouldn't like to be videotaped" or that it would destroy the patient's feeling of safety. It has been my experience that most patients do not mind being videotaped and, in fact, may welcome this sign that the therapist works to improve and enhance his/her clinical expertise. Most patients quickly forget about the videotape and adjust to the situation. In fact, I have found that when I fail to record the session of a patient whom I typically record, I am quickly reminded.

Equipment

The cost of videotaping equipment is reasonable enough now that it truly is affordable for all therapists and should be viewed as an essential tool in clinical practice. In group settings or clinics, this equipment can be shared, further reducing the cost. Basic equipment includes a camera, tripod, monitor, and playback machine. The cost of videotapes is nominal. In hospital or university settings, an audiovisual laboratory with state-of-the-art equipment is a vital part of training and research. In large facilities, an audiovisual technician is often needed to coordinate the use of the equipment and can even be used to operate one camera for the therapist and another one for the patient.

Patient Protocol

Some clinicians decide to videotape all their short-term psychotherapy cases; others are more selective. I highly recommend videotaping the extended session of each new patient and the termination session, at the very least. Reviewing the case at its onset is an excellent way of focusing the treatment, especially for therapists with limited access to supervision. Some cases should be videotaped from beginning to end, and the process should be reviewed, in order to observe the various phases of therapy. One can learn a great deal from observing the full course of treatment.

Before a clinician can begin videotaping, he/she must procure a signed consent form from the patient. I generally explain that I videotape all STDP therapy and then describe the purposes for which I might use the material: follow-up, review, supervision, training, and research. The patient has the right to decide that he/she does not want to be videotaped. At no time should the clinician pressure his/her patient into this. I tell some hesitant patients that if they feel at any time that the videotaping interferes with their comfort, they may ask me to turn it off. This has occurred on a few occasions. Patients in sensitive jobs with the government or in the public eye seem to be the ones who are uncomfortable with taping and may ask to limit the use of the material for follow-up. Some even erase the tapes following termination.

The safety and confidentiality of videotapes should be maintained as with any other clinical material, and this should be communicated to the patient. If tapes are to be used for research or training, written permission must be obtained. Also, the therapist should be judicious in presenting videotapes of local patients in supervisory or training forums.

Tapes should be coded without the patient's name and kept in a locked cabinet. Provisions for the safe disposal of the tapes in case of the death or incapacity of the clinician should be determined ahead of time. In institutional settings, the hospital research committee should develop guidelines for the use and maintenance of these tapes and establish an archive where this material can be used by psychotherapy researchers and trainees. Consent agreements must be signed by all taped patients.

Follow-Up Interviews

Most psychotherapists do not conduct follow-up interviews. I hope that readers of this book will consider doing so with at least a sample of their short-term cases. Follow-up interviews, since they are a part of the format for consolidating treatment gains and determining the need for another block of treatment, are billable services. If the follow-up is for research purposes, then I do not charge the patient. There are different methods of conducting follow-up studies, with varying levels of sophistication. I have included some suggestions that will make the use of these follow-up interviews worth the time and trouble of conducting them.

Follow-up procedures are an excellent technique for consolidating patient gains and getting direct feedback about the impact of the treatment. Most patients respond enthusiastically to the recommendation of scheduling a 6-month follow-up interview. In 6 months, enough time has elapsed to ascertain whether the core issues have been adequately resolved or whether there are residual issues that need to be addressed. If residual issues do emerge, a few more sessions or an extended block can be scheduled. Telephone follow-up interviews, which are more for research purposes and the therapist's development, can also be conducted (Dornelas et al., 1996). There is no comparison, however, to a face-to-face follow-up interview. The live interview allows the therapist to see how the patient looks, expresses him/herself, and relates interpersonally.

Prescheduled Follow-Up Interview[1]

The follow-up interview should be scheduled at the termination of treatment, and, of course, the function should be explained to the patient. The thought of one more appointment at a later date provides a segue from the intensity of the therapeutic relationship to life without the therapist. I have been told that it also functions to help the patient hold onto the positive aspects of the therapy and the therapist and promotes the internalization of healthy self-concept.

Follow-Up Interview and Review of Audiovisual Recordings

If the therapist has videotaped a patient's extended session or more, the therapist can play back predetermined or random selections for review with the patient. Either the therapist or the patient can stop the tape at any time and discuss specific issues. This is a powerful experience for the patient, especially when that patient has already made significant characterological change. Patients often report that the person they see on the screen seems like someone else altogether. It is a valuable opportunity for the patient to take stock of the enormous change that has occurred and to relish his/her accomplishments. It is also painful in that the patient is confronted with his/her former pain and must acknowledge the futility of his/her discarded character defenses. This serves to reinforce the patient's empathy for him/herself.

Telephone Follow-Up Interview

Telephone follow-up interviews are another way for the therapist to get direct feedback from the patient. The therapist must first ask the patient if the call has been made at a good time; if it has not, the therapist should schedule a more convenient time for the telephone interview.

Follow-Up Interview with an Independent Evaluator

When the therapist works as part of a team or has a willing associate, the therapist can have another therapist conduct the follow-up interview with the patient. This, when videotaped, can provide insight into the mechanism and dynamic of the patient's change.

Mechanics of the Follow-Up Interview

The format of the follow-up interview will vary, depending on the manner in which it is conducted and the amount of time allocated for the interview. Basically, the format is as follows:

1. *Review clinical case material and identify the goals of treatment prior to meeting with the patient.* The clinician should review the clinical material with special attention to the problems that were targeted for change.

2. *Explain the purpose of the interview and obtain the patient's consent.* For example, "The purpose of my call (or session) is to conduct a follow-up to see how you are doing and how you felt about the treatment." If this follow-up is by phone, the patient should be asked to indicate a convenient time for the call. If a review of videotape is part of the follow-up, the patient should be told this.

3. *Review portions of the extended interview.* The clinician should have the video monitor set up and ready to play. The patient should be told that he/she can stop the videotape at any time to discuss his/her reactions, thoughts, or feelings.

4. *Review the patient's problem list and assess degree of change.* Following the review of the videotape, the clinician should recapitulate the patient's problem list and have the patient rate and discuss the degree of change from the beginning of treatment until the present time.

5. *Determine whether there are further problems that the patient wants to address.* If there is evidence in the interview that more working through is required, the patient and therapist can determine the number of sessions needed to finalize the treatment. If there are no further issues, the patient and therapist can share their feelings at parting and say good-bye.

In the following sections, I report the prescheduled 6-month follow-up session with *The Case of the Woman Who Was Always a Victim* where treatment gains are maintained and continue with a 2-year telephone follow-up. Next, I present the research protocol of *The Case of the Man with the Skeletal View,* where the treatment outcome was marginal.

Prescheduled Six-Month Follow-Up

The patient is obviously pregnant and very excited. She has been off medication since the second month of treatment and reports a positive mood. "I may get down a little bit but not depressed. . . . I find myself standing up for myself a lot more."

THERAPIST: Can you give me an example of an incident in which you were more assertive?

PATIENT: Yeah, I was going for an *in vitro* [fertilization]. The first time I went there, I waited over an hour for this man. Nobody told me he was running late or anything. I spoke to him when he was through. I said, in the future I would like to know when you're running late. I would never have done that before; I would have sat there and gotten mad and not said anything. He was joking about it, like, "Oh, there is only one of me." And I looked at him and said, "Well you know there is only one of me too, and I have things to do." The next time he came in he was very pleasant and said, "I'm only 2 minutes late."

THERAPIST: So you were appropriately assertive because in the past you had tremendous difficulty with authority figures. You let them walk all over you.

PATIENT: Especially men. I had another incident with my father. He was furious and rude and really nasty with us. Later I called him and explained to him how I felt. He denied everything. I would have never done that with him. I would have buried my anger.

The patient reports her anxiety is manageable and does not hold her back. Her original issues are summarized and she says, "It's hard to remember things when they aren't bothering you any more." She reports the first 3 months of pregnancy were like having PMS, but she and her husband survived it.

THERAPIST: If we review where you were when you started treatment, you started therapy very depressed and suicidal on medication, severe panic, generalized anxiety, and a tremendous concern about your body image. How did you feel about the therapy?

PATIENT: Great. We did great work in a short period of time. I really appreciate what I got out of it. It's great not being on medication and not worrying about things all the time. It's weird being happy most of the time. We had spoken about when things are going really well I can't deal with it, but I catch myself doing that.

THERAPIST: Would you say that your relationship is better with your parents?

PATIENT: Yes, because I know how to deal with it better. I can just leave. I don't have to stay there, and if they look at that as running away, well fine; my sanity is important to me at this point. And it is a little sad: We are having a child, and it would be nice if they were involved. But God, I don't want anybody to go through what I did with them.

The patient was contacted by phone 2 years after the termination of her treatment. She reported that she continues to do well and is medication-free. She felt that the therapy had made a tremendous difference in her life.

Research Protocol: Two-Year Follow-Up

To further illustrate the flow of the follow-up interview and what can be learned from this process, I return to *The Case of the Man with the Skeletal View* from Chapter 10.

This patient was seen for a follow-up interview approximately 2 years after his treatment was terminated. The first phase of his treatment consisted of defensive restructuring, and the second phase was an empathic model, using more cognitive restructuring. The purposes of the follow-up interview were to get his view of the short-term treatment and to see how he had fared since termination. The follow-up interview lasted 45 minutes and was audiovisually recorded. Abbreviated transcripts follow.

The interviewer presents the purpose of the follow-up evaluation as described previously in this chapter.

PATIENT: Well, things are going pretty well. I changed responsibilities. (*describes his job transfer and says that he likes his work*)

THERAPIST: I remember from the past that deadlines and pressure seemed to be very difficult for you. How do you cope with that now?

PATIENT: I find it very easy. I feel absolutely no tension or pressure on it at all. I'm very confident in my ability to get the job done.

THERAPIST: How did the transfer go for you?

PATIENT: It wasn't long after I stopped seeing you . . . (*discusses his transfer, job responsibilities, and his feelings of competence and satisfaction*)

THERAPIST: So it sounds like you're very satisfied with your job.

PATIENT: Yeah, I think it's ideal. There is not much I want to change. (*describes how he functions independently*)

THERAPIST: So, from where you were when you came in to see me and where you are now, there has been a dramatic improvement in the satisfaction that you get out of your job. What percent improvement?

PATIENT: I would say 0 to 100.

THERAPIST: I remember there were times that you would sit at your desk and write and then cross things out.

PATIENT: Yeah, I'd write, "HELP."

THERAPIST: There was a time when you were suffering tremendously on the job. Do you have periods like that anymore?

PATIENT: No, there are like seconds where it's a little panic or something but no periods where I panic about doing anything. In some ways, my work is not that different.

THERAPIST: Now, in terms of your depression, where is that compared to where it was when you first came in to see me?

PATIENT: I don't have periods where I feel incapacitated. I should say I do take medication. [He was placed on a variety of medications with limited effect.] I take Prozac. In the past, I've taken a variety of things. It could be better; I don't feel great a lot of the time. There have been some periods, in the last few years, when I've felt more like getting out and trying to meet people, and it's like I don't really want to be bothered. It's like I'm uncomfortable with groups of people, and I don't really want to be bothered. In some ways, I've sort of decided I'm really comfortable by myself. A lot of social contact, if there is no structure or no business purpose, is stressful to me, so I'm avoiding it. We talked about an issue of motivation, and you can't change me if I don't want to change. So, right now, I'm sort of at a point where things are fine. Maybe at some point I'll say I'll really be better off if I worked on being more social.

THERAPIST: It sounds like there is a greater level of self-acceptance, that you know some of your limitations, you understand them, and you have a greater acceptance of them.

PATIENT: I think the most important thing I got out of therapy, and I think particularly seeing you, is being aware of my feelings and almost being able to know what feelings are, and list them, and have some consciousness of them, and particularly be aware of discomfort around people and why it's happening. If I want more I can work to get it, but it's enough.

THERAPIST: But what about in terms of your marital situation?

PATIENT: Maybe a truce, that sex was an issue. I sort of wanted more, different things. In truth, I find a lot of things I want are not all that great.

The patient discusses that his sexual relationship is limited and that he and his wife have not had intercourse for about 1 year. He says that he is bothered by the fact that his wife is not affectionate, and this diminishes his sexual interest. He then describes an incident: His wife had gotten a call that her father would die in an hour. The patient thought they should go to him immediately and encouraged such action. They did so, and his wife sat with her father while he died. His wife was grateful for his assertiveness in the situation and willingness to go late in the night.

PATIENT: It sounds like you have a greater understanding of emotional reactions and psychological needs.

THERAPIST: I wouldn't make a big deal out of it.

He then discusses his relationship with his daughter, which is very positive. She sits on his lap while they work on the computer. He generally gives her a bath and has an affectionate relationship with her. He reads stories to her and tucks her in. She looks forward to spending time with him.

PATIENT: How was your experience with short-term therapy?

THERAPIST: Some of the best things in the long run were an occasional concrete suggestion. For example, when you suggested I go out and do something with my father. Like, I never would have thought of that. The short-term stirred up a lot of stuff. I don't know if that served to help stir things up later.

THERAPIST: It seemed, at the time, that it made you feel worse instead of better. [It had seemed to increase his sense of inadequacy for being unable to respond, and he had often appeared frozen.]

PATIENT: It's almost like I miss it a little. Even when it seemed like I wasn't doing anything whatsoever, I was feeling was very intense. I remember feeling like I was pushing down [referring to a period when he physically pushed down his arms]. It sort of was an interesting period. My gut feeling is that it was helpful. It was a memorable time. It's sort of hard to know what difference it would have made without it.

The patient seems grateful for the work that was accomplished. He relates to the evaluator in a direct way and seems emotionally fluid. There is evidence of some sadness.

PATIENT: Work was the initial problem that brought me in here and sort of the thing that really kicks off the stress.

THERAPIST: How are you feeling right now?

PATIENT: I sense it's time to go. A little sad. My father is ill. He apparently has colon cancer. The other thing is he apparently has Alzheimer's disease.

He talks about the loss of his father and how he might react, but it is clear that he is at peace with this.

Although this is a rather complex case, I think much can be gained from treating and reviewing cases of patients with attachment disorders. Many of these patients have never made a sufficiently positive early human bond, and each developmental step is burdened by the quintessential struggle: "Do I have the right to exist?" This case highlights the following issues, which have been discussed in previous chapters: the use of psycho-pharmacological agents to mend developmental defects, the use of follow-up interviews, the use of consultation, ways of dealing with treatment stagnation, shifting to a longer-term model, and multimodal treatment.

CONCLUSION

I hope I have demonstrated how the incorporation of audiovisual technology and the follow-up interview can be excellent ways to work on continuous improvement. Learning and perfecting the techniques of STRP require a commitment to both review and follow-up procedures. Patients and clinicians gain much from this process. Even those in independent practice can conduct effective psychotherapy outcome with minimal effort.

■ CHAPTER 13

Future Challenges

Psychotherapy is probably ten to twenty years away from its heyday.
. . . Fortunately, as society begins to turn more and more to behavior
changes and lifestyle changes as the best preventions and interventions
for many health problems, psychology is likely to replace biology as
the hottest science, just as biology once surpassed chemistry.
—PROCHASKA AND DiCLEMENTE (1992, pp. 328–329)

The future of long-term psychoanalysis as a viable treatment modality for those seeking personality change in the current *zeitgeist* of managed care and reduced reimbursement for psychotherapy seems dim. Sifneos (1990) wrote that the question as to whether focalized dynamic treatment has application to more disturbed patients is unanswered. I hope that this book is another step in the direction of unequivocally answering this question. STDP may be the best alternative in-depth treatment for those seeking to modify their personality. Although up to 40 sessions may not be considered short-term by the current standards used by managed care, it is a short period of time in which to treat long-standing characterological distur-bances. In comparison to years of costly psychoanalysis, 40 sessions is indeed short-term. I predict that STDP will be vitally important to the future of psychoanalytic treatment.

The future of psychodynamic therapy rests in the hands of those willing to design and carry out research proving the efficacy of this treatment with various clinical conditions—with personality disorders being one of the most complex and challenging applications. As I have said before, we are entering an era in which undocumented treatments will not be reimbursed by insurance companies. Only the approaches that have documented their effectiveness with certain disorders, such as cognitive-behavioral therapy for anxiety disorders and interpersonal psychotherapy for depression, will be reimbursed. It is incumbent upon the current generation of psychodynamic therapists to develop and document the effectiveness of STDP or risk losing this important contribution.

THE POSSIBILITY OF QUANTUM CHANGE

Clinicians who witness dramatic examples of change often refer to these as "outliers or fabrications." "Yet numerous observations suggest that relatively sudden and profound changes can and do occur, at least occasionally, in the organized and enduring patterns of behavior usually regarded as personality" (Miller & C'deBaca, 1994, p. 276). I cannot stress this point enough. There is much work to be done in this area, as summarized by these authors.

> Science typically proceeds beyond description by hypothesizing principles for organizing and predicting observations. Who undergoes such transformations, under what conditions? Are there precursors of quantum change? Are there consistent patterns or types? Which changes endure, and why? ... If, as seems to be the case, these are often profoundly positive developmental events, is it possible to facilitate them? Could therapeutic strategies be designed to trigger quantum change? The reorganization of personality is, after all, an historic objective of long-term psychotherapy. (p. 277)

Theodore Millon (1996), one of the seminal workers in the field of nosology, described personology as a rapidly evolving area of scientific interest that will show major advances in the next 50 years. As its importance becomes evident to politicians, businesspersons, and the public, this area will attract much attention. This renewed interest in personology provides psychotherapists with an unusual opportunity to combine two previously nonintersecting fields: short-term therapy and the study of personality.

PERSONALITY DISORDERS AND THEIR TREATMENT

I believe it is time to develop innovative treatment programs that incorporate multimodal treatments on "rapid change units," which should be affiliated with hospitals and outpatient facilities. Some very exciting steps toward this end have already been taken with the application of Linehan's dialectic behavior therapy. This therapy has been successfully applied to patients on inpatient units for the treatment of bipolar disorder.

Rapid change units could provide short-term psychotherapy using extended sessions and also incorporate other modalities of brief treatment in modules. STDP is an excellent modality for treatment centers, because patients are not bound by the usual weekly time schedule. Patients could work with intensity for brief time frames and then return for modules of treatment, allowing enough time between sessions to maximize the treatment gains before return. These units could also serve as training and research centers where new methods are developed.

CALL FOR PREVENTIVE MEASURES

As economic conditions worsen and the trend toward family breakdown continues, we can predict an increase in the incidence of personality disorders. We know the roots of these disorders are a complex interaction of biogenic and psychogenic factors combined with societal influences. Family therapists have already researched the repetitive generational patterns of many dysfunctional families. There is every indication that personality disorders are "handed down" as well.

> PDs are associated with crime, substance abuse, disability, increased need for medical care, suicide attempts, self-injurious behavior, assaults, delayed recovery from Axis I and medical illness, institutionalization, underachievement, underemployment, family disruption, child abuse and neglect, homelessness, illegitimacy, poverty, STDs, misdiagnosis and mistreatment of medical and psychiatric disorder, malpractice suits, medical and judicial recidivism, dissatisfaction with and disruption of psychiatric treatment settings, and dependency on public support. (Ruegg & Frances, 1995, pp. 16–17)

Current societal conditions such as the exposure of young children to random violence, family disruption, child abuse and various conditions resulting from poverty will ensure another generation of people suffering from personality disorders that will, in turn, tax our country's dwindling resources. What can be done?

Certainly we must continue to develop effective treatments for those who suffer from these disturbances, but early intervention is imperative. We now have a wealth of clinical and research evidence that indicates some of the factors in children that predispose them to developing personality disorders as adults. This is an area that would benefit from additional research.

Pediatricians are the first line of defense, but most are not trained to identify characterological disturbances. Simple screening tests and training in danger signs should be developed and implemented so that referrals for appropriate interventions can be made early.

School psychologists, counselors, and social workers are the second line of defense. Parents and educators should be taught about the conditions that cause and exacerbate personality problems. For therapists, each personality disordered patient we help reduces the negative impact of such people and their families on society. However, we need psychotherapists who are willing to accept the challenge of treating personality disorders instead of looking for easy ways out or by copping out and saying they are untreatable, especially in short-term formats. We also need psychotherapists who are willing to advance their training in an era when many are cutting back on education and training.

TRAINING

Mastering a complicated effort such as psychotherapy is a lifelong commitment and endeavor. Without access to training and research opportunities, it is very difficult to advance one's skills beyond a certain level. This is particularly so for those who treat personality disorders. In this section, I will discuss some of the training formats available for those who want to advance their knowledge and skill.

Cautionary note: Therapists untrained in the application of the techniques of defense analysis to the treatment of the severe personality disorders should not attempt treatment without proper training and supervision. Although there is little danger in applying a time-limited model, which activates the grief process, use of the anxiety-arousing, defense analysis techniques should not be undertaken lightly. Nonsystematic defense analysis can have serious negative consequences and should be attempted only after sufficient experience and mastery of less anxiety-arousing methods.

Current State of Training

Currently, there are no training programs widely advertised that offer a certificate program at a postdoctoral level for those who want to learn STDP. This does not mean that such programs do not exist, only that they are not promoted in the places where one might find, for example, programs in psychoanalytic psychotherapy or psychoanalysis. Further, at this time, there is no central credentialing body that certifies practitioners at a basic or advanced level of competence in the practice of STDP. This makes it difficult for those who desire training to find it. There are a number of free-standing training programs that offer workshops and supervised training. The potential trainee must investigate the quality of each one for him/herself. Despite the lack of readily available programs, there are a number of ways to find desired training.

University Medical-School-Affiliated Training Programs

A number of research centers, primarily on the east and west coasts of the United States and in Europe, currently conduct research in STDP. Finding one's way into one of these centers might be a way to receive training.

Free-Standing Training Programs in STDP

There have been a number of free-standing programs that are not affiliated with institutions. As a consumer, the potential trainee should investigate the qualifications and training of the supervisors. The trainee also must be wary of advocates of one particular school of thought to the exclusion of others. There are many points of view, and they tend to compete with each other for followers. Remember, no one approach provides the solution for all cases!

The format used for training should include group audiovisual supervision as well as individual supervision with an experienced practitioner. Expect to spend at least 2 years to acquire a basic competency in STDP. Advanced training will require many more years.

Workshops and Seminars

There are numerous workshops that provide a broad overview of basic concepts. There are limitations to what one will learn in a workshop format, even a lengthy one, and it is no substitute for clinical supervision or organized training.

Reviewing the Videotapes of the Pioneers

It is possible to view the videotapes of the pioneers of STDP at conferences and symposia. I strongly encourage those who are interested to pursue this course. The tapes provide a tremendously interesting opportunity to witness the masters at work, as they develop and refine their techniques.

Individual Clinical Supervision

Individual supervision with an experienced practitioner is another way to learn STDP. For those who cannot find a suitable training program in their area, this is probably the next best alternative.

Group Supervision

An excellent forum for learning STDP is to organize a supervisory group of others who are interested in learning the approach. The group can meet with an experienced practitioner on a regular basis and also do peer review to increase comfort with videotape and develop a collaborative spirit.

Personal STDP

As with traditional psychoanalytic training, undergoing STDP oneself is an excellent way to resolve unconscious issues that interfere with one's analytic work. Also, even a modicum of character change will positively affect one's professional as well as personal life. Understanding the process from "the other side of the couch" is an excellent experience for any practitioner.

Current Training Needs

As you may have deduced from this section on training, there is a need for well-designed, advanced clinical training programs to prepare clinicians for the challenges of the 21st century, when cost-effective and documented treatment protocols will be required. Without accessible clinical training programs, the subspecialty of STDP is in danger of losing its place in clinical practice and from further evolving its effectiveness. Also, the need for manualized treatment has become more apparent as a criterion for efficacy research and standardized training.

Manualized Treatment

The development and incorporation of manualized treatment have become increasingly necessary for research and training (Binder, 1993; Binder et al., 1993; Luborsky, 1993). Manualized treatment formats provide a step-by-step description of the treatment process, including technical interventions. Although there is controversy regarding the use of treatment manuals for STDP (Osimo, 1994) and some evidence of an inverse relationship between adherence to a manual and successful outcome (Hoglend, 1993), the trend is that most psychotherapy researchers advocate manualized treatment. These manuals have been developed and have been successful in increasing technical adherence to a particular method of treatment and are used by some to assess therapist competency. Moras (1993) found limited evidence from controlled studies that supports the conclusion that treatment manuals markedly improve the training process. However, he believes, and I concur, that

> manuals are likely to increase teaching efficiency for the novice psycho-
> therapist for two reasons. First, a well-specified manual is a systematic,
> focused, and goal-oriented base for teaching. Second, a well-specified
> manual provides a common conceptual frame of reference for the
> supervisor–trainee dyad's work. (p. 583)

Although treatment manuals can never fully capture or convey the art of therapy, there is an elegance and intellectual rigor inherent in any approach that can be described in a manual. Laikin and Winston (1988), for instance, have produced a treatment manual for STDP that emphasizes the defense challenging approach, primarily based on Davanloo's model. Pollack, Flegenheimer, Kaufman, Pereira, and Sadow (1988) have also developed a manual for brief adaptive psychotherapy based on the approach developed by Sifneos. Sifneos (1987) has also manualized his treatment method. Strupp and Binder (1984) produced a guide for their time-limited psycho-therapy.

Although treatment manuals represent an important advancement in the development of psychotherapy, STDP may not lend itself as easily to manualization as the cognitive-behavioral approaches. Nevertheless, manu-als do provide worthwhile information on the various approaches, and it is probable that reimbursement will be denied for nonmanualized and unsupported therapeutic approaches in the foreseeable future.

CONCLUSION

I believe that practicing psychotherapy is a privilege as well as an extremely demanding endeavor. I am concerned about the future of psychotherapy. Effective psychotherapy does not take place when the clinician is worried about paying the rent. I think that advancing as a psychotherapist is very difficult, especially in the current sociopolitical and economic atmosphere where issues of survival seem to dominate everyone's thinking. I am discouraged when I see endless conferences on marketing and business practices, where in the past one would have seen clinically stimulating topics. I think psychotherapists need to have opportunities to think about their work and confer with others. I also believe that life experiences broaden one's approach and style. When survival is threatened, professional reading as well as extracurricular activities often go by the wayside. This occurred in the field of psychotherapy in the former Soviet Union upon the advent of communism. In a recent workshop, I described the similarity to what happened in the communist countries before the Iron Curtain fell, and repression was lifted, to what psychotherapists are currently experiencing. Psychotherapy was banned, for political reasons, and those who wanted to keep the practice alive would occasionally plan conferences in the mountains, literally in tents. I received correspondence following this workshop from a psychiatrist who said he appreciated the opportunity to join me in the tent. I invite you all to pitch tents.

Notes

CHAPTER 1

1. The passive–aggressive personality disorder has been moved to the DSM-IV Appendix for further research corroboration.

2. Comormidity refers to the existence of independent psychiatric disorders.

3. I use "character armor" here but will use the term "character defenses" in the future to describe what Reich observed as the chronic hardening of the defenses into a kind of armor.

4. In a study of naturally occurring quantum change experiences, the authors conducted in-depth interviews and administered a battery of tests to 55 subjects. Overall, the findings corroborated the subjects' reports of personal transformation. The authors state, "It is conceivable that quantum changes represent a major and enduring reorganization of behaviors triggered by highly significant discrepancies, involving goals that are central to meaning and identity" (p. 273).

5. The Symptom Checklist (SCL-90) is a commonly used measure of patient reported symptoms used in many psychotherapy outcome studies.

CHAPTER 2

1. Trait is defined as "the propensity to use particular defenses, or *defensive style*" (Soldz, Budman, Demby, & Merry, 1995, p. 357).

2. Although Freud is noted for his development of psychoanalysis, which is a lengthy procedure (3 to 6 years), he originally treated a number of cases using short-term analysis. For instance, he treated Gustav Mahler for impotence in a single extended session of 4 hours. Freud also treated a number of analysts in as few as 2 months. It is interesting to note that the concept of extended interviews or *trial therapy* made famous by David Malan and Habib Davanloo were experimented with by Freud.

3. Pine (1990) discusses the three waves of psychoanalysis: drive theory, ego psychology, and object relations. Ego psychology (Hartmann, 1939) is intimately tied to drive theory but emphasizes capacities for adaptation. That is how defense mediates the inner world of fantasy, instincts, and affects with the demands of reality. Although this represents a major development in psycho-

analytic thinking, because of its strong tie with drive theory we will not present this separately, which historically speaking, is inaccurate. We will rely quite heavily on these concepts in the assessment section.

4. For those seeking an in-depth overview of the topic of narcissism, the reader should consider Morrison's (1986) book *Essential Papers on Narcissism.*

5. As I review later, the derepression of the unconscious through defense analysis is not appropriate for patients suffering from developmental psychopathology because the basis for their personality exists at the level of disturbance in early object relations, so that structuralization of the psychic agencies has not taken place (York, Wiseberg, & Freeman, 1989).

6. This approach has much in common with the experiential psychotherapy (client centered) developed by Rogers (1957), where the curative aspects of treatment derive from optimal therapeutic conditions. These aspects of the therapeutic relationship include genuineness, acceptance, nonjudgmentalness, empathy, and prizing. This has also been termed "empathic attunement." These are considered aspects of what occurs in normal childrearing to help synthesize emotional reactions and develop a strong self (Stern, 1985).

7. Annie Reich (1960) explains the relationship between narcissism and self-esteem in a seminal paper entitled *Pathologic Forms of Self-Esteem Regulation*: "In the course of growing up, we must learn to evaluate our potentialities and accept our limitations. Continued hope for the impossible represents an infantile wish, revealing a basic lack of ability to face inner and outer reality. Self-esteem thus depends on the nature of the inner image against which we measure our own self, as well as on the ways and means at our disposal to live up to it" (quoted in Morrison, 1986, p. 45).

8. Malan's brief psychotherapy (BP) is probably the most similar to Davanloo's but does not as heavily confront the defensive system.

9. Sandor Ferenczi was an early proponent of "active therapy."

10. Deutsch (1949) developed a similar form of treatment, which he termed "sector therapy."

11. These comments were contained in an introduction to a conference entitled *The Future of Psychotherapy,* sponsored by the New England Educational Institute of which Robert Guerette, M.D., is the Director. They are reprinted with his permission.

12. Pine (1990) states, "The concept of structure is the one most often used in psychoanalytic theorizing to subsume those phenomena that make for stability and continuity over time." He believes that the concept eludes definition and prefers "the somewhat softer terms *stability* or *organization*" (p. 100).

13. York et al. (1989) use the term "macrostructure" to describe the main psychic agencies: id, ego, and superego. "Microstructures" are aggregates of drives, affects, cognitions, and defenses that become synthesized and achieve permanence within the personality. These make up attitudes, behavior, and relationships.

14. A good definition of psychopathology is provided by Brown (1977) who defines it as: "the development and maintenance of patterns which [*sic*] limit a person's potential for growth, pleasure, and happiness" (p. 1).

15. The current cognitive approaches recognize the importance of establishing and working through these core structures.

CHAPTER 3

1. Presented by Wolpe (1973) in *Behavior Therapy*. He felt knowledge of the magnitude of the patient's anxiety was indispensable in effective systematic desensitization.

2. Clinicians who treat mental health professionals are more likely to encounter patients who express a desire to do characterological reconstruction, but, because of their intellectualized defenses, they are often highly resistant to treatment nevertheless.

3. I like Rogers's (1942) definition of insight: "It involves the reorganization of the perceptual field. It consists in seeing new relationships. It is the integration of accumulated experience. It signifies a reorientation of the self" (p. 206).

4. Linehan (1993) discusses this in her book *Cognitive-Behavioral Treatment of Borderline Personality Disorder* and suggests that managing the self-destructive behavior of the chronically suicidal patient must be the first order of business.

5. Although most patients will agree to these expectations, it is unlikely that the personality disordered patient will adhere to them because of the nature of these patients' resistances. However, they should be explained. When resistances ensue, defense restructuring techniques are called for to identify the system.

6. It must be understood that a "personality disorder" is a concept and does not represent a real entity. It is a heuristic device that provides a system for classifying "personality" and making certain generalizations that can be used to guide the treatment process.

CHAPTER 4

1. This is also referred to as the "core genetic structure," which emphasizes the early relationship characteristics with caregivers, their dynamics, and developmental influences affecting character development.

2. Reik (1949) believed psychologists "are born, not made." He likened the gift for psychological observation akin to mathematical or musical talent: "Where it is not present, nothing—not even courses, lectures, and seminars—will produce it. . . . Talent alone is not enough; but work and industry alone, without talent, are nothing" (p. 3).

3. I like the way Pine (1990) explains the importance of oedipal issues: "The biological facts of having been born of two parents and of being born as one

sex only (in a two-sex world), coupled with the sociopsychological fact of having (ordinarily) been reared by two parents, lead to immensely significant positions, desirings, and rivalings vis-à-vis the parents in the life and mind of the growing child" (p. 185).

CHAPTER 6

1. I often use this defense restructuring approach with impaired professionals, as this group of patients generally possesses both sufficient ego-strength and motivation to progress rapidly.

2. This list is not an exhaustive compendium of defenses that have been identified by workers in the field. It draws from various theoretical schools. The most recent additions were developed by the self psychologists. Some of the defenses that I did not include, such as self-assertion, self-observation, and affiliation, seem more indicative of ego adaptive capacities and not necessarily defenses in the way I would define them, as attempts to ward off or manage anxiety. Other defenses that were not included were cases where the defense seemed superfluous. Jacobson et al. (cited in Vaillant, 1992) have listed defenses such as turning against the self as a defense. I do not think this is really the case, as all defenses involve some turning against the self.

CHAPTER 7

1. The first session is considered to be a consultation because, until a collaborative agreement has been reached, therapy has not yet begun.

2. As developed by Trad, previewing is a method that allows the patient undergoing the rapid change of short-term therapy to acclimate to the change once the conflict is resolved or to predict "imminent developmental change and therefore overcome the transition in an adaptive manner" (p. 66). The therapist might ask the patient to imagine and predict how his/her life would be if he/she left behind characterological problems and symptoms. "The therapist would encourage the patient to envision the cognitive, emotional, social and motivational implications that a specific change might precipitate" (p. 68). Previewing can help the patient predict the emotional consequences of future events. For example, at the onset of treatment, the therapist can ask the patient to predict what will happen if he/she continues to resist making an honest attempt to understand and resolve his/her problems, and vice versa, such as "If we are unsuccessful, I will feel sad."

3. There is some good research evidence that indicates that overzealous use of transference interpretations can be detrimental to treatment, especially with patients who are rated high on object relations (Piper, Azim, Joyce, & McCallum, 1991). They may regard the overuse of interpretation as critical. However, patients rated low on object relations seemed to respond more positively. This

seems to fit the clinical data. Patients who are more syntonic require and appreciate more active and vigorous interpretation.

4. Some of the books I recommend that have been very helpful include *The Drama of the Gifted Child* (Miller, 1983), which is a very compelling description of how narcissistic injuries affect development of the self. *In Search of the Real Self* (Masterson, 1988) helps patients understand the causes of their behavior patterns and can reduce their belief that they alone suffer with issues of abandonment, attachment, and fear of intimacy. *Trauma and Loss* (Herman, 1992) is especially useful for women with posttraumatic stress syndrome.

5. Maine describes father hunger as "a deep, persistent desire for emotional connection with the father that is experienced by all children. When this normal craving is satisfied, children are likely to grow up feeling confident, secure, strong and 'good enough.' Often, however, this yearning is not acknowledged and the child's hunger and need for a bond with the father grows" (p. 3).

CHAPTER 8

1. Although "classification is at the heart of any science" (Barlow, 1988, p. 319), the polemics concerning diagnostic classification is ongoing. Beutler and Clarkin (1990) state: "On a conceptual and scientific basis, the organization of Axis II is a messy short story in need of a good editor. A review of individual criteria reveals that the items do not represent the same level of abstraction, they are not intercategorically consistent, and there is much interdiagnostic item overlap" (p. 53). For this reason, many patients are found to have multiple Axis II diagnoses. This is evident to those of us in clinical practice who rarely encounter a clearcut case of an Axis II disorder. This is why I believe that the characterological system of psychoanalysis has more flexibility and explanatory value. However, we are in the position of having to fit our patients into DSM categories to satisfy the requirements of third party payors. McWilliams (1994) states: "The essential character structure of any human being cannot be understood without an appreciation of two distinct and interacting dimensions: developmental level of personality organization and defensive style within that level" (p. 40). DSM is a starting point; sophisticated treatment demands a system with finer discrimination, especially in the rapid-fire pace of short-term psychotherapy.

2. Some words and phrases used by the clinician during defense analysis are adapted from the work of Davanloo (1980, 1990).

3. As much as possible, the therapist should attempt to get to the more primary and at times primitive affect and impulses underneath the secondary emotions, as this increases the power of the derepression.

4. The therapist should not be squeamish about using words such as rage, murderous feelings, kill, and so on, as this reduces the patient's fear that his/her impulses are horrendous and cannot be let out in the open. As we will observe

in the following chapters, this type of language would not be appropriate with patients whose ego capacities are weak.

5. It should be noted that many professional patients suffer from personality disorders that are not evident to others except those closest to them. They often function adequately or are even overachievers at work. However, upon closer inspection of their personal life, many of these patients reveal life-long and chronic interpersonal, sexual, and emotional disturbances. A thorough assessment will reveal these conditions so that appropriate treatment can be initiated.

6. The importance of directly inquiring about the patient's sexual functioning cannot be understated and will often elicit important material that might be withheld because of embarrassment. Timing, tact, and sensitivity are required, of course.

CHAPTER 9

1. I think the previous therapy with this patient laid the groundwork for a short-term approach. In fact, her previous therapy probably moved her along the structural spectrum from a borderline to a lower neurotic level of functioning. So we cannot isolate the contribution of previous psychotherapy and must give credit to the work of the previous therapists. It is a tribute to the solid work that was done previously that this patient is not being presented in the section of this chapter on "Borderline Phenomenon."

CHAPTER 12

1. Prescheduled follow-up interviews are the only follow-up protocols that the patient should be charged for. The last two categories are considered research protocols even though they can be useful for the patient in providing an opportunity to reflect on the treatment experience and outcome.

References

Aguayo, R. (1991). *Dr. Deming: The American who taught the Japanese about quality.* New York: Simon & Schuster.

Akhtar, S. (1992). *Broken structures: Severe personality disorders and their treatment.* Northvale, NJ: Jason Aronson.

Alexander, F. G., & French, T. M. (1946). *Psychoanalytic therapy: Principles and applications.* New York: Ronald Press.

American Psychiatric Association. (1987). *Diagnostic and statistical manual of mental disorders* (3rd ed., rev.). Washington, DC: Author.

American Psychiatric Association. (1994). *Diagnostic and statistical manual of mental disorders* (4th ed.). Washington, DC: Author.

Austad, C. S., & Hoyt, M. F. (1992). The managed care movement and the future of psychotherapy. *Psychotherapy, 29*(1), 109–118.

Austin, L., & Inderbitzin, L. B. (1983). Brief psychotherapy in late adolescence: A psychodynamic and developmental approach. *American Journal of Psychotherapy, 37*(2), 202–209.

Balint, M. (1992). *The basic fault: Therapeutic aspects of regression.* Evanston: Northwestern University Press. (Original work published 1969)

Barlow, D. (1988). *Anxiety and its disorders: The nature and treatment of anxiety and panic.* New York: Guilford Press.

Basch, M. F. (1988). *Understanding psychotherapy: The science behind the art.* New York: Basic Books.

Bauer, G. P., & Kobos, J. C. (1984). Short-term psychodynamic psychotherapy: Reflections on the past and current practice. *Psychotherapy, 21*(2), 153–170.

Bauer, G. P., & Kobos, J. C. (1987). *Brief therapy: Short-term psychodynamic intervention.* Northvale, NJ: Jason Aronson.

Beck, A. T., Rush, A. J., Shaw, B., & Emery, G. (1979). *Cognitive therapy of depression.* New York: Guilford Press.

Beck, A. T., Freeman, A., & Associates. (1990). *Cognitive therapy of personality disorders.* New York: Guilford Press.

Benjamin, L. S. (1993). *Interpersonal diagnosis and treatment of personality disorders.* New York: Guilford Press.

Bennett, M. J. (1983). Focal psychotherapy—terminable and interminable. *American Journal of Psychotherapy, 37*(3), 365–375.

Berenbaum, H. (1969). Massed time-limited psychotherapy. *Psychotherapy: Theory, Research and Practice, 6,* 54–56.

Beutler, L. E., & Clarkin, J. F. (1990). *Systematic treatment selection: Toward targeted therapeutic interventions.* New York: Brunner/Mazel.

Binder, J. L. (1993). Observations on the training of therapists in time-limited psychotherapy. *Psychotherapy, 30*(4), 592–598.

Binder, J. L., Bongar, B., Messer, S., Strupp, H. H., Lee, S. S., & Peake, T. H. (1993). Recommendations for improving psychotherapy training based on experiences with manual-guided training and research: Epilogue. *Psychotherapy, 30*(4), 599–600.

Blatt, S. J. (1991). A cognitive morphology of psychopathology. *Journal of Nervous and Mental Disease, 179*(8), 449–457.

Blatt, S. J., & Felsen, I. (1993). Different kinds of folks may need different kinds of strokes: The effect of patients' characteristics on therapeutic process and outcome. *Psychotherapy Research, 3*(4), 245–259.

Borden, E. (1979). The generalizability of the psychoanalytic concept of the working alliance. *Psychotherapy, 16,* 252–260.

Bowlby, J. (1973). *Attachment and loss: Vol. 2. Separation: Anxiety and anger.* New York: Basic Books.

Brack, G., Brack, C. J., & Zucker, A. (1992). Time perception and time processing as an aspect of the therapeutic process. *Psychotherapy, 29*(3), 336–343.

Brown, M. (1977). *Psychodiagnosis in brief.* Dexter, MI: Huron Valley Institute.

Buckley, P. (Ed.). (1986). *Essential papers on object relations.* New York: New York University Press.

Budman, S. H. (Ed.). (1981). *Forms of brief therapy.* New York: Guilford Press.

Budman, S. H. (1994). *Treating time effectively: The first session in brief therapy* [Videotape and manual]. New York: Guilford Press.

Budman, S. H., & Gurman, A. S. (1988). *Theory and practice of brief therapy.* New York: Guilford Press.

Budman, S. H., Hoyt, M. F., & Friedman, S. (Eds). (1992). *The first session in brief therapy.* New York: Guilford Press.

Burke, J. D., White H. S., & Havens, L. L. (1979). Which short-term therapy? *Archives of General Psychiatry, 36,* 177–186.

Clarkin, J. F., & Lenzenweger, M. (Eds.). (1996). *Major theories of personality disorders.* New York: Guilford Press.

Cooper, A. (1986). Narcissism. In A. P. Morrison (Ed.), *Essential papers on narcissism* (pp. 112–143). New York: New York University Press.

Cooper, A. M., Frances, A. J., & Sacks, M. H. (Eds.). (1986). *The personality disorders and neuroses.* New York: Basic Books.

Crits-Christoph, P., & Barber, J. P. (Eds.). (1991). *Handbook of short-term dynamic psychotherapy.* New York: Basic Books.

Cummings, N. (1991). Intermittent therapy throughout the life cycle. In C. S. Austad & W. H. Berman (Eds.), *Psychotherapy in managed care.* Washington, DC: American Psychological Association Press.

Davanloo, H. (Ed.). (1980). *Short-term dynamic psychotherapy.* New York: Jason Aronson.

Davanloo, H. (1987). Unconscious therapeutic alliance. In P. Buirski (Ed.), *Frontiers of dynamic psychotherapy* (pp. 64–88). New York: Brunner/Mazel.

Davanloo, H. (1990). *Unlocking the unconscious.* Chichester: Wiley.

Davis, D. M. (1991). Review of the psychoanalytic literature on countertransference. *International Journal of Short-Term Psychotherapy, 6*(3), 131–143.

Davison, W. T., Pray, M., & Bristol, C. (1990). Mutative interpretation and close process monitoring in a study of psychoanalytic process. *Psychoanalytic Quarterly, 59,* 599–629.

Della Selva, P. C. (1993). The significance of attachment theory for the practice of intensive short-term dynamic psychotherapy. *International Journal of Short-Term Psychotherapy, 8*(4), 189–206.

Della Selva, P. C. (1996). *Intensive short-term dynamic psychotherapy: Theory and tecnique.* New York: Wiley.

Deming, W. E. (1986). *Out of the crisis* (2nd ed.). Cambridge, MA: MIT Center for Advanced Engineering Study.

Deutsch, A. (1949). *The mentally ill in America* (2nd ed.). New York: Columbia University Press.

Deutsch, F. (1965). *Neuroses and character types: Clinical psychoanalytic studies.* New York: International Universities Press.

Deutsch, F., & Murphy, W. F. (1955). *The clinical interview* (2 vols.). New York: International Universities Press.

Dobyns, L., & Crawford-Mason, C. (1991). *Quality or else.* New York: Houghton Mifflin.

Dornelas, E. A., Correll, R. E., Lothstein, L., Wilber, C., & Goethe, J. W. (1996). Designing and implementing outcome evaluations: Some guidelines for practitioners. *Psychotherapy, 33*(2), 237–245.

Eisenstein, S. (1986). Franz Alexander and short-term dynamic psychotherapy. *International Journal of Short-Term Psychotherapy, 1*(3), 179–191.

Ekman, P. (1972). The analysis of movement behavior during the clinical interview. In A. Siegman & B. Pope (Eds.), *Studies in dyadic communication.* New York: Pergamon Press.

Ekman, P., & Davidson, R. J. (Eds.). (1994). *The nature of emotions: Fundamental questions.* New York: Oxford University Press.

Ekman, P., & Friesen, W. V. (1969). Nonverbal leakage and clues to deception. *Psychiatry, 32,* 88–106.

Ezriel, H. (1952). Notes on psychoanalytic group therapy: Interpretation and research. *Psychiatry, 15,* 119–126.

Fairbairn, W. R. D. (1954). *An object-relations theory of personality.* New York: Basic Books.

Farber, B. A., Lippert, R. A., & Nevas, D. B. (1995). The therapist as attachment figure. *Psychotherapy, 32*(2), 204–212.

Fenichel, O. (1945). *The psychoanalytic theory of neurosis.* New York: Norton.

Ferenczi, S., & Rank, O. (1925). *The development of psychoanalysis.* New York: Nervous and Mental Diseases Publishing Co.

Flegenheimer, W. V. (1993). *Techniques of brief psychotherapy.* Northvale, NJ: Jason Aronson.

Fosha, D. (1992). The interrelatedness of theory, technique and therapeutic stance: A comparative look at intensive short-term dynamic psychotherapy and accelerated empathic therapy. *International Journal of Short-Term Psychotherapy, 7*(3), 157–176.

Fosha, D. (1995). Technique and taboo in three short-term dynamic psychotherapies. *Journal of Psychotherapy Practice and Research, 4,* 297–318.

Frances, A., Clarkin, J., & Perry, S. (1984). *Differential therapeutics in psychiatry: The art and science of treatment selection.* New York: Brunner/Mazel.

Freedheim, D. K. (Ed.). (1992). *History of psychotherapy.* Washington, DC: American Psychological Association.

Freud, S. (1953). Introductory lectures on psycho-analysis. In *Standard edition* (Vol. 15–16, pp. 1–482). London: Hogarth Press. (Original work published 1916–1917)

Freud, S. (1957). The future prospects of psychoanalytic therapy. In *Standard edition* (Vol. 11, pp. 1–56). London: Hogarth Press. (Original work published 1910)

Frieswyk, S. H., Allen, J. G., Colson, D. B., Coyne, L., Gabbard, G. O., Horowitz, L., & Newsom, G. (1986). Therapeutic alliance: Its place as a process outcome variable in dynamic psychotherapy research. *Journal of Consulting and Clinical Psychology, 54*(1), 32–38.

Frommer, J., Reissner, V., Tress, W., & Langenbach, M. (1996). Subjective theories of illness in patients with personality disorders: Qualitative comparison of twelve diagnostic interviews. *Psychotherapy Research, 6*(1), 56–69.

Gatson, L., Piper, W. E., Debbane, E. G., Bienvenu, J.-P., & Garant, S. (1994). Alliance and technique for predicting outcome in short- and long-term analytic psychotherapy. *Psychotherapy Research, 4*(2), 121–135.

Gaylin, W. (1979). *Feelings: Our vital signs.* New York: Harper & Row.

Gendlin, E. T. (1986). What comes after traditional psychotherapy research? *American Psychologist, 41*(2), 131–136.

Goldberg, A. (1973). Psychotherapy of narcissistic injuries. *Archives of General Psychiatry, 28,* 722–726.

Goldenson, R. M. (1970). *The encylopedia of human behavior: Psychology, psychiatry, and mental health* (Vol. 1). New York: Doubleday.

Greenberg, L. S., Rice, L. N., & Elliott, R. (1993). *Facilitating emotional change: The moment-by moment process.* New York: Guilford Press.

Guerette, R. (1995, February 24–26). Keynote address. In *The future of psychotherapy.* Symposium conducted by the New England Educational Institute, Orlando, FL.

Gustafson, J. P. (1986). *The complex secret of brief psychotherapy.* New York: Norton.

Gustafson, J. P. (1995). *Brief versus long psychotherapy: When, why, and how.* Northvale, NJ: Jason Aronson.

Hager, D. (1992). Chaos and growth. *Psychotherapy, 29*(3), 378–384.

Hammer, E. (1990). *Reaching the affect: Style in the psychodynamic therapies.* Northvale, NJ: Jason Aronson.

Harper, R. G., Wiens, A. N., & Matarazzo, J. D. (1978). *Nonverbal communication: The state of the art.* New York: Wiley.

Harriman, P. L. (1947). *The new dictionary of psychology.* New York: Philosophical Library.

Hartmann, H. (1939). *Ego psychology and the problem of adaptation.* New York: International Universities Press.

Havens, L. (1989). *A safe place.* New York: Ballantine Books.

Heatherton, T. F., & Nichols, P. A. (1995). Conceptual issues in assessing whether personality can change. In T. F. Heatherton & J. L. Weinberger (Eds.), *Can personality change?* (pp. 3–18). Washington DC: American Psychological Association.

Heatherton, T. F., & Weinberger, J. L. (1995). *Can personality change?* Washington, DC: American Psychological Association.

Herman, J. L. (1992). *Trauma and recovery.* New York: Basic Books.

Hill, C. E. (1996). Dreams and therapy. *Psychotherapy Research, 6*(1), 1–15.

Hill, E. F. (1987). The dynamics and treatment of the "detached" patient. *Psychotherapy in Private Practice, 5*(2), 81–88.

Hjelle, L. A., & Ziegler, D. J. (1976). *Personality theories: Basic assumptions, research, and applications.* New York: McGraw-Hill.

Hoglend, P. (1993). Transference interpretations and long-term change after dynamic psychotherapy of brief to moderate length. *American Journal of Psychotherapy, 47,* 494–507.

Horner, A. J. (Ed.). (1994). *Treating the neurotic patient in brief psychotherapy.* Northvale, NJ: Jason Aronson.

Horner, A. J. (1995). *Psychoanalytic object relations therapy.* Northvale, NJ: Jason Aronson.

Horney, K. (1937). *The neurotic personality of our time.* New York: Norton.

Horney, K. (1939). *New ways in psychoanalysis.* New York: Norton.

Horney, K. (1950). *Neurosis and human growth.* New York: Norton.

Horowitz, M., Marmar, C., Krupnick, J., Wilner, N., Kaltreider, N., & Wallerstein, R. (1984). *Personality styles and brief psychotherapy.* New York: Basic Books.

Horowitz, M. J., Marmar, C. R., Weiss, D. S., Kaltreider, N. B., & Wilner, N. R. (1986). Comprehensive analysis of change after brief dynamic psychotherapy. *American Journal of Psychiatry, 143*(5), 582–589.

Howard, K. I., Kopta, S. M., Krause, M. S., & Orlinsky, D. E. (1986). The dose–effect relationship in psychotherapy. *American Psychologist, 41,* 159–164.

Hoyt, M. F. (1985). Therapist resistances to short-term dynamic psychotherapy. *Journal of the American Academy of Psychoanalysis, 13*(1), 93–112.

Hoyt, M. F. (Ed.). (1994). *Constructive therapies.* New York: Guilford Press.

James, W. (1981). *The varieties of religious experience* (5th ed.). New York: Macmillan. (Original work published 1890)

Johnson, S. M. (1985). *Characterological transformation: The hard work miracle.* New York: Norton.

Johnson, S. M. (1991). *The symbiotic character.* New York: Norton.

Johnson, S. M. (1994). *Character styles.* New York: Norton.

Jones, E. E., Parke, L. A., & Pulos, S. M. (1992). How therapy is conducted in the private consulting room: A multidimensional description of brief psychodynamic treatments. *Psychotherapy Research, 2*(1), 16–30.

Jordan, J. V. (1995). Female therapists and the search for a new paradigm. In M. B. Sussman (Ed.), *A perilous calling: The hazards of psychotherapy practice* (pp. 259–272). New York: Wiley.

Kalpin, A. (1993). The use of the countertransference in the evaluation of the therapeutic alliance. *International Journal of Short-Term Psychotherapy, 8*(1), 23–28.

Karen, R. (1992, February). Shame. *Atlantic Monthly.*

Keltner, D., Moffitt, T. E., & Stouthamer-Loeber, M. (1995). Facial expressions of emotion and psychopathology in adolescent boys. *Journal of Abnormal Psychology, 104*(4), 644–652.

Kernberg, O. (1984). *Severe personality disorders: Psychotherapeutic strategies.* New Haven: Yale University Press.

Kernberg, O. (1986). Further contibutions to the treatment of narcissistic personalities. In A. P. Morrison (Ed.), *Essential papers on narcissism* (pp. 245–292). New York: New York University Press.

Kertay, L., & Reviere, S. L. (1993). The use of touch in psychotherapy: Theoretical and ethical considerations. *Psychotherapy, 30*(1), 32–40.

Kiesler, D. J. (1982). The interpersonal circle: A taxonomy for complementarity in human transactions. *Psychological Review, 90,* 185–214.

Klein, M. (1948). *Contributions to psychoanalysis, 1921–1945.* London: Hogarth Press.

Klein, M. (1957). Envy and gratitude. In *Envy and gratitude and other works, 1946–1963* (pp. 176–235). New York: Free Press.

Kohut, H. (1971). *The analysis of the self.* New York: International Universities Press.

Kohut, H. (1977). *The restoration of the self.* New York: International Universities Press.

Kolden, G. G., & Klien, M. H. (1996). Therapeutic process in dynamic therapy for personality disorders: The joint influence of acute distress and dysfunction and severity of personality pathology. *Journal of Personality Disorders, 10*(2), 107–121.

Laikin, M., & Winston, A. (1988). *Short-term dynamic psychotherapy manual (STDP)* (Social and Behavioral Sciences Documents Abstracts, number 18). Washington, DC: American Psychological Association.

Laikin, M., Winston, A., & McCullough, L. (1991). Intensive short-term dynamic psychotherapy. In P. Crits-Christoph & J. P. Barber (Eds.), *Handbook of short-term dynamic psychotherapy* (pp. 80–109). New York: Basic Books.

Lambert, M. J. (1992). Psychotherapy outcome research: Implications for integrative and eclectic therapists. In J. C. Norcross & M. R. Goldfried (Eds.), *Handbook of psychotherapy integration* (pp. 94–129). New York: Basic Books.

Lambert, M. J., Shapiro, D. A., & Bergin, A. E. (1986). The effectiveness of psychotherapy. In S. L. Garfield & A. E. Bergin (Eds.), *Handbook of psychotherapy and behavior change* (3rd ed., pp. 157–212). New York: Wiley.

Langs, R. (1989). *The technique of psychoanalytic psychotherapy* (Vols. 1 & 2). NJ: Jason Aronson.

Langs, R. (1990). *Psychotherapy: A basic text*. Northvale, NJ: Jason Aronson.

Lazarus, R. S. (1991). *Emotion and adaptation*. New York: Oxford Press.

Leary, T. (1957). *Interpersonal diagnosis of personality: A functional theory and methodology for personality evaluation*. New York: Ronald Press.

Lemaire, A. (1994). *Jacques Lacan*. London: Routledge. (Original work published 1970)

Linderman, E. (1944). Symptomatology and management of acute grief. *American Journal of Psychiatry, 51*, 141–148.

Linehan, M. M. (1993). *Cognitive-behavioral treatment of borderline personality disorder*. New York: Guilford Press.

Livesley, W. J., Schroeder, M. L., Jackson, D. N., & Jang, K. L. (1994). Categorical distinctions in the study of personality disorder: Implications for classification. *Journal of Abnormal Psychology, 103*(1), 6–17.

Loewald, H. (1960). On the therapeutic action of psychoanalysis. In G. I. Fofel (Ed.), *The work of Hans Loewald: An introduction and commentary* (pp. 15–59). Northvale, NJ: Jason Aronson.

Luborsky, L. (1984). *Principles of psychanalytic psychotherapy: A manual for supportive-expressive treatment*. New York: Basic Books.

Luborsky, L. (1993). Recommendations for training therapists based on manuals for psychotherapy research. *Psychotherapy, 30*(4), 578–580.

Luborsky, L., Crits-Christoph, P., Mintz, J., & Auerbach, A. (1988). *Who will benefit from psychotherapy? Predicting therapeutic outcomes*. New York: Basic Books.

Magnavita, J. J. (1993a). The treatment of passive–aggressive personality disorder: A review of current approaches. Part 1. *International Journal of Short-Term Psychotherapy, 8*(1), 29–41.

Magnavita, J. J. (1993b). The evolution of short-term dynamic psychotherapy. *Professional Psychology: Research and Practice, 24*(3), 360–365.

Magnavita, J. J. (1993c). On the validity of psychoanalytic constructs in the 20th century. *Professional Psychology: Research and Practice, 25*(3), 198–199.

Magnavita, J. J. (1994a). Premature termination of short-term dynamic psychotherapy. *International Journal of Short-Term Psychotherapy, 9*(4), 213–228.

Magnavita, J. J. (1994b). [Review of the book *Character–styles*. (S. M. Johnson 1994)]. *Psychotherapy, 31*(4), 744–745.

Maher, B. A., & Maher, W. B. (1994). Personality and psychopathology: A historical perspective. *Journal of Abnormal Psychology, 103*(1), 72–77.

Main, M. (1991). *Father hunger: Fathers, daughters, and food*. Carlsbad, CA: Gürze Books.

Malan, D. H. (1963). *Brief study of psychotherapy*. New York: Plenum Press.

Malan, D. H. (1976). *The frontier of brief psychotherapy: An example of the convergence of research and clinical practice*. New York: Plenum Medical.

Malan, D. H. (1979). *Individual psychotherapy and the science of psychodynamics*. London: Butterworth.

Malan, D. H., & Osimo, F. (1992). *Psychodynamics, training, and outcome in brief psychotherapy*. Oxford: Butterworth–Heinemann.

Mann, J. (1973). *Time-limited psychotherapy*. Cambridge, MA: Harvard University Press.

Mann, J., & Goldman, R. (1982). *A casebook in time-limited psychotherapy.* New York: McGraw-Hill.

Masterson, J. F. (1988). *The search for the real self: Unmasking the personality disorders of our age.* New York: Free Press.

McCrae, R. R., & Costa, P. T., Jr. (1994). The stability of personality: Observations and evaluations. *Current Directions in Psychological Science, 3*(6), 173–175.

McCullough, L., Winston, A., Farber, B. A., Porter, F., Pollack, J., Laikin, M., Vingiano, W., & Trujillo, M. (1991). The relationship of patient–therapist interaction to outcome in brief psychotherapy. *Psychotherapy, 28,* 525–533.

McGinn, L. K., & Sanderson, W. C. (1995). The nature of panic disorder. *In Session: Psychotherapy in Practice, 1*(3), 7–19.

McWilliams, N. (1994). *Psychoanalytic diagnosis: Understanding personality structure in the clinical process.* New York: Guilford Press.

Meissner, W. W. (1981). Meissner's glossary of defenses. In H. I. Kaplan & B. J. Sadock (Eds.), *Modern synopsis of comprehensive textbook of psychiatry* (3rd ed., pp. 137–138). Baltimore: Williams & Williams.

Menninger, K. (1958). *Theory of psychoanalytic technique.* New York: Basic Books.

Merikangas, K. R., & Weissman, M. M. (1986). Epidemiology of DSM-III Axis II personality disorders. In A. J. Frances & R. E. Hales (Eds.), *Psychiatric update: The American Psychiatric Association annual review* (Vol. 5). Washington, DC: American Psychiatric Press.

Messer, S. B. (1996). A psychodynamic perspective on resistance in psychotherapy: Vive la resistance. *In Session: Psychotherapy in Practice, 2*(1), 25–32.

Messer, S. B., & Warren, C. S. (1995). *Models of brief psychodynamic therapy.* New York: Guilford Press.

Milbrath, C., Bauknight, R., Horowitz, M. J., Amaro, R., & Sugahara, C. (1995). Sequential analysis of topics in psychotherapy discourse: A single-case study. *Psychotherapy Research, 5*(3), 199–217.

Miller, A. (1983). *The drama of the gifted child.* New York: Noonday Press.

Miller, A. (1990). *For your own good.* New York: Noonday Press.

Miller, W. R., & C'deBaca, J. (1994). Quantum change: Toward a psychology of transformation. In T. F. Heatherton & J. L. Weinberger (Eds.), *Can personality change?* (pp. 253–280). Washington DC: American Psychological Association.

Millon, T. (1981). *Disorders of personality: DSM-III, Axis II.* New York: Wiley.

Millon, T. (1992, June 22–26). *Understanding personality disorders.* New England Educational Institute, Cape Cod Summer Symposium.

Millon, T., & Davis, R. D. (1996). *Disorders of personality: DSM-IV and beyond* (2nd ed.). New York: Wiley.

Millon, T., Everly, G., & Davis, R. D. (1993). How can knowledge of psychopathology facilitate psychotherapy integration? A view from the personality disorders. *Journal of Psychotherapy Integration, 3*(4), 331–352.

Millon, T., & Klerman, G. L. (Eds.). (1986). *Contemporary directions in psychopathology: Toward the DSM-IV.* New York: Guilford Press.

Monsen, J. T., Odland, T., Faugli, A., Daae, E., & Eilertsen, D. E. (1995). Personality disorders: Changes and stability after intensive psychotherapy focusing on affect consciousness. *Psychotherapy Research, 5*(1), 33–48.

Moore, B. E., & Fine, B. D. (Eds.). (1990). *Psychoanalytic terms and concepts.* New Haven: The American Psychoanalytic Association and Yale University Press.

Moras, K. (1993). The use of treatment manuals to train psychotherapists: Observations and recommendations. *Psychotherapy, 30*(4), 581–586.

Morrison, A. P. (Ed.). (1986). *Essential papers on narcissism.* New York: New York University Press.

National Advisory Mental Health Council. (1995). Basic behavioral science research for mental health. *American Psychologist, 50*(10), 838–845.

Nemiah, J. C. (1975). Denial revisited: Reflections on psychosomatic theory. *Psychotherapy and Psychosomatics, 26,* 140–147.

Norcross, J. C., & Goldfried, M. R. (1992). *Handbook of psychotherapy integration.* New York: Basic Books.

Norville, R., Sampson, H., & Weiss, J. (1996). Accurate interpretations and brief psychotherapy outcome. *Psychotherapy Research, 6*(1), 16–29.

Noy, P. (1977). Metapsychology as a multimodal system. *International Review of Psychoanalysis, 4,* 1–12.

Osimo, F. (1994). Method, personality and training in short-term psychotherapy. *International Journal of Short-Term Psychotherapy, 9,* 173–187.

Overholser, J. C. (1995). Elements of the socratic method: IV. Disavowal of knowledge. *Psychotherapy, 32*(2), 283–292.

Paris, J. (1994). The etiology of borderline personality disorder: A biopsychosocial approach. *Psychiatry: Interpersonal and Biological Processes, 57*(4), 316–325.

Patrick, J. (1985). Therapeutic ambiance in the treatment of severely disturbed narcissistic personality disorders. *American Journal of Psychoanalysis, 45*(3), 258–267.

Perry, J. C. (1990). Perry's defense rating scale. In G. E. Vaillant (Ed.), *Ego mechanisms of defense: A guide for clinicians and researchers* (pp. 253–259). Washington, DC: American Psychiatric Press.

Pine, F. (1990). *Drive, ego, object, and self: A synthesis for clinical work.* New York: Basic Books.

Pinsker, H., Rosenthal R., & McCullough, L. (1991). Dynamic supportive psychotherapy. In P. Crits-Christoph & J. P. Barber (Eds.), *Handbook of short-term dynamic psychotherapy* (pp. 220–247). New York: Basic Books.

Piper, W. E., Azim, H. F., Joyce, A. S., & McCallum, M. (1991). Transference interpretations, therapeutic alliance, and outcome in short-term individual psychotherapy. *Archives of General Psychiatry, 48,* 946–953.

Pollack, J., Flegenheimer, W., Kaufman, J., Pereira, P., & Sadow, J. (1988). *Brief adaptive psychotherapy manual (BAP).* (Social and Behavioral Sciences Documents Abstracts, number 18). Washington DC: American Psychological Association.

Pollack, J., & Horner, A. (1985). Brief adaptation-oriented psychotherapy. In A. Winston (Ed.), *Clinical and research issues in short-term dynamic psychotherapy.* Washington DC: American Psychiatric Press.

Pollack, M. H., Otto, M. W., Rosenbaum, J. F., & Sachs, G. S. (1992). Personality disorders in patients with panic disorders: Association with childhood anxiety disorders, early trauma, comorbidity, and chronicity. *Comparative Psychiatry,* *33,* 78–83.

Prochaska, J. O., & DiClemente, C. C. (1992). The transtheoretical approach. In J. C. Norcross & M. R. Goldfried (Eds.), *Psychotherapy integration* (pp. 300–334). New York: Basic Books.

Prochaska, J. O., DiClemente, C. C., & Norcross, J. (1992). In search of how people change: Applications to addictive behaviors. *American Psychologist, 47,* 1102–1114.

Rank, O. (1945). *Will therapy and truth and reality.* New York: Knopf.

Rank, O. (1947). *Will therapy: An analysis of the therapeutic process in terms of relationship.* New York: Knopf.

Rank, O. (1973). *The trauma of birth.* New York: Harper & Row. (Original work published 1929)

Rapaport, D., & Gill, M. M. (1967). The points of view and assumptions of metapsychology. In M. M. Gill (Ed.), *The collected papers of David Rapaport* (pp. 795–811). New York: Basic Books.

Reich, A. (1960). Pathologic forms of self-esteem regulation. *Psychoanalytic Study of the Child, 15,* 215–232.

Reich, W. (1945). *Character analysis* (3rd. ed.). New York: Noonday Press.

Reik, T. (1941). *Masochism and modern man.* New York: Farrar & Rinehart.

Reik, T. (1949). *Listening with the third ear.* New York: Farrar, Straus.

Robins, C. J. (1993). Implications of research in the psychopathology of depression for psychotherapy integration. *Journal of Psychotherapy Integration, 3*(4), 313–330.

Rogers, C. R. (1942). *Counseling and psychotherapy: Newer concepts in practice.* Boston: Houghton Mifflin.

Rogers, C. R. (1957). The necessary and sufficient conditions of therapeutic personality change. *Journal of Consulting Psychology, 21,* 95–103.

Rowe, C. E., Jr., & Mac Isaac, D. S. (1991). *Empathic attunement: The "technique" of psychoanalytic self psychology.* Northvale, NJ: Jason Aronson.

Ruegg, R., & Frances, A. (1995). New research in personality disorders. *Journal of Personality Disorders, 9*(1), 1– 48.

Safran, J. D. (1993). Breaches in the therapeutic alliance: An arena for negotiating authentic relatedness. *Psychotherapy, 30*(1), 11–24.

Safran, J. D., & Greenberg, L. S. (Eds.). (1991). *Emotion, psychotherapy, and change.* New York: Guilford Press.

Safran, J. D., & Muran, J. C. (1995). Introduction: The therapeutic alliance. *In Session Psychotherapy Practice, 1*(1), 3–5.

Sandler, J., with Freud, A. (1985). *The analysis of defense.* New York: International Universities Press.

Schafer, R. (1968). *Aspects of internalization.* New York: International Universities Press.

Schulte, D. (1995). How treatment success could be assessed. *Psychotherapy Research, 5*(4), 281–296.

Seinfeld, J. (1991). *The empty core: An object relations approach to psychotherapy of the schizoid personality.* Northvale, NJ: Jason Aronson.

Seivewright, N., Ferguson, B., & Tyrer, J. (1992). The general neurotic syndrome:

Co-axial diagnosis of anxiety, depression and personality disorders. *Acta Psychiatrica Scandianavica, 85,* 201–206.

Shapiro, D. (1989). *Psychotherapy of neurotic character.* New York: Basic Books.

Shea, M. T., Pilkonis, P. A., Beckham, E., Collins, J. F., Elkin, I., Sotsky, S. M., & Docherty, J. P. (1990). Personality disorders and treatment outcome in the NIMH Treatment of Depression Collaborative Research Program. *American Journal of Psychiatry, 147,* 711–718.

Sifneos, P. E. (1972). *Short-term psychotherapy and emotional crisis.* Boston: Harvard University Press.

Sifneos, P. E. (1981). Short-term anxiety-provoking psychotherapy: Its history, technique, outcome, and instruction. In S. H. Budman (Ed.), *Forms of brief therapy* (pp. 45–81). New York: Guilford Press.

Sifneos, P. E. (1984a). The current status of individual short-term dynamic psychotherapy and its future: An overview. *American Journal of Psychotherapy, 38*(4), 472–482.

Sifneos, P. E. (1984b). Short-term dynamic psychotherapy of phobic and mildly obsessive–compulsive patients. *American Journal of Psychotherapy, 34*(3), 314–322.

Sifneos, P. E. (1987). *Short-term dynamic psychotherapy: Evaluation and technique* (2nd ed.). New York: Plenum Medical.

Sifneos, P. E. (1990). Short-term anxiety-provoking psychotherapy (STAPP): Termination outcome and videotaping. In J. K. Zeig & S. G. Gilligan (Eds.), *Brief therapy: Myths, methods, and metaphors* (pp. 318–326). New York: Brunner/Mazel.

Sifneos, P. E. (1995, February 24–26). Short-term dynamic psychotherapy with Peter Sifneos. In *The future of psychotherapy.* Symposium conducted by the New England Educational Institute, Orlando, FL.

Singer, J. L. (1971). Theoretical implications of imagery and fantasy techniques. *Contemporary Psychoanalysis, 8*(1), 82–96.

Slakter, E. (1987). *Countertransference.* Northvale, NJ: Jason Aronson.

Small, L. (1971). *The briefer psychotherapies.* New York: Brunner/Mazel.

Smith, M. L., Glass, G. V., & Miller, T. I. (1980). *The benefits of psychotherapy.* Baltimore: Johns Hopkins University Press.

Soldz, S., Budman, S., Demby, A., & Merry, J. (1995). The relation of defensive style to personality pathology and the big five personality factors. *Journal of Personality Disorders, 9*(4), 356–370.

Stadter, M. (1996). *Object relations brief therapy: The therapeutic relationship in short-term work.* Northvale, NJ: Jason Aronson.

Stanton, M. (1991). *Sandor Ferenczi: Reconsidering active intervention.* Northvale, NJ: Jason Aronson.

Stern, D. (1985). *The interpersonal world of the infant: A view from psychoanalysis and developmental psychology.* New York: Basic Books.

Stierlin, H. (1968). Short-term vs. long-term psychotherapy in the light of a general theory of human relationships. *British Journal of Medical Psychology, 41,* 357.

Stiles, W. B., Shapiro, D. A., & Elliott, R. (1986). Are all psychotherapies equivalent? *American Psychologist, 41*(2), 165–180.

Stone, M. H. (1980). *The borderline syndromes.* New York: McGraw-Hill.

Stone, M. (1993). *Abnormalities of personality: Beyond and within the realm of treatment.* New York: Norton.

Straker, M. (1980). Crisis intervention: An overview. In H. Davanloo (Ed.), *Short-term dynamic psychotherapy* (pp. 222–236). Northvale, NJ: Jason Aronson.

Strupp, H. H. (1978). Psychotherapy research and practice: An overview. In S. L. Garfield & A. E. Bergin (Eds.), *Handbook of psychotherapy and behavior change* (2nd ed., pp. 3–22). New York: Wiley.

Strupp, H. H., & Binder, J. L. (1984). *Psychotherapy in a new key: A guide to time-limited dynamic psychotherapy.* New York: Basic Books.

Strupp, H. H., Hadely, S. W., & Gomes-Schwartz, B. (1977). *Psychotherapy for better or worse: The problem of negative effects.* New York: Jason Aronson.

Sullivan, H. S. (1953). *The interpersonal theory of psychiatry.* New York: Norton.

Svartberg, M., Seltzer, M. H., & Stiles, T. C. (1996). Self-concept improvement during and after short-term anxiety-provoking psychotherapy: A preliminary growth curve study. *Psychotherapy Research, 6*(1), 43–55.

Svartberg, M., & Stiles, T. C. (1994). Therapeutic alliance, therapist competence, and client change in short-term anxiety-provoking psychotherapy. *Psychotherapy Research, 4*(1), 20–33.

Talley, P. F., Strupp, H. H., & Butler, S. F. (Eds.). (1994). *Psychotherapy research and practice: Bridging the gap.* New York: Basic Books.

Trad, P. V. (1992). Mastering developmental transitions through prospective techniques. *International Journal of Short-Term Psychotherapy, 7*(2), 59–72.

Trad, P. V. (1993). Expressive cues and previewing behaviors during short-term psychotherapy part II: Clinical evidence. *International Journal of Short-Term Psychotherapy, 8*(4), 167–187.

Tuttman, S. (1982). Regression: Curative factor of impediment in dynamic psychotherapy. In S. Slipp (Ed.), *Curative factors in dynamic psychotherapy.* New York: McGraw Hill.

Tryon, G. S., & Kane, A. S. (1995). Client involvement, working alliance, and type of therapy termination. *Psychotherapy Research, 5*(3), 189–198.

Vaillant, G. E. (Ed.). (1992). *Ego mechanisms of defense: A guide for clinicians and researchers.* Washington, DC: American Psychiatric Press.

Vaillant, L. (1994). The next step in short-term dynamic psychotherapy: A clarification of objectives and techniques in an anxiety-regulating model. *Psychotherapy, 31*(4), 642–654.

Van Denburg, T. F., & Kiesler, D. J. (1996). An interpersonal communication perspective on resistance in psychotherapy. *In Session: Psychotherapy in Practice, 2*(1), 55–66.

Viederman, M. (1991). The real person of the analyst and his role in the process of psychoanalytic cure. *Journal of the American Psychoanalytic Association, 39,* 451–489.

Watson, D., & Clark, L. A. (1994). Introduction to the special issue on personality and psychopathology. *Journal of Abnormal Psychology, 103*(1), 3–5.

Webster's New World Dictionary (V. Neufeldt, Ed.). (1990). New York: Simon & Schuster.

Weissman, M. M. (1993). The epidemiology of personality disorders: A 1990 update. *Journal of Personality Disorders, 7,* 44–62.

Wells, M., & Glickauf-Hughes, C. (1993). A psychodynamic–object relations model for differential diagnosis. *Psychotherapy Bulletin, 28*(3), 41–48.

Westen, D. (1986). What changes in short-term dynamic psychotherapy? *Psychotherapy, 23*(4), 501–512.

Widiger, T. A., & Costa, P. T., Jr. (1994). Personality and personality disorders. *Journal of Abnormal Psychology, 103*(1), 78–91.

Winnicott, D. (1949). Hate in the countertransference. *International Journal of Psycho-Analysis, 30,* 69–74.

Winnicott, D. W. (1965). *The maturational processes and the facilitating environment.* New York: International Universities Press.

Winnicott, D. W. (1986). *Home is where we start from: Essays by a psychoanalyst.* New York: Norton.

Winston, A., Laikin, M., Pollack, J., Samstag, L. W., McCullough, L., & Muran, C. (1994). Short-term psychotherapy of personality disorders. *American Journal of Psychiatry, 151*(2), 190–194.

Winston, A., Pollack, J., McCullough, L., Flegenheimer, W., Kestenbaum, R., & Trujillo, M. (1991). Brief psychotherapy of personality disorders. *Journal of Nervous and Mental Disease, 179*(4), 188–193.

Winston, B., Samstag, L. W., Winston, A., & Muran, J. C. (1994). Patient defense/therapist interventions. *Psychotherapy, 31*(3), 478–491.

Wolf, A., & Kutash, I. (1991). *Psychotherapy of the submerged personality.* Northvale, NJ: Jason Aronson.

Wolman, B. (1968). *The unconscious mind: The meaning of Freudian psychology.* Englewood Cliffs, NJ: Prentice Hall.

Wolpe, J. (1973). *The practice of behavior therapy.* New York: Pergamon Press.

Woody, R. H. (1991). *Quality care in mental health: Assuring the best clinical services.* San Francisco: Jossey-Bass.

Wright, F. (1987). Men, shame and antisocial behavior: A psychodynamic perspective. *Group, 11*(4), 238–246.

Wright, F. (1992, October 9). *The many faces of shame in psychotherapy.* Annual symposium conducted by Hartford Hospital Department of Psychiatry, Hartford, CT.

Wright, F., O'Leary, J., & Balkin, J. (1989). Shame, guilt, narcissism, and depression: Correlates and sex differences. *Psychoanalytic Psychology, 6*(2), 217–230.

York, C., Wiseberg, S., & Freeman, T. (1989). *Development and psychopathology: Studies in psychoanalytic psychiatry.* New Haven: Yale University Press.

Young, J. E. (1990). *Cognitive therapy for personality disorders: A schema-focused approach* (rev. ed.). Sarasota, FL: Professional Resource Press.

Author Index

Subject Index

"Triangle of conflict," 24, 34–36
  case vignette, 36
  and cognitive restructuring, 127
  and core issues, 69, 70
  and defensive restructuring, 105, 106
  elements of, 34, 35
"Triangle of persons," 24, 32–36
  case vignette, 36
  and cognitive restructuring, 127
  and core conflict, 69, 70
  and defensive restructuring, 105, 106
  elements of, 32, 33
  and interpretation, 33, 34
Twelve-step programs, 286

Unconscious
  and anxiety-arousing techniques, 83, 84
  and length of treatment, 15, 16

middle treatment phase interpretations, 145, 146
short-term dynamic psychotherapy foundation, 19
Uncovering of defenses, 111
Unresolved grief, 142, 231

Videotapes, 281, 282, 295–299
  credentialing tool, 297
  feedback to patient, 281, 282
  and follow-up interview, 300
  format, 297, 298
  patient protocol, 298, 299
  research use, 294, 297
  in treatment enhancement, 295
Visual behavior, 82

Women, emotional expression, 125, 126
Workshops, 311